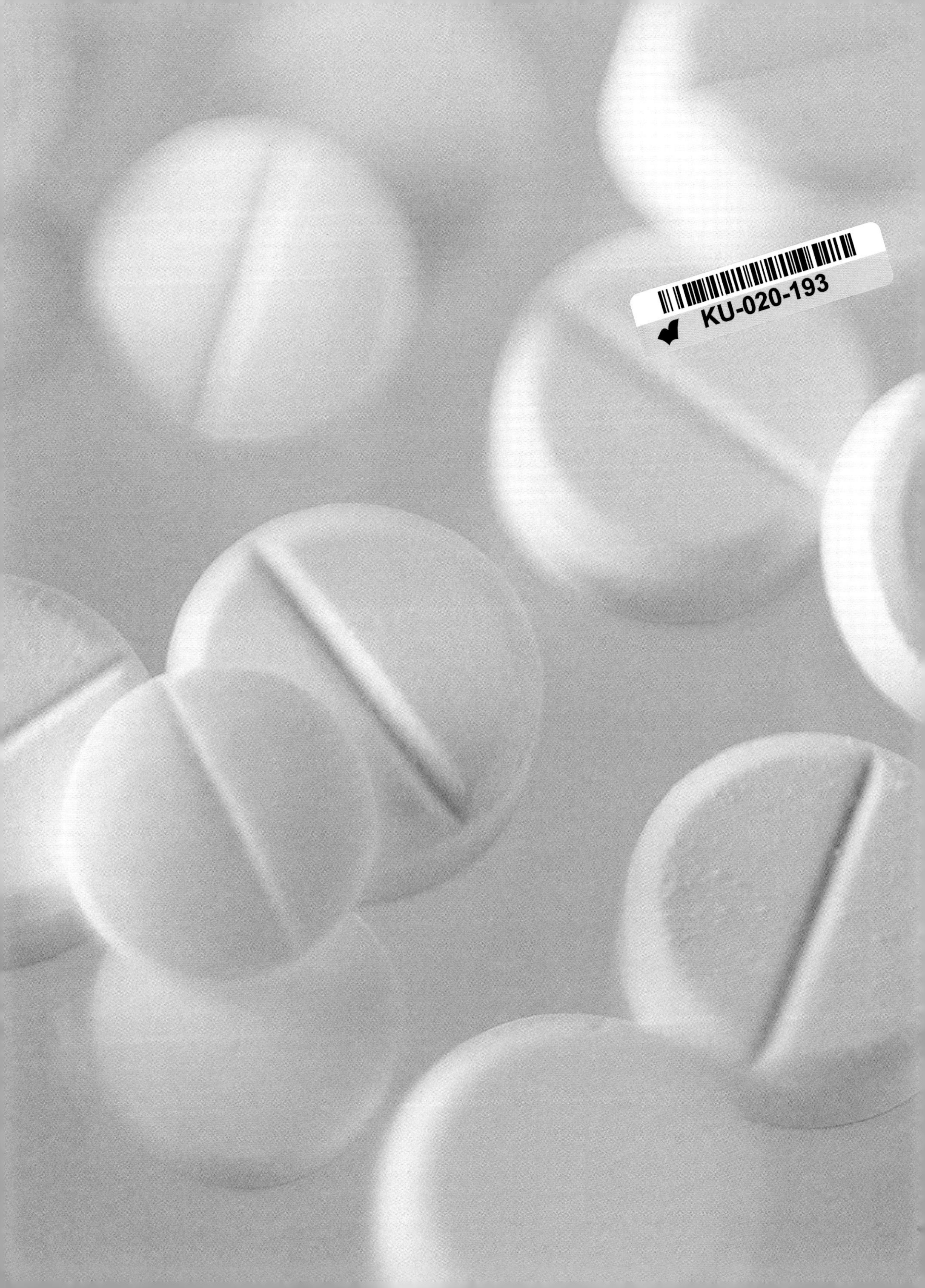

MEDICAL
BREAKTHROUGHS
2003

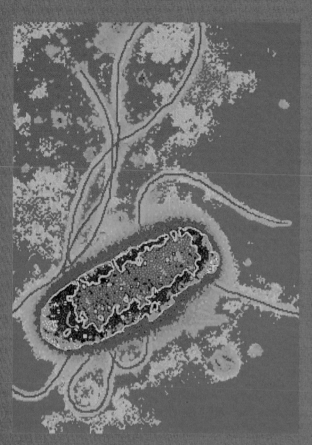

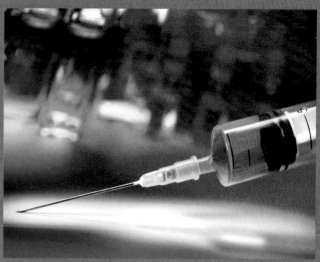

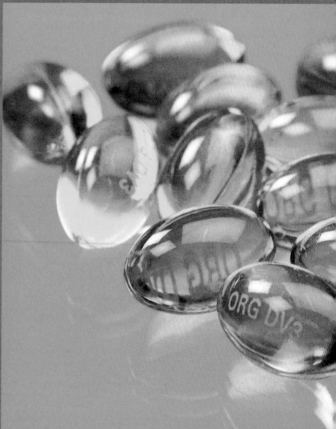

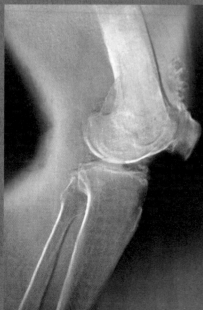

MEDICAL
BREAKTHROUGHS
2003

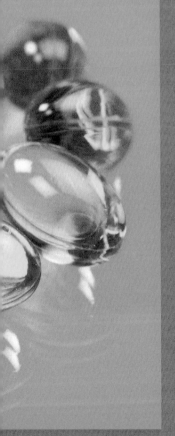

The year's most important
health developments
and how they can improve
and extend your life

Published by
The Reader's Digest Association Limited
London • New York • Sydney • Montreal

READER'S DIGEST PROJECT STAFF

Consultant
Dr. Vince Forte

Project editor
Rachel Warren Chadd

Assistant editors
Alison Candlin
Celia Coyne
Helen Spence

Art editor
Kate Harris

Editorial assistant
Rachel Weaver

Indexer
Marie Lorimer

READER'S DIGEST GENERAL BOOKS

Editorial Director
Cortina Butler

Art Director
Nick Clark

Executive Editor
Julian Browne

Development Editor
Ruth Binney

Managing Editor
Alastair Holmes

Picture Resource Manager
Martin Smith

Style Editor
Ron Pankhurst

Book Production Manager
Fiona McIntosh

Pre-press Account Manager
Penelope Grose

Origination
Colour Systems Limited, London
Printing and Binding
MOHN Media, Germany

Medical Breakthroughs 2003 was originated by
the editorial team of the Reader's Digest Association, Inc., USA

This edition was adapted and published by
The Reader's Digest Association Limited, London

First edition Copyright © 2003
The Reader's Digest Association Limited,
11 Westferry Circus, Canary Wharf,
London E14 4HE

We are committed to both the quality of our products and the service we provide to our customers. We value your comments, so please feel free to contact us on 08705 113366 or via our web site at: www.readersdigest.co.uk If you have any comments or suggestions about the content of our books, email us at: gbeditorial@readersdigest.co.uk

Any references in this book to any products or services do not constitute or imply an endorsement or recommendation.

ISBN 0 276 42728 9
BOOK CODE 440-103-01
CONCEPT CODE IE 0088A/IC

READER'S DIGEST USA

PROJECT STAFF

Senior Editor
Marianne Wait

Senior Designer
Susan Welt

Contributing Designers
Stephanie Koslow
Jennifer Tokarski

Production Technology Manager
Douglas A. Croll

Manufacturing Manager
John L. Cassidy

CONTRIBUTORS

Editor
Jeff Bredenberg

Writers
Bruce Beans, Linda Carroll, Jack Croft,
Kelly Garrett, Debra Gordon, Matthew
Hoffman, Linda Mooney, Nissa Simon,
Carol Svec

Copy Editor
Janice Fisher

Indexer
Ann Cassar

Design
Wendy Talvé Reingold

Picture Research
Carousel Research, Inc.
Laurie Platt Winfrey, Van Bucher, Mary
Teresa Giancoli, Cristian Pena

MEDICAL ADVISORS

Charles Atkins, M.D.
Medical Director, Western Connecticut
Mental Health Network;
Assistant Professor, Yale University
School of Medicine, New Haven,
Connecticut

Lawrence W. Bassett, M.D.
Iris Cantor Professor of Breast Imaging,
David Geffen School of Medicine at
UCLA, Los Angeles, California

Lawrence C. Brody, Ph.D.
Senior Investigator, Head, Molecular
Pathogenesis Section, National Human
Genome Research Institute, National
Institutes of Health, Bethesda, Maryland
(contributions rendered as an individual,
not in the name of the U.S. government)

Nicholas A. DiNubile, M.D.
Orthopaedic Consultant, Philadelphia
76ers Basketball and Pennsylvania
Ballet; Clinical Assistant Professor,
Department of Orthopaedic Surgery,
Hospital of the University of
Pennsylvania, Philadelphia

Marygrace Elson, M.D.
Associate Clinical Professor of
Obstetrics and Gynecology, University
of Iowa Hospital and Clinics, Iowa City

Bradley Fenton, M.D.
General Internist, Clinical Associate
Professor, Thomas Jefferson University
Hospital, Philadelphia, Pennsylvania

Enrique Garcia-Valenzuela, M.D, Ph.D.
Assistant Professor of Ophthalmology,
Emory University School of Medicine;
Chief of the Retina Service, Atlanta
Veterans Administration Medical
Center, Atlanta, Georgia

Malcolm H. Gottesman, M.D.
Chief, Division of Neurology, Winthrop
University Hospital, Mineola, New York;
Associate Professor of Neurology,
SUNY at Stony Brook

Jonathan A. Haas, M.D.
Clinical Assistant Professor of
Radiation Oncology, SUNY at Stony
Brook; Attending Physician, Division
of Radiation Oncology, Winthrop
University Hospital, Mineola, New York

Joel A. Kahn, M.D.
President, WorldCare Global Health
Plan Ltd., Boston, Massachusetts

Douglas S. Katz, M.D.
Director, Body Computed Tomography,
and Vice Chair, Clinical Research and
Education Department of Radiology,
Winthrop University Hospital, Mineola,
New York; Associate Professor of Clinical
Radiology, SUNY at Stony Brook

Steven Alan Lerner, M.D.
Private Practice, Gastroenterology,
Los Angeles, California

Jerre Lutz, M.D.
Associate Professor of Cardiology,
Emory Clinic, Emory University School
of Medicine, Atlanta, Georgia

Barry Make, M.D.
Director, Emphysema Center,
National Jewish Medical and Research
Center; Professor of Medicine, University
of Colorado School of Medicine,
Denver, Colorado

Douglas E. Mattox, M.D.
Professor and Chair, Department
of Otolaryngology—Head & Neck
Surgery, Emory University School
of Medicine, Atlanta, Georgia

Eric Ravussin, Ph.D.
Douglas L. Gordon Endowed Chair
in Diabetes & Metabolism and Head,
Pennington Biomedical Research Center,
Health & Performance Enhancement
Division, Baton Rouge, Louisiana

Gregory Smith, M.D.
Private Practice, Hematology and
Medical Oncology, St. Helena Hospital,
Deer Park, California

Louis Vogel, M.D.
Clinical Faculty, Department of
Dermatology, New York University
School of Medicine, New York City

Contents

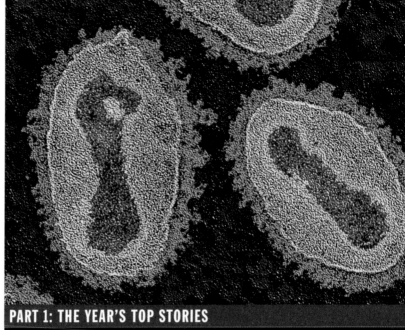

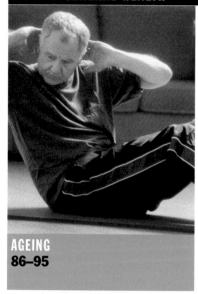

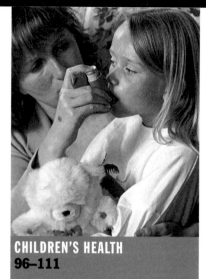

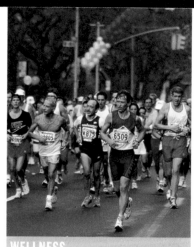

AGEING
86–95

CHILDREN'S HEALTH
96–111

WELLNESS
112–123

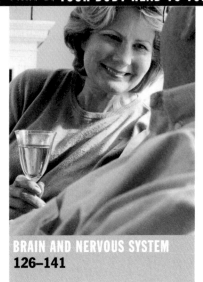

BRAIN AND NERVOUS SYSTEM
126–141

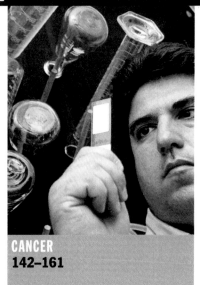

CANCER
142–161

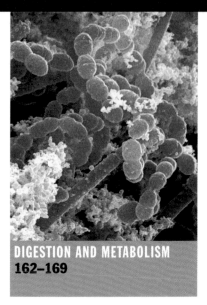

DIGESTION AND METABOLISM
162–169

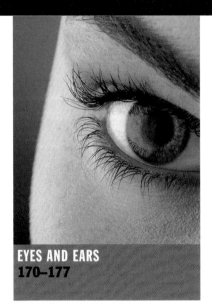

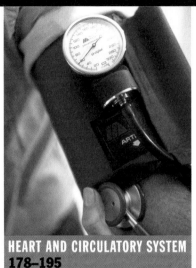

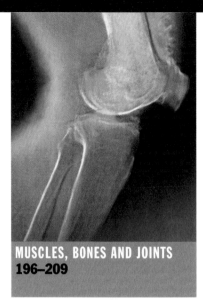

EYES AND EARS
170–177

HEART AND CIRCULATORY SYSTEM
178–195

MUSCLES, BONES AND JOINTS
196–209

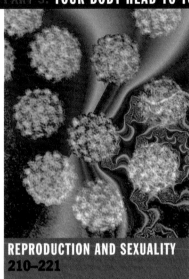

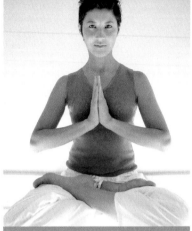

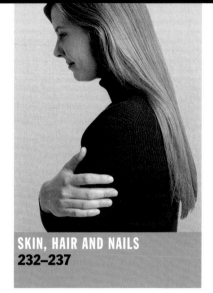

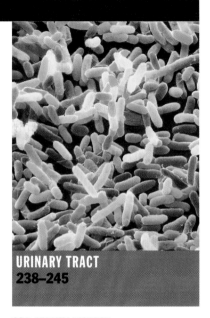

**URINARY TRACT
238–245**

AILMENT AND CONDITION LOOKUP

About this book

Some people pore over the day's financial pages. Others scour the sports section for the latest cricket or football scores. Still others are addicted to the gossip columns. But one thing that brings us all together – what everyone needs to know – is the latest health news. This brand new annual *Medical Breakthroughs 2003* is your ultimate guide to a full year's worth of important scientific discoveries and cutting-edge medical advances.

Among the highlights: the development of a smart cane to help blind people 'see', an amazing experimental treatment for Parkinson's disease, and new reasons to think about taking a statin drug – even if your cholesterol levels are normal.

The book is divided into three parts. Turn to Part I (The year's top stories) to read in depth about the most important medical issues to touch our lives in the past year, from the fascinating new research into proteins that may hold the key to many diseases, to the controversy now overshadowing hormone replacement therapy, to what scientists are doing to guard the population against bioterror threats such as anthrax and smallpox.

For general health updates that could benefit you and your family, Part II contains sections on general wellness, children's health and ageing. If you are concerned about the possibility of developing Alzheimer's disease, see page 88 to discover which simple vitamin could help you to hold this devastating disease at bay. And find out on page 115 why it's more vital than ever to comply with the law and ensure that your back-seat passengers wear their car seatbelts.

Finally, Part III is packed with news about specific medical conditions. If you have osteoporosis and are suffering the awkward regime involved in taking daily pills, you'll want to read about the annual injection that offers the same protection (see the Muscles, Bones and Joints chapter, page 196). If you're suffering the effects of the menopause or its male equivalent, you'll want to know how to relieve the symptoms (see Reproduction and Sexuality, page 210). To learn about a new vaccine that combats hay fever, look at the chapter on the Respiratory System, page 222, and get the low-down on the wrinkle smoothing 'beauty poison' in Skin, Hair and Nails, page 232.

Medical Breakthroughs 2003 presents all the latest, most important health developments in one volume – unlike any other reference book. Our panel of 19 leading medical experts has ensured that every word is accurate. And our editors have taken pains to present the information as clearly as possible in plain English.

One important reminder: although *Medical Breakthroughs 2003* comprises the newest advances in medicine, it isn't necessarily the kind of reference book that you open to discover how to manage any condition that you suffer from now; more orthodox, treatments that are already available, could well be the best way to tackle your particular illness.

The new tests and treatments described here may become standard one day but some are not yet available to the general public. It often takes years of testing for a new drug or technique to gain government approval. But you may not have to wait; you might be eligible to take part in a clinical trial that tests the efficacy of new treatments. Ask your specialist or consult the web site: www.2from.com – a small consultancy which endeavours to match volunteers to suitable trials in their area. However, it is important to discuss this with your GP or specialist so that together you can determine the best course for you.

Medical Breakthroughs 2003 presents all the latest, most important health developments in one volume.

Finally, don't keep the valuable information in this book to yourself. To order an extra copy of *Medical Breakthroughs 2003* for a friend or loved one, call 08705 113366. And watch for next year's edition, for sequels to these stories and more exciting discoveries in the extraordinary world of modern medical science.

Tomorrow's medicine today

Doctors and researchers are constantly extending the frontiers of medicine, demanding new progress, new options, new hope. Our advisors have been exploring the new territory and are very excited by what they see. That's great news for patients, the ultimate beneficiaries.

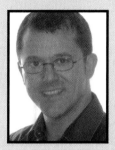

'This was a tremendously exciting project. While researching the state of the art of British medical science for this book, I was amazed to discover the breadth and scope of the developments now underway. Many of them have barely reached mainstream medical literature, or have done so in a quiet and unannounced way which belies the huge impact they will have in years to come. In spite of being immersed in medical writing for several years, much of the newest scientific work was a revelation. It's great to see a high-quality book at the cutting edge of patient information.'

DR. VINCE FORTE, consultant for this book, trained at Cambridge and London Universities. He is a qualified GP, although the focus of his clinical work is now forensic medicine. Dr. Forte has written more than 500 articles, published a medical text book *Symptom Sorter* and has appeared as a resident doctor on Anglia TV.

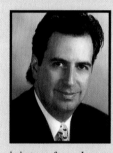

'There has never been a more exciting time, in terms of innovation and progress, for orthopaedic surgery and musculoskeletal related issues. We have new promising options for repairing ligaments and joint surface damage, treating and preventing arthritis and osteoporosis and promoting fracture healing. We have entered the Bone and Joint Decade (www.bonejointdecade.org), which is a global initiative to improve the health-related quality of life for people with musculoskeletal disorders, focusing on education, prevention, treatment and research related to these disabling conditions. The future is very bright.'

DR. NICHOLAS A. DINUBILE is currently Orthopaedic Consultant, Clinical Assistant Professor, Department of Orthopaedic Surgery, Hospital of the University of Pennsylvania.

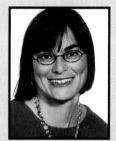

'It's an exciting time to be practising medicine, especially in my field of general obstetrics and gynaecology. Scientific advances, especially in the areas of genetics and immunology, as well as better medical imaging and interventional radiology, improve the understanding of disease processes and expand a woman's treatment options. Assisted reproductive technology has undergone tremendous refinement in helping infertile couples achieve a successful pregnancy. Modern technology allows us instant global communication. Today's practitioner can't be content to just do things "the way I've always done them", but must endeavour to practise scientific, evidence-based medicine. But the best practitioners will keep the human side of medicine foremost – the empathy and compassion which drew most of us into the medical profession in the first place.'

DR. MARYGRACE ELSON is Associate Clinical Professor of Obstetrics and Gynaecology, University of Iowa Hospital and Clinics, Iowa.

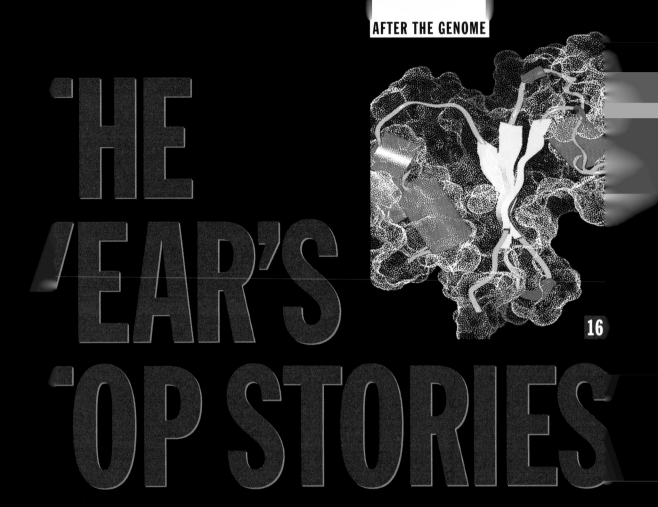

THE YEAR'S TOP STORIES

16

ealth issues have grabbed headlines throughout the year. The

go-ahead was given to establish Europe's first stem cell bank in

fordshire, fuelling hot debate about cloning and gene treatment.

areas of vital interest to women – hormone replacement therapy

mammography – came under fire, raising controversy and

tions. The fear of terrorist anthrax attack drove scientists to

ch for solutions to this and other potential biological threats.

Britain teetered on the brink of an obesity epidemic, with around

the population officially overweight and numbers ever rising.

's an in-depth look at these and other top health stories

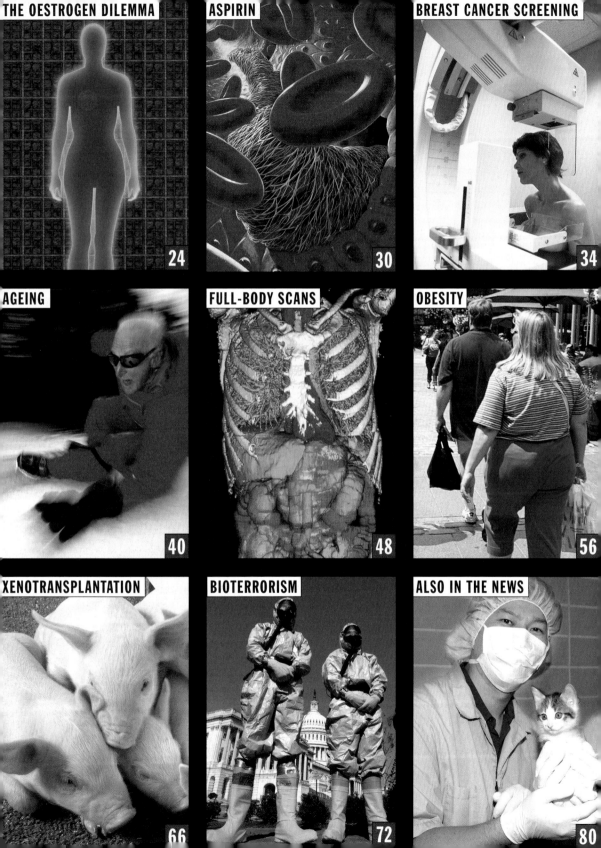

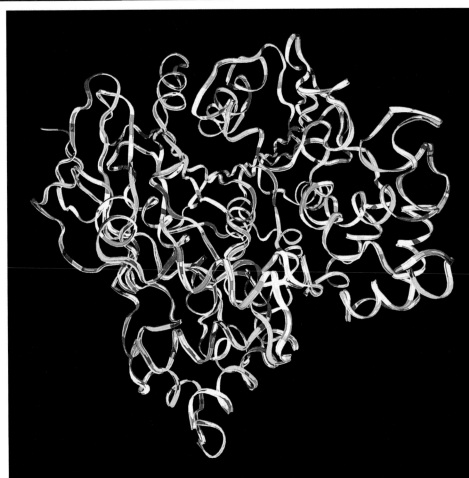
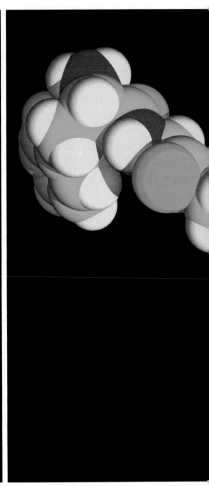

Human proteins take centre stage

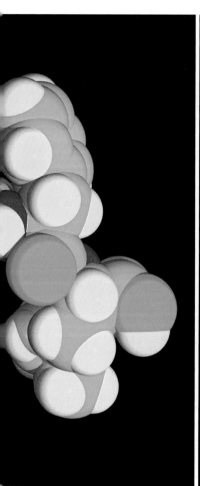

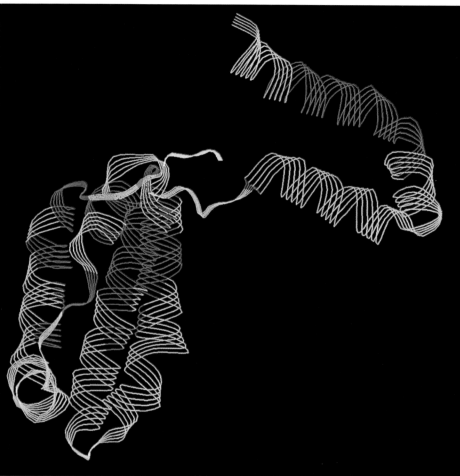

▲ Proteins, in their myriad forms, perform many of the body's functions. From left to right, we see the loose ribbon-like structure of lipase, a digestive enzyme; the clustered spheres of enkephalin, a pain mediator; and the crystalline spirals of interleukin 10, which plays a key role in the immune system. Understanding how proteins work – and why they malfunction – will help us cure the diseases of mankind.

B ack in 2001, the medical community announced to great fanfare that scientists had completed the first draft of the human genome – the sequence of all the genes that go into creating a human being. They had also figured out for the first time roughly how many genes the human body contains – somewhere in the region of 30,000 or 40,000. Impressive? Actually, the humble sweetcorn is believed to contain some 50,000 genes.

So what makes humans any more sophisticated? In that answer may lie the future of medicine.

For although human genes provide a kind of blueprint for the body, blueprints don't actually do anything. As an analogy, when building a car it's fine to start with the blueprint but you'll need parts to construct it and make it run. Likewise, genes provide instructions, but they don't perform most of the tasks that get done in the human body.

'More than 98 per cent of disease is caused by something wrong with proteins.'

The real 'engines', 'transmissions', 'carburettors' and other working components are complex molecules called proteins, which perform most life functions and even make up the majority of our cellular structures.

Mapping the human genome was merely a warm-up to mapping the more complex human proteome, loosely defined as a catalogue of all the proteins present in a cell at a given time. Once that project is completed, scientists will be one huge step closer to solving the mysteries of life – how we grow, mature and age, and why we get sick and die – and to fighting or preventing our greatest scourges, including cancer, diabetes, heart disease and even ageing itself.

What's so special about proteins?

'More than 98 per cent of disease is caused by something wrong with proteins,' says Young-Ki Paik, Ph.D., president of the Korean Human Proteome Organization (KHUPO). 'When you look at the gene sequence, you will never know anything about the disease – it doesn't say anything about cause. The most direct information about disease is in proteins.'

Dive down to the biological core of life – down to the level of the cell – and you'll find genes contained in DNA, the familiar double helix that holds the blueprints for our bodies. Each gene holds instructions for making 5, 20 or even 100 different variants of a single protein, or even different proteins, each able to perform a different function.

For those who grew up thinking that protein was just something we ate in steak and eggs, the idea that proteins perform may be surprising. In fact, they perform countless functions. Proteins form

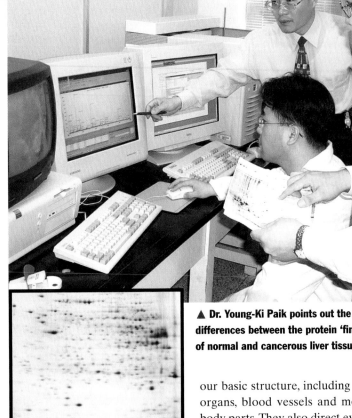

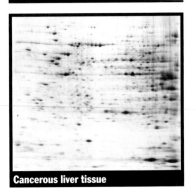

Normal liver tissue

Cancerous liver tissue

▲ **Dr. Young-Ki Paik points out the differences between the protein 'fingerprints' of normal and cancerous liver tissue.**

our basic structure, including our skin, organs, blood vessels and most other body parts. They also direct every body process and run the day-to-day operations of the cell. Proteins make up hormones (such as insulin), enzymes (like those that help us digest food), and neurotransmitters (the brain communication chemicals). They help our blood clot so that we don't bleed to death after a minor cut, and they constitute the antibodies our bodies must create to fight off infections.

If a protein mutates or malfunctions, it can't do its job properly. Malfunctions can be caused by faulty genes, invasion by a virus or other harmful microbe, or an environmental influence, such as overexposure to sunlight. One or two bad apples won't ruin the barrel but if enough proteins malfunction, the whole system can fall apart.

Proteins run in networks, so if one protein stops working, then other proteins they interact with may also malfunction, which can affect more proteins. This cascade of problems can, in some cases, lead to disease. With proteomics, scientists can identify which proteins are malfunctioning, work out how they cause the disease, then design drugs to block the harmful activities – attacking the disease at its root cause.

Unfortunately, doctors can't just go in and wipe out a specific bad protein. A single protein has more than one task, so removing a problem protein may have devastating effects elsewhere in the body. One of the challenges of proteomics, therefore, is to understand not only the specific proteins involved in various diseases but also their roles and functions in the body.

Mutating molecules add to the puzzle

What makes proteins unique is their 3D structure. Chemical attractions between molecules cause the chain of amino acids that makes up a protein to bend, fold and twist into a messy-looking tangle. But there is method to this madness. The shape of the protein is vitally important to its function. Like jigsaw puzzle pieces, the irregular surface area of one protein connects with one or more other proteins, creating a larger protein complex or activating the protein the way a car key connected to the ignition activates an engine.

Although each cell has the same genes, they don't simply pump out a steady stream of identical proteins; a stomach cell and a brain cell make different proteins, for example. Also, the type and number of proteins a cell makes can change depending on time of day, how hungry you are, how much alcohol you drink, whether you have a disease or any number of other factors. In addition, existing proteins can change into different proteins through 'post-translational modifications', alterations that occur after the protein is created. This means that the protein in your body is no longer the same protein created by your DNA. Many factors, including heat, oxidation, radiation, chemicals and even foods you eat, can cause proteins to change.

Tackling the impossible?

The magnitude of all this activity and change makes proteomics an exceptionally challenging field for researchers. Just explaining proteomics is tough, even for experts like Norman G. Anderson, Ph.D., chief scientist at Large Scale Biology Corporation in Germantown, Maryland, USA, the man many scientists call the father of proteomics.

'The essence of an explanation is to say *this* is like *that*, comparing the unknown to something you know about,' says Dr. Anderson. 'Proteomics is a *this* for which there is no *that*. There's nothing like it…. Imagine an aeroplane that flies along and changes all its parts – because all of our proteins turn over all the time. We're making them and throwing them away. Nuts and bolts drop out of this plane and new ones grow in their place. When you increase the load, the wings grow. When you decrease the number of people aboard, the wings decrease in size.'

The ability that proteins have to transform their nature and numbers in this way makes mapping the human proteome nearly impossible. 'It's a little

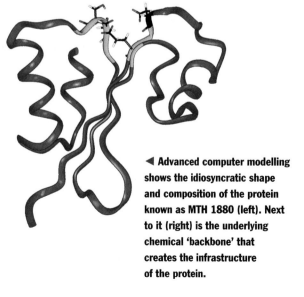

◄ **Advanced computer modelling shows the idiosyncratic shape and composition of the protein known as MTH 1880 (left). Next to it (right) is the underlying chemical 'backbone' that creates the infrastructure of the protein.**

5.00
4.00
3.00
2.00
1.00
0.00
−1.00
−2.00
−3.00
−4.00
−5.00

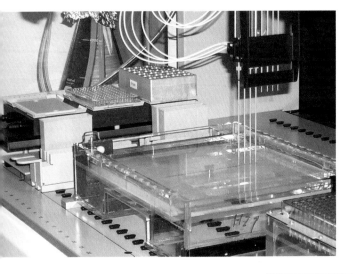

naive to say we can map the proteome,' says Dr. Joshua LaBaer, Ph.D., director of the Institute of Proteomics at Harvard Medical School, 'because there is no single proteome. There are essentially an infinite number of proteomes.'

So unlike the genome project, mapping the human proteome will not be a race to the finish by any one team – especially since, with a potentially infinite number of proteins, no one knows where the finish line is. Instead, most scientists in the field focus on proteins in just one part of the body, or on one type of disease. Major efforts are under way to understand human heart, brain, and liver proteins. Specialized research is focused on the problems of malaria, tuberculosis, cancer, heart disease, diabetes and pain, among others.

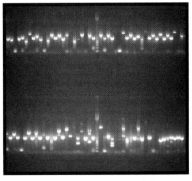

▲Robots like this (top picture) are helping Dr. Joshua LaBaer and his team at Harvard's Institute of Proteomics build a repository containing a template of every human protein. The robot places genetic material into a gel that sorts by weight, separating genes from impurities. The top scan shows unpurified genetic material. In the one below, the purified genes can be seen distinctly, four to a set.

Mapping protein pathways

Building on the mapping of the human genome, a biotechnology firm is mapping the pathways along which proteins inside cells interact with one another. This information could help pharmaceutical companies create drugs to interrupt or alter a signal's pathway, alleviating or stopping disease symptoms with few side effects.

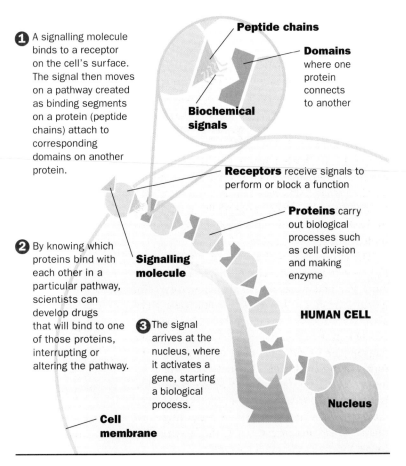

① A signalling molecule binds to a receptor on the cell's surface. The signal then moves on a pathway created as binding segments on a protein (peptide chains) attach to corresponding domains on another protein.

② By knowing which proteins bind with each other in a particular pathway, scientists can develop drugs that will bind to one of those proteins, interrupting or altering the pathway.

③ The signal arrives at the nucleus, where it activates a gene, starting a biological process.

Peptide chains

Domains where one protein connects to another

Biochemical signals

Receptors receive signals to perform or block a function

Proteins carry out biological processes such as cell division and making enzyme

Signalling molecule

HUMAN CELL

Nucleus

Cell membrane

A group effort

Especially encouraging is the unprecedented cooperation by proteomics scientists around the world. Corporations, government agencies, disease foundations and academic institutions are meeting and talking about common ground. In late 2001, an international group of scientists founded the not-for-profit Human Proteome Organization (HUPO), whose mission is to encourage research by promoting the sharing of resources and technology, facilitating technology development, and creating laboratory standards and databases.

Region-specific proteome organizations include KHUPO in Korea, Asian and Oceanian HUPO, the Swiss Proteomics Society, the German Society of Proteome Research, and other major centres in Japan, France and Russia. In Britain, which has four members on the HUPO council, the British Society for Proteome Research was established in 2002 (evolving from the British Electrophoresis Society) to help promote and coordinate proteome research efforts and to address diseases of special concern. The US Food and Drug Administration (FDA) and the National Cancer Institute (NCI) have already joined forces to form a joint proteomics programme to translate laboratory work into effective tools to diagnose and treat cancer.

Fingerprinting cancer

There are two main ways to conduct proteomics research. The most common is called abundance-based or expression proteomics. First, samples of diseased tissue, such as cancer cells, are taken from the body and analysed to see which proteins are in those cells and in what quantities. The results show a protein pattern for that disease. Then healthy cells are analysed the same way. Finally, the pattern from the diseased cells is compared with the pattern from the healthy cells. The differences clearly show which proteins are involved in the disease.

This information can be used in a couple of ways. If, for example, a particular protein is three times more common in cancer cells than in normal cells, more research on that protein could yield clues about how to treat the cancer. Typically, however, no single protein stands out. Instead, the important nugget of information is the pattern of proteins found in diseased cells. That pattern, formed by hundreds or even thousands of different proteins, is as distinctive as a fingerprint. It can be used to diagnose or screen for diseases by comparing a test sample to the protein pattern. If the fingerprint is found, the disease culprit is caught.

One example of expression proteomics is the research being conducted by the FDA-NCI Clinical Proteomics Program. They analyse proteins in cancer cells from hundreds of patients, then run the results through a powerful computer to look for common patterns.

Emanuel Petricoin, Ph.D., at the FDA's Center for Biologics Evaluation and Research, and the co-director of the Clinical Proteomics Programme, says they have already identified over 500 proteins

TOOLS OF THE TRADE

Scientists finally have tools that are powerful enough to let them study thousands of proteins at a time. The most commonly used tools are explained below.

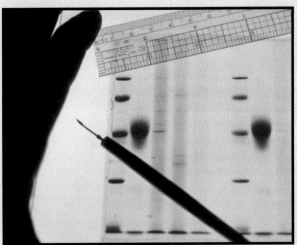

Analysing the distribution of different proteins within a cell using electrophoresis.

■ **2-D GEL ELECTROPHORESIS** is used to separate proteins. In a cell, thousands of proteins are mixed together rather like ingredients in a soup. The 'soup' is applied to a thin gel and then run through a machine that separates the proteins according to molecular charge and molecular mass. The result looks like a splatter of dots, with each dot representing a different protein.

■ **MASS SPECTROMETRY** reveals the details of the cell, including which proteins are there, what they look like, and whether they are functioning. This process can expose the 'fingerprint' pattern of proteins in a sample of cells, as well as identify specific proteins and their interactions. One way scientists visualize the results is by a computer-generated picture of a protein pattern.

■ **NUCLEAR MAGNETIC RESONANCE IMAGING** gives information about the structure of a molecule, similar to the way in which magnetic resonance imaging scans give information about internal body tissue. The result is a 3D computer diagram of a single protein molecule.

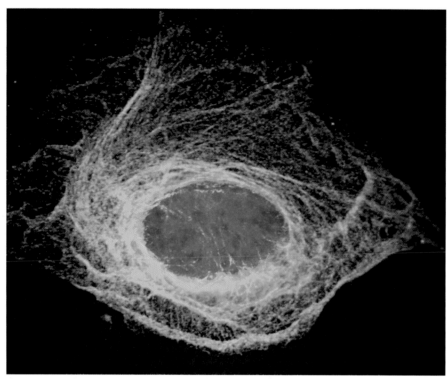

▲ A fluorescent antibody specific to the protein cytokeratin 19 highlights that protein (green) in this breast cancer cell. Proteins in this cell can be compared to those of healthy cells.

in ovarian, prostate, breast, colon, lung, oesophageal and pancreatic cancer that were found in different amounts in the cancers compared to controls.

'We can take normal cells, pre-cancerous cells, and cancer cells all from the same patient and compare them – almost take a timeline of the history of cancer progression – and see what proteins went up and down.'

Their results offer the first real-world use for proteomics – they have discovered a protein pattern for ovarian cancer that allows them to diagnose the cancer from a small blood sample. At present, a woman with suspicious symptoms might be sent for an ultrasound and then perhaps a needle biopsy, and finally surgery. 'All that takes a tremendous amount of time, especially when you consider that ovarian cancer grows extremely rapidly,' says Dr. Petricoin.

'It's thought that in a period of about 18 months, you can go from nothing at all there to stage III (advanced) cancer, which is why it's scary, because of how fast it can go. Just a couple of months of

prevarication and going to see this specialist and this other specialist – that can translate into deaths.'

Early diagnosis means a better chance of recovery. The protein-pattern test for ovarian cancer is undergoing clinical trials with women who have gene mutations that increase their risk of the cancer. Protein profiles are also being developed for prostate, lung, colon, breast and pancreatic cancers. Blood tests based on these profiles may be available within 5 to 10 years.

Other research involving expression proteomics is equally impressive. John R. Yates, Ph.D., at the Scripps Research Institute in La Jolla, California, is looking at the proteins involved in the different stages of malaria. His goal is to locate a good target for a vaccine for this killer disease. In Australia researchers are searching for a vaccine and drug treatments for tuberculosis. And Gary Sweeney, Ph.D., of York University in Toronto, Canada is using proteomics to find better treatments for type 2 diabetes and to locate the protein-related causes of obesity.

The second approach to proteomics research is function-based proteomics. Rather than looking at amounts of proteins, here the goal is to understand what proteins do and how they interact. The basic idea is to add or remove proteins from cells, and then see the reaction. If the additions or deletions cause the cells to act abnormally, then those proteins are good candidates for further investigation.

The promise of personalized medicine

The investigation of proteins and their functions is just the beginning. The ultimate goal is to find ways to prevent or block malfunctioning proteins with medications. It is conceivable that treatments for cancer may someday be as easy and effective as taking an antibiotic for an ear infection. 'It's going

It is conceivable that treatments for cancer may some day be as easy and effective as taking an antibiotic for an ear infection.

to be a few years, but there's no doubt that proteomics is going to have a profound impact on the generation of new drugs, and also on the ability to do what's called personalized medicine,' says Michael Moran, Ph.D., chief science officer at MDS Proteomics in Toronto. 'That's the ability to design the therapeutics to each individual's version of a disease they may have.'

For example, monoclonal antibodies are drugs created to bind to a specific target protein on diseased cells. Once attached, the antibodies prevent the cells from growing and dividing. One way the drugs are developed is by looking at the target protein's 3D structure, then creating an antibody that will bind with the protein, fitting like a puzzle piece into the protein's grooves.

Proteomics will eventually provide a shortcut when it comes to developing new drugs. 'There's so much attrition in the drug discovery process, so many failures along the way,' says Dr. Moran. 'That's what drags the time period out and makes it so expensive.'

The typical drug discovery process is a hit-or-miss scenario in which the developers are basically flying blind. Drugs that seem as if they should work end up failing, and drugs often have unexpected side effects. With proteomics, scientists will know their targets and be able to design drugs to hit those targets like precision bombs. The bottom line – new drugs will get from the laboratory to prescription faster.

As a rule, researchers tend to downplay the value of their work for fear of raising expectations too high or too soon. Proteomics researchers, on the other hand, have difficulty hiding their enthusiasm.

'We're at the point of a new era for cardiac research,' says Peipei Ping, Ph.D., a lead researcher for the Cardiac Proteome Project. 'We're going to gain information that will potentially benefit generations to come. I think major breakthroughs [in preventing and treating heart attacks] will happen within five years, if not sooner.'

Proteomic discoveries in disease diagnosis and personalized medicines are already being tested. It is just possible that some day doctors will no longer talk of 'cures' because proteomics will have revealed the secrets of preventing disease in the first place.

WHAT DOES IT MEAN TO YOU?

Working out which proteins are involved in a certain disease may one day lead to better diagnosis and drugs that target the root cause of the disease. The protein profile for ovarian cancer has been generated and its accuracy and value as a screening tool for women at high risk of the disease are now being tested in clinical trials. Other hot areas of research:

■ **LIVER AND BREAST CANCER** Korean researchers have isolated proteins that may be used to diagnose and monitor the treatment of liver cancer. Other researchers are using cells taken from breast ducts to look for protein patterns that might allow easy diagnosis of breast cancer.

■ **ALZHEIMER'S DISEASE** In an attempt to better understand the causes of Alzheimer's, researchers from New Zealand have found up to 125 malfunctioning proteins in the brains of people with the disease, with different proteins affected in different parts of the brain.

■ **HEART DISEASE** Researchers are investigating what makes a person's heart vulnerable to heart disease, with the goal of developing drugs to treat or prevent heart attacks.

■ **CYSTIC FIBROSIS** One of the dangers of cystic fibrosis is that serious bacterial infections can develop and cause permanent lung damage. Researchers at Proteome Systems Ltd in Australia have teamed up with the Cystic Fibrosis Foundation in the USA to develop a home test to signal when protein patterns in sputum match patterns of infection. This will help patients identify infections early so they can start taking antibiotics immediately.

■ **DRUG FUNCTION** Prescribing medications for many illnesses is a hit-or-miss process. A drug is given and doctors and patients wait weeks or months to see if it works. If not, a new drug is tried. With the help of proteomics, future doctors will be able to analyse the response of proteins in disease cells almost immediately, dramatically reducing the time it takes to cure the disease.

■ **AGEING** Proteomic study of ageing is just beginning. Scientists know that free radicals or oxidation molecules are produced in our cells and, over time, cause or lead to changes in proteins associated with ageing. That's why antioxidant nutrients are so important, because they are thought to block the harmful effects of free radicals. Some researchers are investigating exactly how antioxidant drugs interfere with oxidation and what protein molecules they might target for therapeutic intervention to slow the ageing process.

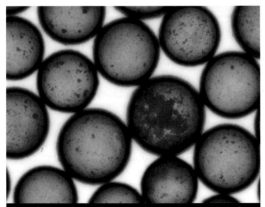

Tiny microcarrier beads are used to capture proteins of interest from cells. The rest of the cell is washed away. A blue dye that binds to proteins highlights the results.

Hormone replacement therapy loses its appeal

For more than 50 years, doctors have been encouraging women to take oestrogen after the menopause. At first, the hormone was promoted as a virtual fountain of youth. It could quell symptoms of menopause such as hot flushes and night sweats, keep skin supple, prevent wrinkles and increase sexual desire. Then, over a decade ago, US and British doctors began to urge women to take hormone replacement therapy (HRT) – oestrogen or a combination of oestrogen and progesterone – for other health reasons: to protect against brittle bones and especially against stroke and heart disease.

But disturbing news began to emerge from laboratories and universities. Much to the surprise of many doctors, data published in 1998 showed that oestrogen did *not* reduce the overall risk of heart attack or the risk of dying from coronary heart disease. In 2001 even newer research confirmed these findings, and a 2001 study examining the effects of HRT on stroke again found no benefit. Then, in July 2002, America's National Heart, Lung, and Blood Institute (NHLBI) announced that it was halting a major clinical trial early because results showed an increase in breast cancer, heart disease, stroke and blood clots.

Such research has prompted the American Heart Association (AHA) to change its guidelines on HRT. The new ones advise against prescribing hormones to women with heart disease to prevent heart attacks or stroke. The British Heart Foundation has recommended

► **Natural oestrogen may stave off heart disease in younger women but does HRT help later in life?**

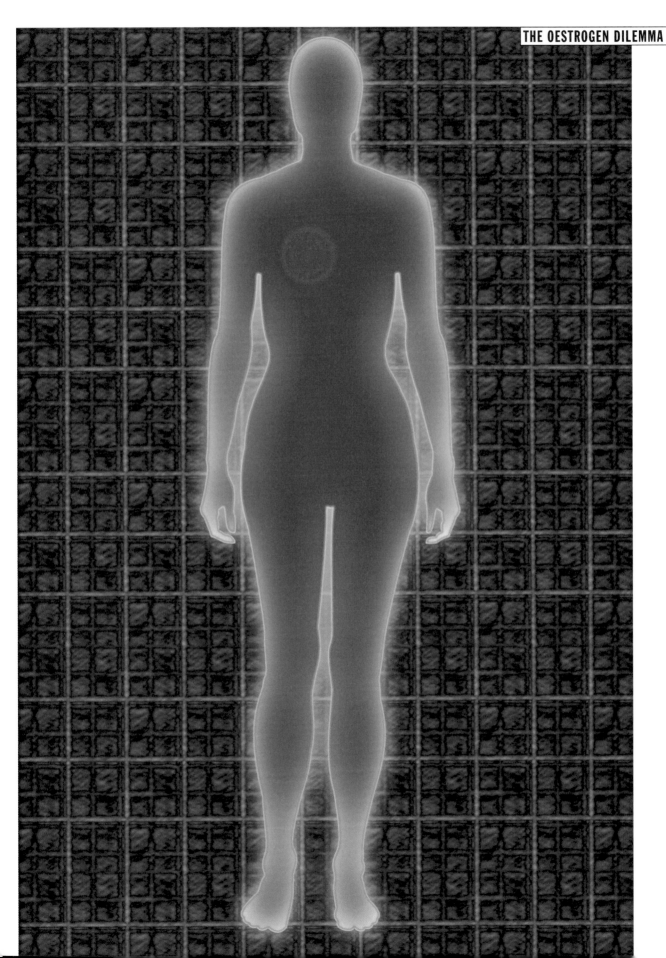

that HRT should not be prescribed solely to reduce the risk of coronary heart disease. But neither organization has advised women with heart disease to stop taking HRT if they are already on it or if they have osteoporosis or severe menopausal symptoms. And the £20 million 'Wisdom' study – the Women's International Study of Long Duration Oestrogen after the Menopause – funded by the Medical Research Council, the Department of Health and the British Heart Foundation, will continue investigating the effects of HRT on cancers, heart disease, Alzheimer's, osteoporosis and other age-onset diseases as long as the women taking part are fully informed about known risks.

Background to HRT hopes

It helps to know why scientists first thought that HRT was good for the heart. Several large studies had shown that women who took hormones were less likely than other women to develop clogged arteries. In addition, the researchers found that HRT improved cholesterol levels. LDL ('bad') cholesterol levels went down, while HDL ('good') cholesterol levels went up. But this research

A nagging question arose: Did the women who chose HRT benefit from the oestrogen itself or from something else? Perhaps they were healthier to begin with; maybe they exercised more ...

depended on 'observational' studies, the kind that involved women who chose to take hormones. It became evident that these women were younger, better educated, and more health conscious than those who decided not to take oestrogen.

A nagging question arose: Did the women who chose HRT benefit from the oestrogen itself or from something else? Perhaps they were healthier to begin with; maybe they exercised more or didn't smoke, or had better health care, or ate plenty of fruit and vegetables.

The only way to test the potential protective powers of oestrogen was to devise large, 'double-blind' clinical trials in which post-menopausal women whose arteries were already clogged with athero-sclerotic plaque could be randomly assigned either oestrogen or a placebo. (The studies are called double-blind because neither researchers nor participants would know which group of women took which kind of pill until the results were in.)

Several such studies concluded that HRT was far from being the magic bullet for heart disease that doctors had once thought. One of the largest US studies, the Heart Estrogen/Progestin Replacement Study (HERS), published in 1998, reported that HRT did not prevent further heart attacks or death from coronary heart disease. (HERS involved more than 2,700 postmenopausal women at an average age of 67, who were treated for about four years.) Even worse, in the first year of the study, those who took hormones were 50 per cent *more* likely to have heart attacks and die. After women had undergone several years of HRT the trend reversed itself, and ultimately the women taking the

CUSTOMIZED HORMONES

Keen to find alternatives to HRT, pharmaceutical companies have begun to develop drugs that provide the benefits of oestrogen without the drawbacks. These drugs, known as selective oestrogen receptor modulators, are often called 'designer oestrogens'.

The drugs take advantage of the fact that the chemical structure of oestrogen receptors varies from tissue to tissue. They are formulated to bond with the oestrogen receptors of some tissues, like bone, but not with breast tissue. Thus they hold out the promise of helping a woman keep her heart and bones healthy without risking breast cancer.

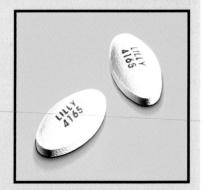

Raloxifene mimics oestrogen to prevent and treat osteoporosis.

One such drug, called tamoxifen, is used to treat some breast cancers because it blocks oestrogen in breast tissue. It also mimics oestrogen's beneficial effect on bone. Raloxifene, a newer version, also has an oestrogen-like effect on bones but not on breast tissue. Another drug, lasofoxifene, is currently being tested in the USA.

'These drugs are the wave of the future,' says Dr. JoAnn Z. Pinkerton, director of Mid-Life Health and associate professor of obstetrics and gynaecology at the University of Virginia in Charlottesville. 'We believe we'll soon be able to offer an individualized, tailored approach to each woman that will take into account her menopausal symptoms and specific risk factors, such as bone loss or breast cancer.'

hormones were having fewer heart attacks but experienced more blood clots and gallbladder disease. Overall, oestrogen had not helped. Two more studies published in 2001 found similar results.

Results from studies on stroke painted the same bleak picture. In one major clinical trial called the Women's Estrogen for Stroke Trial (WEST), reported in the *New England Journal of Medicine* in October 2001, researchers kept track of more than 600 postmenopausal women with a history of strokes. The study concluded that HRT was not effective in preventing a further stroke. In fact, compared to women who took a placebo, women who took oestrogen had a higher risk of a fatal stroke and more severe impairments after a stroke.

Its link to breast cancer also reduced oestrogen's appeal. Adding progesterone to the formulation did not eliminate that risk. Then in April 2002, Swedish research found that the risk of ovarian cancer was also higher in women who took HRT. This was not the first time scientists had examined the risk of ovarian cancer in women on HRT. In March 2001, researchers reported that post-menopausal women using HRT for a decade or more had an increased risk of dying from the disease.

The study halted by the NHLBI involved more than 16,000 women aged between 50 and 79. That study also showed increased risk of breast cancer among the women taking oestrogen plus progesterone, as well as an increased risk of heart disease, stroke and blood clots. The women on HRT had *lower* rates of colon cancer and bone fractures, but the researchers decided that these did not outweigh the potential risks, so they stopped the study.

Could age be the answer?

But the news about HRT is not all bad. Recent research argues that oestrogen does help prevent heart attacks – but not in everyone.

While the WEST study showed that oestrogen provided no cardiac benefit to its 600 postmenopausal subjects, when researchers looked only at younger women with healthy arteries, the results were different. In fact, several recent reports have

suggested that HRT may stave off heart disease and stroke in these women. Some researchers believe this may be because oestrogen isn't potent enough to help arteries that are already clogged but may keep plaque from overwhelming healthy arteries.

A study reported in the *Annals of Internal Medicine* in December 2001 found that women who had relatively clear arteries and began taking HRT when they reached menopause were less likely to accumulate artery-clogging plaque than similar women who took no hormones.

In another, the Estrogen in the Prevention of Atherosclerosis Trial (EPAT), researchers found that women who didn't take hormones had twice as much arterial thickening as those who did. The study's lead author, Dr. Howard N. Hodis, associate professor of medicine and preventive medicine at the University of Southern California in Los Angeles, says that this degree of thickening could double or triple the risk of a heart attack.

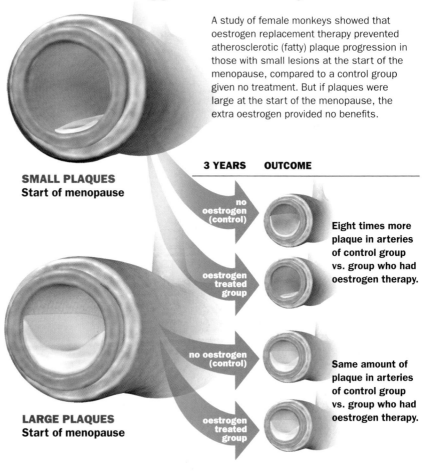

Clogged arteries study

A study of female monkeys showed that oestrogen replacement therapy prevented atherosclerotic (fatty) plaque progression in those with small lesions at the start of the menopause, compared to a control group given no treatment. But if plaques were large at the start of the menopause, the extra oestrogen provided no benefits.

**SMALL PLAQUES
Start of menopause**

3 YEARS **OUTCOME**

no oestrogen (control)

oestrogen treated group

Eight times more plaque in arteries of control group vs. group who had oestrogen therapy.

**LARGE PLAQUES
Start of menopause**

no oestrogen (control)

oestrogen treated group

Same amount of plaque in arteries of control group vs. group who had oestrogen therapy.

Clogged arteries block protection

One reason scientists find it difficult to assess HRT's influence is that heart disease can take decades to develop after menopause, which is when women generally begin taking hormones. In a foolproof study, researchers would have to randomly assign menopausal women to HRT or a placebo, then wait for two or three decades to find the answers.

Take action

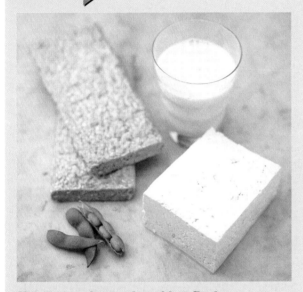

How to combat and cool hot flushes

Now, it seems, women **can** protect their hearts and bones and cool off hot flushes at the same time. Recent research shows that a diet rich in soya protein eases hot flushes while lowering cholesterol and staving off bone loss. 'A lot of studies show that soya helps to control cardiovascular risk factors,' says Mary S. Anthony, Ph.D., assistant professor of pathology and public health sciences at Wake Forest University School of Medicine in Winston-Salem, North Carolina. 'You need about 25g of soya each day, the amount in a third of a cup of roasted soya nuts or a soya protein beverage.'

Many women also turn to herbs such as dong quai, ginseng, black cohosh and liquorice root to quell menopausal symptoms. But experts say that these herbs may not be risk-free, so proceed with caution. Research published in March 2002 revealed that in test-tube studies, these herbs encouraged the growth of cancer cells. Whether they will have the same effect in humans needs further investigation.

Both aerobic and weight-bearing exercise can decrease the severity of hot flushes and also strengthen bone and keep cholesterol levels in check, helping to prevent heart disease.

In the USA, animal studies are supplementing the work on humans. Researchers at Wake Forest University Medical Center in Winston-Salem, North Carolina, looked at the effect of hormone therapy in postmenopausal monkeys. First, they tested tissue samples from the monkeys' arteries, then they put the apes on an artery-clogging diet.

After three years they checked the monkeys again. Their report, presented to the annual meeting of the American College of Cardiology in March 2002, revealed that while the oestrogen worked to keep arteries clear in those monkeys with the least amount of plaque, it had almost no effect on the monkeys whose arteries were clogged at the start of the study.

The study's lead researcher Mary S. Anthony, Ph.D., assistant professor of pathology and public health sciences, suspects that plaque blocked the effects of oestrogen. 'When arteries have plaque lesions, the oestrogen receptors don't work as well,' she says. 'This would explain the differences we've seen between observational studies and clinical trials. In nearly all the observational studies, the women started taking oestrogen at menopause. In the clinical trials, the women already had quite a lot of atherosclerosis and were older.'

A number of other studies will soon yield more results, but none will come close to a perfect clinical trial that enrols women just as they enter menopause, says Dr. Richard H. Karas, Ph.D., director of the Women's Heart Center at Tufts Medical Center in Boston. In an editorial in the journal *Circulation* in November 2001, he argues that data from studies like HERS should not be taken to mean that HRT has no place in preventing heart disease. 'Oestrogen may be able to help maintain healthy blood vessels but may not be strong enough to take on those that are already highly diseased and turn them back into healthy ones,' he says.

No easy answers

At this point, experts simply aren't sure about the best advice to give women, and they don't expect matters to change for several years. But oestrogen does have some unquestionable advantages. Used for three to five years, it can safely ease the hot flushes and night sweats associated with the menopause. It may also turn out to be the female equivalent of Viagra. 'Oestrogen not only helps to relieve vaginal dryness, it has an impact on orgasm,' says Dr. Marianne J. Legato, founder and director of the Partnership for Women's Health at Columbia Presbyterian Medical Center in New York City.

'If a woman has experienced problems with breast tenderness or bleeding on the standard dose of oestrogen, then she might benefit from a lower dose.'

After the menopause, she says, 'Without oestrogen, women find orgasms more difficult to achieve and the intensity tends to decrease.'

Oestrogen also slows the loss of bone and preserves bone mineral density. There's even a possibility that HRT can help to prevent mental decline. Several studies have suggested that oestrogen may reduce the risk and also delay the onset of Alzheimer's disease, and a study published in the journal *Neurology* in December 2001 found that women who took HRT retained memories better than those who never took oestrogen.

Ultimately, the oestrogen decision may depend on family history. If a woman is worried about thinning bones or wants extra insurance against heart disease or mental decline, she may choose to take oestrogen. New low-dose formulations, to be launched this year, may help women to decide. The new lower doses can protect bones while minimizing unpleasant side effects, according to several studies completed in 2001 and early 2002. And there may be other advantages.

'If a woman has experienced problems with breast tenderness or bleeding on the standard dose of oestrogen, then she might benefit from a lower dose,' says Dr. Margery Gass, director of the Menopause and Osteoporosis Center at the University of Cicinnati College of Medicine. 'Bone density is, however, related to dose, so higher doses may provide greater benefits.'

Another problem women face is deciding how long to stay on HRT. 'We currently have more questions than answers about the long-term safety and efficacy of HRT,' says Dr. JoAnn Z. Pinkerton, associate professor of obstetrics and gynaecology at the University of Virginia. 'We just don't have definitive data yet.' That is why some doctors now recommend that women should stay on HRT only long enough to treat menopausal symptoms.

Given the current uncertainties and the lack of a one-size-fits-all answer, the best thing you can do is sit down with your doctor and go over the pros and cons of HRT as it relates to your own health, then make the decision that you feel is best for you.

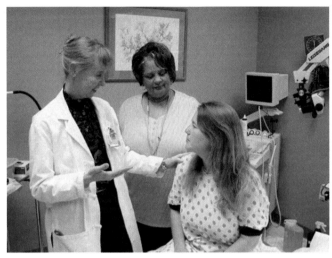

▲ **Dr. JoAnn Pinkerton discusses the finer points of hormone therapy with one of her patients.**

WHAT DOES IT MEAN TO YOU?

Should you consider hormone replacement therapy (HRT) or stay on it if you've already started? There is, unfortunately, no simple answer. You have to weigh the risks and benefits and decide what's right for you.

■ Oestrogen effectively reduces the incidence and severity of hot flushes and night sweats, and using it for anywhere from three to five years seems to pose no risk. After that, the picture becomes murkier.

■ When it comes to heart disease, it seems that HRT can protect blood vessels from artery-clogging plaque – but only if you begin taking it at menopause when arteries are still clear. If you wait, the chances of having a heart attack or stroke may increase.

■ Although HRT can lower levels of LDL ('bad') cholesterol and raise HDL ('good') cholesterol, the American Heart Association does not recommend using it as an alternative to cholesterol-lowering drugs such as statins, which greatly reduce the risk of heart attacks and stroke.

■ HRT can help to protect against bone loss and increase bone density, but if you're worried about developing breast cancer, you may opt for a more targeted substitute known as a 'designer oestrogen' (see Customized hormones, page 34).

■ Your doctor can help you sort through the pros and cons of HRT as it relates to your own health. But in the end, the decision comes down to one that you must be comfortable with.

Aspirin – the wonder drug?

I t's sitting in every medicine cabinet, buried in the bottoms of handbags, tucked into desk drawers. It's long been the first thing to reach for when treating headaches, pain or fever. But recently this popular cure-all has been tipped for star status, as evidence emerges of aspirin's beneficial effects on more serious, or even life-threatening, diseases such as heart disease and cancer.

The reason for aspirin's newfound respect? Quite simply: a reduction in heart attacks. The results of an Italian study of patients with at least one risk factor for cardiovascular disease, but no history of heart problems, were published in *The Lancet* in January 2001. They showed that a low daily dose of aspirin (100mg a day) reduced the patients' risk of death from cardiovascular causes by a staggering 44 per cent and also reduced the risk of experiencing non-fatal cardiovascular events, such as heart attack.

An American medic, Dr. M. Pignone, evaluated the results of several large studies on the topic, and found that an aspirin a day could reduce the risk of heart attacks in healthy people, too. British doctors are hesitant in prescribing aspirin to healthy patients, but healthcare professionals in the United States are convinced, and are being encouraged to talk about the benefits (and dangers) of aspirin with patients at increased risk of cardiovascular disease.

How it works wonders

Aspirin's cardiovascular benefits are ascribed to its effects on platelets – tiny blood cells that are partly responsible for forming clots, which cause heart attacks and strokes. Aspirin reduces the clotting ability of blood by making the platelets less sticky (called the antiplatelet effect). Scientists have also recently learned that tissue inflammation plays a significant role in heart disease, and they report that aspirin's anti-inflammatory qualities help to protect inflamed and inflexible blood vessels, like those in patients with atherosclerosis (narrowed arteries).

Inflammation is the immune system's first line of defence against injury or infection. It's caused by an increase in blood flow and a mass movement of immune cells into the damaged tissue. But even mild inflammation, which may occur with common ailments such as colds, can also harm tissue by causing changes in blood vessels that are similar to those seen in people at high risk for heart disease. In people with atherosclerosis, inflammation is part of an ongoing cycle of injury and healing in plaque-lined arteries, that can lead to clot formation. Aspirin works to interrupt this chain of events.

But aspirin's strength may also be its weakness. Because it inhibits clotting, aspirin increases the danger of gastro-intestinal bleeding, either from an ulcer or gastritis (stomach inflammation).

▶ Aspirin is so widely used that 35,000 tonnes is produced worldwide each year: enough to make more than 100 billion tablets.

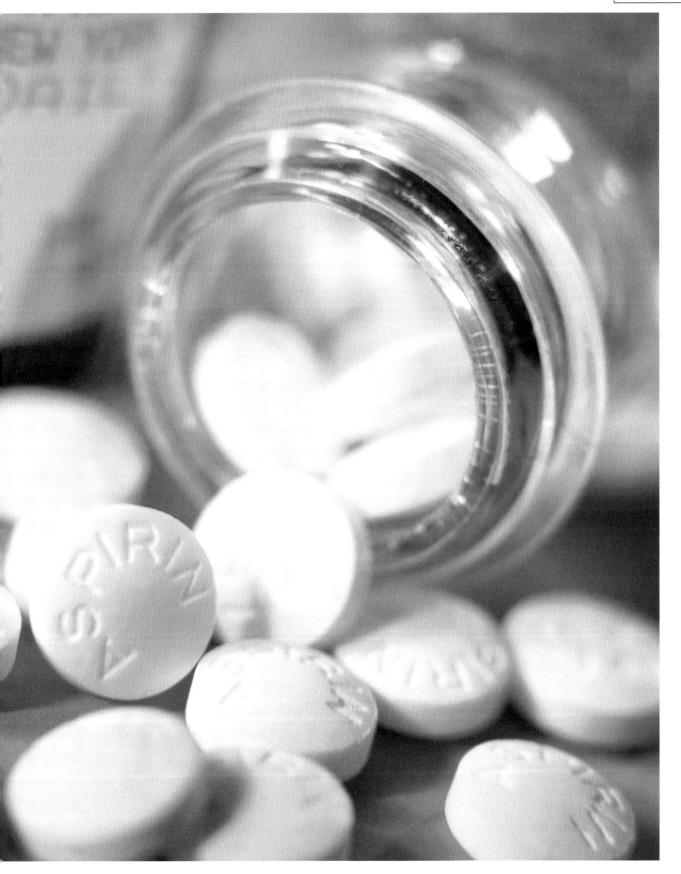

It also raises the odds of a rare form of stroke, known as haemorrhagic stroke, caused by bleeding in the brain, and GPs in the UK fear that these risks may outweigh the preventative benefits of taking aspirin if a patient does not demonstrate a clear-cut clinical risk of cardiovascular disease.

Dr. Pignone measured aspirin's benefits against all its potential downsides and, although his British counterparts may disagree, sums it up this way: 'Once you're over 50, unless you have absolutely pristine blood pressure and cholesterol and none of the other risk factors for heart disease, you should talk to your doctor about taking a daily low-dose aspirin.' If you're under 50 and have any risk factors for heart disease – you smoke, have diabetes, are overweight, or rarely exercise, for example – you should also consider the drug, he claims. People with uncontrolled high blood pressure, however, should bring their pressure under control first.

People under 50 with a low risk of heart disease probably don't need it, as the risks for them may be greater than the benefits. So does he take a daily aspirin? 'No. I'm 35, have normal blood pressure and cholesterol, I exercise, don't smoke, and don't have diabetes,' he reports. 'My risk of developing cardio-vascular disease in the next five years is very low.'

Unfortunately, many people who would benefit from aspirin therapy – patients with a history of heart attack or stroke, or clinical evidence of a risk of heart disease – are not getting it, perhaps misled by its familiarity into doubting its powers. Only 30 to 40 per cent of the people who have most to gain from the drug are taking it and British medical efforts are focussed on addressing this shortfall before broadening the drug's use.

Aspirin the cancer fighter

In addition to its heart-protective properties, a growing body of research suggests that aspirin may help to prevent certain cancers, including:

- **Prostate cancer** According to the Mayo Clinic in Rochester, Minnesota, regular use of aspirin, ibuprofen and other nonsteroidal anti-inflammatory drugs (NSAIDs) may help to protect against prostate cancer. In March 2002, *Mayo Clinic Proceedings* published a study that found that men aged 60 and older who used NSAIDs every day cut their risk of prostate cancer by as much as 60 per cent.
- **Bowel cancer** Several recent studies support the claim that taking low dosage aspirin may help to prevent bowel, or colorectal cancer.

Blood clot formation

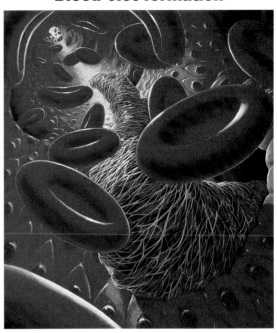

A serpentine clot forms inside a blood vessel as a sticky web of fibrin threads causes the saucer-like red blood cells to clump together. Aspirin helps to prevent such clots.

Research at the Molecular Medicine Unit at the University of Leeds examined the effects of a variety of NSAIDs, including aspirin, on human colorectal cancer cells and found that all stopped the cells spreading. The protective effect may be linked to an enzyme called cyclooxygenase-2 (COX-2), which is elevated in colon cancer. Aspirin and other NSAIDs suppress the production of the enzyme and, in animal studies, have been shown to cause colon tumours to shrink dramatically.

- **Lung cancer** In a New York study published in the July 2002 *British Journal of Cancer*, 14,000 women were questioned about their long-term use of aspirin. The medical histories of 81 women who developed lung cancer were compared with those of more than 800 who didn't. Researchers found that, while smoking was the biggest risk factor, women who took aspirin regularly had less than half the normal risk of non-small-cell lung cancer, the most common form of the disease.

Researchers do not yet know exactly how aspirin protects against these and, possibly, other cancers, but they have several theories. For instance, aspirin and other NSAIDs work to block the production of chemicals called prostaglandins, which cause inflammation and appear to encourage the growth of certain tumours. Aspirin may also prevent some cell division – a particularly important property when dealing with cancer cells, whose main danger is their propensity to divide uncontrollably. Another reason for aspirin's anti-cancer effects may stem from the drug's ability to prevent the production and action of enzymes produced by certain cancer cells. Other possible mechanisms of action include aspirin's apparent power to limit the damaging effects of some cancer-causing carcinogens, such as cigarette smoke and environmental toxins, and to induce apoptosis, or programmed cell death, which kills off tumour cells.

And the benefits don't stop there

In addition to its possible protective effects against cancer and heart disease, aspirin may have other benefits as well, including:

■ **Preventing Alzheimer's disease** In a study published in the November 2001 *New England Journal of Medicine*, Dutch researchers found that people who used NSAIDs for at least two years were only one-sixth as likely to get Alzheimer's as those who didn't. The study found that the timing is important. It appears that the drugs must be taken for at least two years before the onset of any Alzheimer's symptoms. Other trials are under way to test the use of 'super-aspirins' called COX-2 inhibitors (celecoxib, or Celebrex, and rofecoxib, or Vioxx) in Alzheimer's patients. Although scientists don't know exactly how the drugs work in relation to the disease, it is believed that inflammation in the brain is an important factor in the Alzheimer's disease process and they suspect that aspirin's anti-inflammatory actions may play a role.

■ **Extending your life** Preventing a heart attack or cancer would, by definition, extend your life. But a September 2001 article in the *Journal of the American Medical Association* found that people who took aspirin to reduce their risk of heart attack also lowered their risk of dying by one-third during a three-year follow-up. Another study, published in March 2002, found that people who are aspirin resistant (that is, the drug simply doesn't work on them) have a higher risk of dying from heart disease than others.

■ **Preventing headaches** A study conducted through four UK Migraine Clinics showed that mouth-dispersible tablets acted fastest in treating moderate migraine, with relief seen as early as within 30 minutes. However, there is also evidence that an aspirin-a-day seems to prevent as well as treat headaches.

■ **Reducing severity of stroke** A report in the December 2001 issue of the journal *Stroke* found that stroke patients generally had less severe strokes if they had been taking aspirin before the attack than if they hadn't. Aspirin's powers may stem from its antiplatelet effect, which may improve blood circulation in the brain; its antioxidant properties, which may help to reduce tissue damage during a stroke; or some other anti-inflammatory effect that protects the brain.

■ **Preventing obesity-related resistance to insulin** People who are obese often develop an insulin resistance, a precursor of diabetes. Studies in rats, published in *Science* and the *Journal of Clinical Investigation* in August 2001, suggest that by shielding cells from the damage caused by inflammation, aspirin may reduce their resistance to insulin.

Aspirin is also being investigated for its ability to prevent outbreaks of herpes zoster (shingles), pre-eclampsia (a potentially fatal condition in pregnant women), and atherosclerosis.

WHAT DOES IT MEAN TO YOU?

Many people who could benefit from aspirin aren't taking it. Check with your doctor about whether aspirin therapy is right for you. You should avoid aspirin if you have a stomach ulcer or liver disease. Find out how aspirin may affect the action of other drugs you may be taking, including blood thinners (such as warfarin) and blood pressure medication. If you are suitable to start aspirin therapy, here's how you may benefit:

■ If you've already had a heart attack, aspirin may help to prevent another one.

■ If you're 50 or older – even if you're healthy – aspirin may help prevent a future heart attack, and may reduce the likelihood or severity of stroke. Some studies indicate that taking a daily aspirin can cut your heart attack risk by a huge 60 per cent.

■ If you're at increased risk of certain cancers, such as prostate, lung or bowel cancer, starting aspirin therapy may reduce your risk.

Mammograms called into question

I n Britain, women over 50 are routinely invited for a free breast screening scan – or mammogram – every three years. It becomes a regular event, in much the same way as three-yearly cervical smear checks have been for much of their fertile lives. Most women take up the invitation, even though mammograms are a slightly uncomfortable and, for some, embarrassing procedure. We've had the benefits of early detection of breast cancer drilled into us for years: better survival rates, less disfiguring surgery, reduced risk of recurrence. So every mammography appointment kept seems like a good move for our health.

But in late 2001, when the news headlines started raising questions about the medical value of mammograms, the people most affected – millions of women around the world – were left worried and confused.

The articles were prompted by an October 2001 report in the British medical publication *The Lancet* that called into question the benefit of regularly screening women for breast cancer using mammography. The report concluded that several earlier studies – the same ones on which the National Cancer Institute (NCI) in the USA and other groups had based their recommendations concerning mammography screening – didn't clearly establish that the use of mammography resulted in fewer deaths from breast cancer. Although the authors admitted that mammograms could indisputably find some cancers early, they questioned the basic assumption that early detection saves lives.

To cancer doctors, breast cancer survivors and women's health advocates, this was tantamount to the Pope questioning the Virgin birth.

▶ Is having a mammogram still a wise move? Many doctors, and most women, think it is.

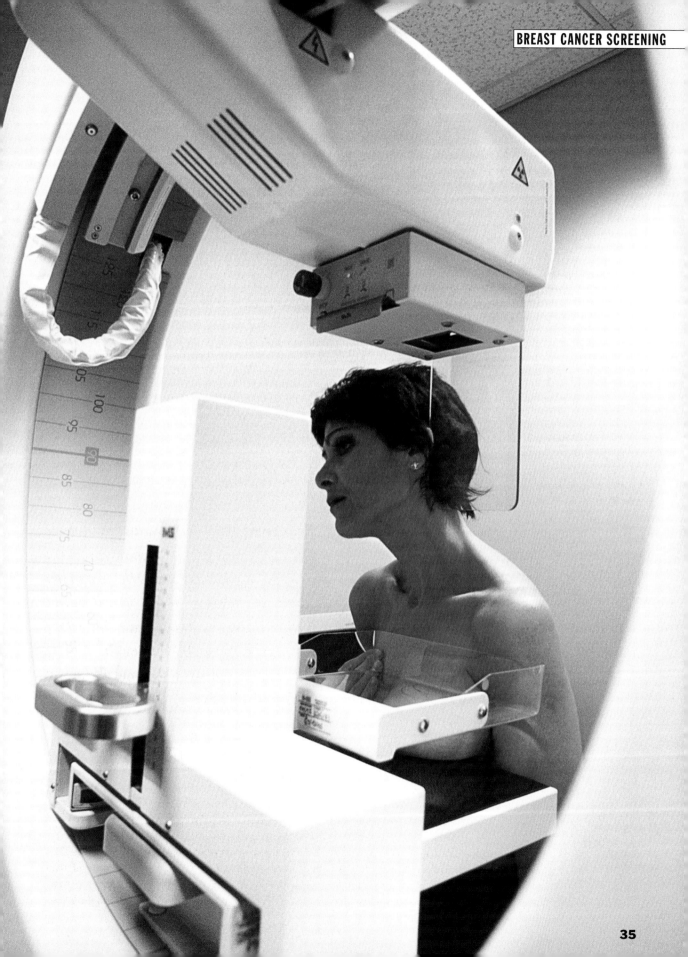

Medical journals, websites and consumer magazines began publishing a plethora of articles designed to calm women's fears and reinforce the importance of mammograms, while trying to put *The Lancet* study in perspective.

'It's a question that comes up every three to four years when someone reanalyses the studies: does mammography save lives, and therefore is it worth the huge investment countries make in screening programs?' says Dr. Beth Deutch, a diagnostic radiologist who specializes in breast cancer in the USA. She has also founded a private screening and breast cancer centre in New Jersey.

Dr. Deutch says the issue of mammography is not an exclusively scientific one; it's political and financial too. For instance, when *The Lancet* study, conducted by two Danish researchers, was released, the Swedish government immediately announced that it would not offer a national screening programme for women. 'Never mind that they never were going to offer it,' she says. It just shows

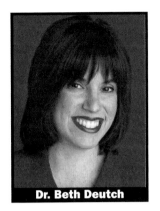

Dr. Beth Deutch

'You can't forget the fact that mammograms cost a lot of money and people would love it not to work so they wouldn't have to pay for it.'

that 'you can't forget the fact that mammograms cost a lot of money and people would love it not to work so they wouldn't have to pay for it.'

And in the USA – which, unlike the UK, Sweden and most other developed countries, does not have a national health service – estimates of the cost-effectiveness of breast screening vary widely. It has been calculated that in the States, where mammograms are recommended for women over the age of 40, screening costs anywhere from £2300 to more than £55,000 per year of life saved. Screening becomes more cost-effective in older women because the incidence of breast cancer increases with age.

But the bottom line is that mammograms do work. In fact, a later study, published in March 2002 in *The Lancet,* re-examined a Swedish study that the Danish researchers had evaluated. That early Swedish study, which followed tens of thousands of women for an average of 29 years, found a 30 per cent reduction in deaths from breast cancer among those who had mammograms. In re-evaluating the Swedish study and removing women included in the mammogram group who, in fact, didn't actually have the test (a crucial flaw in the original study), the later study concluded that the reduction in death rates was closer to 50 per cent – providing a strong argument in favour of mammograms.

Old science, flawed studies

The problem with the ongoing mammogram debate is that it hinges on outdated science and old, less sharp imaging techniques. The Danish researchers, for instance, did not conduct any new studies. Instead, they revisited data from seven large mammography studies conducted between 1963 and 1982. Those studies form the basis for the widely held belief that mammograms reduce deaths from breast cancer by as much as 30 per cent. But *The Lancet* analysis concluded that the studies were flawed and

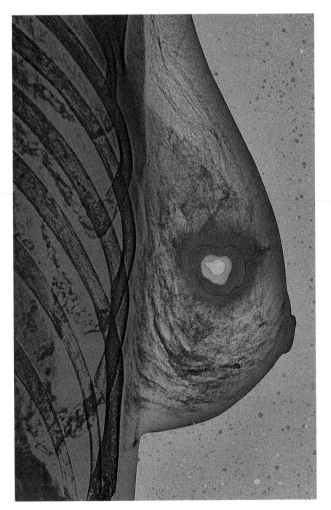

◀ **Mammography can detect much smaller tumours than the ones women discover when they examine their own breasts.**

thus the Danish findings were unreliable. Dr. Deutch agrees that there are serious problems with the studies – not the least of which is the quality of the images themselves. 'If we looked at these mammograms today, we'd refuse to read them,' she says.

In fact, whenever Dr. Lawrence W. Bassett, professor of breast imaging at the University of California's School of Medicine gives a talk about whether mammograms save lives, he projects on to a screen two mammograms, one performed in 1969 and one conducted in 2001 (see images, right). The differences are striking. The older image shows a hazy, poorly defined white area on a black background. It is hard even to identify it as an X-ray of a breast. The 2001 image, however, is so detailed that the pattern of milk ducts is clear. This means that the odds of detecting a tumour at an earlier stage are obviously vastly improved with the current technology.

In the best of all worlds, researchers would recreate those original studies using today's technology and knowledge. However, it's nearly impossible to conduct a randomized, double-blind clinical trial like this today, says Dr. Deutch. Why? Because few women would volunteer for a study in which they might end up in the control group that did not receive mammograms.

Are mammograms harmful?

The controversy gets hotter in the light of claims by some researchers that regular mammograms not only provide little benefit, but may in fact be harmful. Such claims are rooted in the fundamental acknowledgment that mammograms, like nearly everything else in medicine, are not perfect.

If a woman has what looks like a suspicious-looking growth on a mammogram, she will be referred for biopsy. But about 25 per cent turn out not to have cancer, so the test has proved to be a false alarm. According to detractors, this means that mammograms lead to unnecessary biopsies and emotional trauma. But Dr. Deutch finds this claim incredibly paternalistic. 'When you ask most women about this, they say they'll take the 20 minutes of anxiety and discomfort of a biopsy to get definitive reassurance that they don't have breast cancer,' she says. New methods of biopsy are less invasive than in the past. Only if a cancer is found is additional surgery necessary.

To those who say that mammography screenings result in unnecessary biopsies, Dr. Bassett argues that his group found just as many cancers per biopsy when the cancer could be felt as when it was

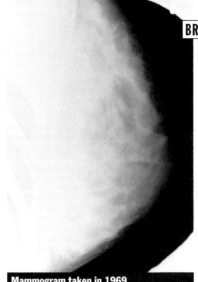

Mammogram taken in 1969

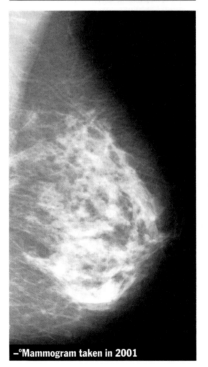

–°**Mammogram taken in 2001**

◀ These two images show just how far mammography has come in the past 30 years. The mammogram taken in 1969 is murky and offers little detail. By contrast, the contemporary mammogram image is crisp and clearly distinguishes structures within the breast, such as the milk ducts or potentially malignant calcifications.

identified only by a mammogram. The difference, however, was in the type of cancers found. Those that had been discovered by physical examination were, on average, 3.7cm long; 33 per cent of them had metastasized (the medical term for a cancer that has spread) to the lymph nodes, and 10 per cent had spread elsewhere.

By contrast, the cancers detected by mammograms were, by and large, less advanced: on average they were only 2cm long, with just 15 per cent having spread to the lymph nodes and none having spread elsewhere. This means that mammography helps to catch breast tumours while they are still in their earlier, more treatable stages.

ALTERNATIVE FORMS OF BREAST SCREENING

Eventually, the debate over mammograms may become irrelevant as new screening tools replace existing technology. For instance, the National Cancer Institute (NCI) in the USA is sponsoring numerous research studies on a variety of screening techniques. These include:

■ MAGNETIC RESONANCE IMAGING
Magnetic resonance imaging, or MRI, uses radiofrequency waves inside a magnetic field to create detailed pictures of the breast without radiation. Since the identification of two genes, BRCA1 and BRCA2, involved in inherited breast cancer, clinical trials are now taking place to compare MRI with regular mammography on women at high risk of carrying the breast cancer genes. The MRI technique could be valuable because young women's breasts are often too dense to be read accurately by mammography. But because MRI is so expensive, it is unlikely to become a routine test in the foreseeable future.

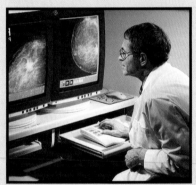

A doctor studies a high-resolution digital mammogram.

■ DIGITAL MAMMOGRAPHY
This technique uses computer enhancement to produce a digital image that can be displayed on high-resolution computer monitors. An ongoing study in the USA of nearly 50,000 women is comparing digital to conventional mammography to determine which works better. One concern is that digital mammography units cost three times as much as conventional units, so there is little economic incentive to use them, says Dr. Douglas S. Katz, associate professor of clinical radiology at the State University of New York.

■ PET SCANS
Positron Emission Tomography or PET scans create computerized images of chemical changes in breast tissue. National Cancer Institute researchers in the USA are exploring how well PET scans detect tumours in dense breasts, and how well they can track the response of a tumour to treatment. But, while this technique may be used to confirm how advanced a cancer is, it is unlikely to be used in breast cancer detection.

■ COMPUTED TOMOGRAPHY
CT (computed tomography) scanning creates a series of detailed X-rays taken from different angles. A computer programme then turns the images into 2 and 3-dimensional pictures. Researchers in the States are exploring the use of a low-dose CT scanner for breast imaging, but in the UK it seems unlikely that it would replace existing screening tools, said a spokesman for Breast Cancer Care.

■ OPTICAL IMAGING
Optical imaging provides information about various chemicals present in tissue. Researchers are looking at superimposing this chemical information on anatomical images such as an MRI of the breast.

■ COMPUTER-AIDED DETECTION
Computer-aided detection or CAD involves the use of computers specially programmed to identify suspicious areas on a mammogram and bring them to the radiologist's attention. It's a bit like running a manuscript through a spellcheck. Ideally, CAD will improve radiologists' ability to interpret mammograms and reduce both the number of missed cancers and the number of women unnecessarily sent for biopsy.

■ ULTRASOUND (SONOGRAPHY)
Ultrasound uses sound waves to see inside the body and is commonly used to identify and characterize breast growths and also to guide doctors during various procedures. It is safe and inexpensive, it does not involve radiation and it complements mammography in the identification of lesions. A few studies suggest that ultrasound may be better than mammography for the detection of potential cancers in women with especially dense breasts.

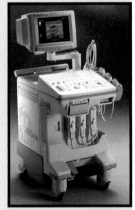

A state-of-the-art ultrasound unit. Could it replace mammograms?

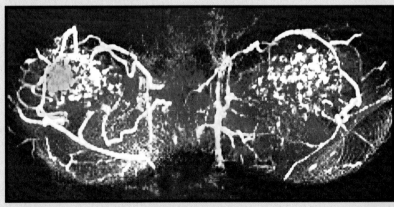

An MRI shows breast tissue (red), blood vessels (yellow) and a tumour (green).

Earlier breast cancer detection

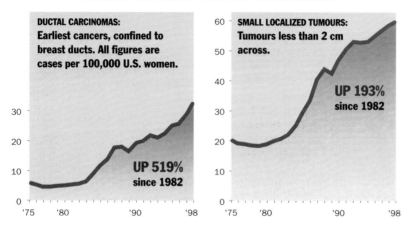

DUCTAL CARCINOMAS:
Earliest cancers, confined to breast ducts. All figures are cases per 100,000 U.S. women.

UP 519% since 1982

SMALL LOCALIZED TUMOURS:
Tumours less than 2 cm across.

UP 193% since 1982

Mammograms allow tumours to be discovered sooner, when they are smaller. In the USA, since mammograms became more common in 1982, five times as many ductal and nearly twice as many small localized tumours have been found.

Another argument against mammograms (if, indeed, the benefits are not as great as once thought) is that mammograms use radiation and that, over the years, that radiation could be potentially harmful. Dr. Deutch disputes this assertion. The radiation dose from an average mammogram, she says, is about what you get from background radiation on a short-haul flight. Only in a very young person – below age 30 – might the lifetime dose of radiation pose a risk. But in Britain regular screening mammograms are not even recommended until women are over 50, and then only every three years.

Tinier cancers discovered

'When I started in 1975, we rarely saw a woman who didn't have a very large cancer,' says Dr. Bassett. 'You could feel them, could see the skin changes.' Today, of course, mammograms find tiny cancers, when they are far easier to treat. But this could be an argument *against* screening mammograms. Some researchers think that mammograms find cancers that are too small – cancers that would either not grow significantly if they were left alone, or would grow slowly but not become a problem, or would be found and treated when they became larger with no difference in outcome. They point to the jump in breast cancers diagnosed early over the past couple of decades but no proportional drop in those diagnosed later.

That misses the bigger picture, says Dr. Bassett. 'People only talk about these studies in terms of mortality reduction. The fact is mammography also changes everything in terms of treatment because now we're finding cancers earlier.'

For instance, in 1975, when he started practising, just 5 per cent of all breast cancers were found in situ, or confined to the milk ducts. Today, that figure is 30 per cent. And it's true that some of those very tiny, very early-stage cancers might not turn into invasive cancers for many years or even in a woman's lifetime. 'We just have to find out which are the bad cancers and which are the ones that are not a threat,' he says. Then there's the added worry that as cancers grow, they tend to become more aggressive, 'so finding them earlier might have other benefits.'

The changes brought about by mammography over the past two decades are, in turn, changing the way doctors classify cancers. A cancer's stage determines its treatment. Now, with more cancers being found earlier, the entire system is being revamped, says Dr. Bassett. 'By working with smaller cancers, it's totally changing the rules. We wouldn't be able to do that without mammograms.'

WHAT DOES IT MEAN TO YOU?

The NHS has no doubt that screening saves lives. Its Cancer Plan, published by the Department of Health in September 2000 plans to:

■ Extend the NHS breast screening programme to cover women from age 50 to age 70. At present, the cut-off age for routine screening is 64 though older women are still entitled to it and can request it via their GP. Women under 50 are not offered routine screening as mammograms seem not to be as effective in premenopausal women.

■ By 2003, all women screened will have two views of the breast taken at every screen instead of, as happens today, just at the first screen. One view will be taken from above and one into the armpit diagonally across the breast. Research shows that this could improve detection rates for the smaller cancers by 43 per cent.

■ UK cancer specialists now recommend that women become what they term 'breast aware', by examining their breasts regularly (such as before a shower or bath) for any change in breast shape, skin texture, or the nipple, and reporting it to their GP. This replaces advice to conduct monthly self-examinations. In a recent survey of 863 women by the British charity Breast Cancer Care about one in seven questioned never checked their breasts and one in three didn't know what to check for.

Can we stop the clock?

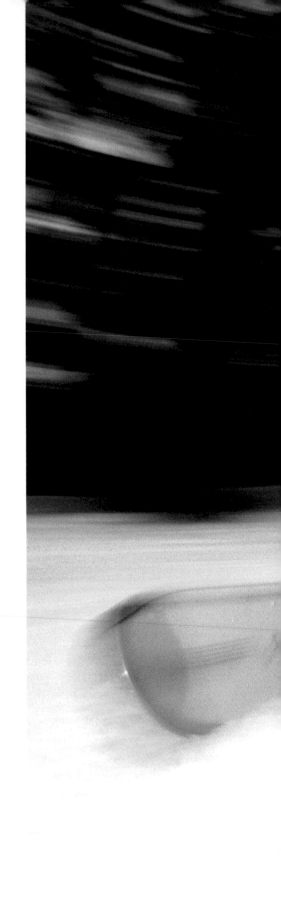

As we begin the 21st century, the human population is living longer than ever before. The world has more centenarians and researchers are fascinated by what these people's genes might reveal about longevity. Several recent studies have pinpointed genetic differences between those who live for a hundred years or more and the rest of us. One such study is run at the Boston Medical Center by Dr. Thomas Perls, who spends most of his time focusing on about 800 men and women who are some 60 years his senior.

▶ Vigorous exercise, a healthy diet, a positive mental attitude and, of course, the gift of good genes can help people to stay active and mentally alert well into old age.

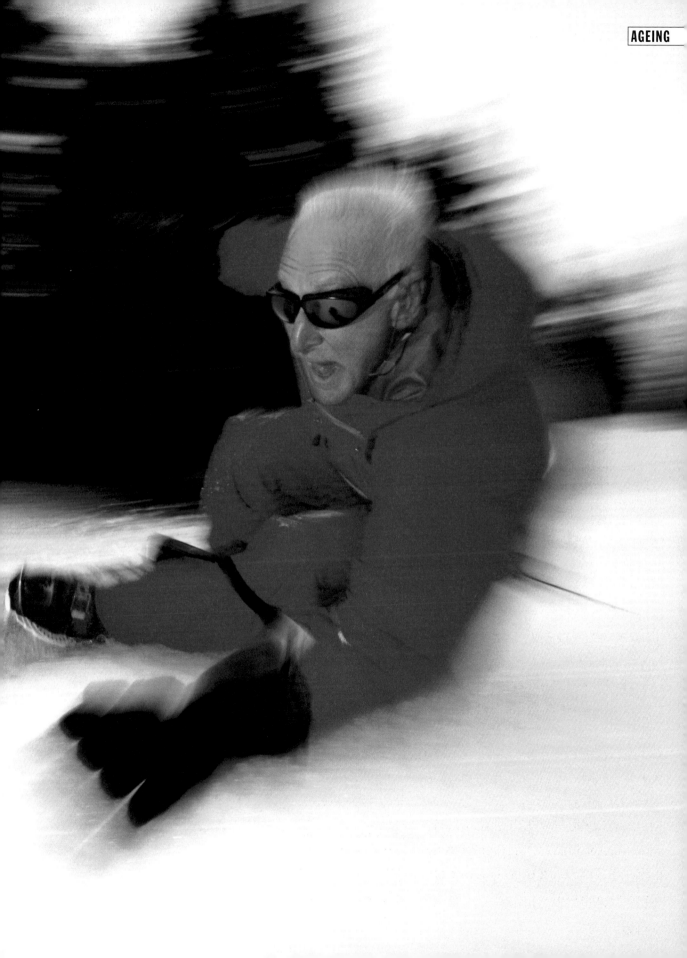

Perls and his colleagues are trying to discover how this special group has managed to avoid – at least for most of their lives – the debilitating ailments that commonly affect older people. His team believes that they are getting closer to solving some aspects of the mystery.

As anyone with a relative who smoked 20 or more cigarettes a day and still lived to a ripe old age will tell you, part of the secret of long life is in the genes. But what our genes give us is an imprecise specification. Genes for longevity do not simply count out our days and then kill us. They give us a particular level of protection against damage. How long we actually keep going is then strongly influenced by things like lifestyle – the foods we eat and the exercise we take – as well as by luck.

A study published in June 2002 by Dr. Perls and his colleagues confirmed that long lives do tend to run in families. The research found, for example, that, compared with the general population, the brothers of centenarians were 17 times more likely, and their sisters at least 8 times more likely, to reach the age of 100.

But what gene gives them their incredible staying power? Tracking down the 'longevity' gene would open the way to finding what Dr. Perls calls 'the fountain of ageing well', in other words, a means of delaying the onset of diseases for as long as possible.

By comparing the DNA of long-lived siblings, the researchers determined that a bit of chromosome 4, which contains somewhere between 100 and 500 genes, is likely to be the site of the one gene associated with extra long life expectancy.

Dr. Perls says that his research team has made tremendous headway and will probably identify the gene within a year. They also believe that, as well as finding the gene that confers longevity, further analysis will expose versions of

Older people on the rise

In the 2001 UK census, 371,269 Britons were aged 90 or over – 288,067 of them women, compared to 83,202 men. The number of people living beyond the age of 100 has also increased dramatically. In 1951 there were fewer than 300 centenarians alive in England and Wales; by 1996 this had risen to about 5,500 and the annual rate of increase is now about 7 per cent.

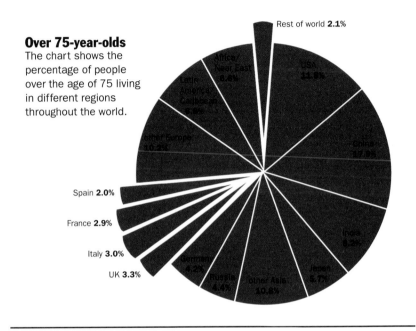

Over 75-year-olds
The chart shows the percentage of people over the age of 75 living in different regions throughout the world.

Rest of world **2.1%**

Africa/Near East **6.6%**

USA **11.9%**

Latin America/Caribbean **5.9%**

Other Europe **10.2%**

China **17.9%**

Spain **2.0%**

France **2.9%**

Italy **3.0%**

UK **3.3%**

Germany **4.2%**

Russia **4.4%**

Other Asia **10.6%**

India **8.2%**

Japan **6.7%**

numerous other genes that enable people to avoid the so-called diseases of ageing such as Alzheimer's disease, stroke, heart disease and cancer.

'Once we find those genes and understand what they do,' says Dr. Perls, 'we hope to develop drugs that can mimic what the centenarians do naturally.' In the meantime, he suggests that people should take advantage of the genes we already know much about. 'Most people could reach their late eighties by exercising more, controlling their weight, not smoking, and eating better,' he says. 'Then, to live 15 or 20 years beyond that, they may need these genetic booster rockets we're looking for – or else a drug that has the same effect.'

Repairing faulty genes

Finding the longevity gene and other genes that guard against the diseases of ageing is just one approach to untangling the secrets of living longer. Researchers are also pursuing another lead. For at least a decade, scientists have suspected that damage to a cell's genes caused ageing, but the precise mechanism has not been clear. Now another piece of the jigsaw has been found: researchers in

Dr. Thomas Perls

'Most people could reach their late 80s by exercising more, controlling their weight, not smoking and eating better.'

Holland have found evidence to suggest that a breakdown in the repair system for DNA plays a major role in ageing.

Professor Jan Hoeijmakers, head of the Institute of Genetics at Erasmus University in the Netherlands, and his colleagues disrupted the way a mouse gene repairs itself. This duplicated a human genetic disorder that causes its victims to become frail and die relatively young. They found that the mice aged much faster than their normal litter mates. Their results were reported in the British journal, *Science*, in April 2002.

Meanwhile, in a laboratory in Atlanta, Georgia, biochemist Paul Doetsch, Ph.D., and his colleagues have patented a group of proteins that may, some day, help corrupted genes to repair themselves.

The damage occurs quite naturally. Chemicals, ultraviolet light and molecules that occur naturally in the body are constantly ravaging DNA, which carries genetic information.

Simply being alive and using oxygen when we breathe or metabolize the food we eat contributes to the production of free radicals – molecules that harm cells. Free radicals have lost an electron, and because electrons are more stable in pairs, free radicals look for a suitable partner to steal from other molecules. This process can spark a chain reaction that causes widespread damage to cells and to their DNA.

'We've discovered some yeast proteins that do a good job recognizing and reversing the DNA damage caused by exposure to sunlight,' says Dr. Doetsch. 'People don't produce these proteins, and

Fighting the attack of free radicals

A stream of free radicals penetrates the nucleus of a cell, damaging the structure of its DNA (the white, ladder-like spiral). Scientists believe that certain yeast proteins may be able to reverse this damage and help to slow the ageing process.

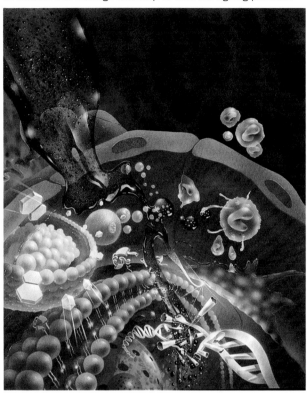

we're trying to find out whether they'll block or reverse sunlight-induced genetic damage if we introduce them into human skin cells.'

The experiments are still at an early stage. The cells Dr. Doetsch is working with are sitting in a solution on a laboratory bench rather than on human skin at the seaside. But Dr. Doetsch can foresee the day when the yeast proteins might be incorporated into a skin cream and applied as routinely as moisturiser. 'In doing this work, we're trying to see if we can eventually block or delay ageing,' Dr. Doetsch explains.

'If it works on skin, it's theoretically possible to target other organs. Some day we may be able to develop a cocktail of different kinds of damage-reversing proteins, each of them good for enhancing the repair of a specific organ.' But don't harbour dreams of regaining the dewy glow of youth once you've lost it. 'If we

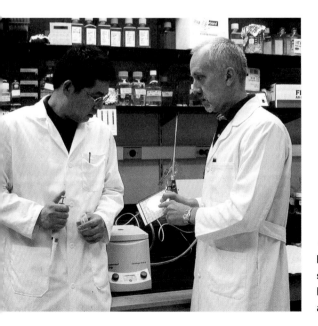

◀ **Dr. Paul Doetsch in the lab with a colleague, studying proteins that may halt the genetic damage associated with ageing.**

Islands of centenarians

Japan has the longest life expectancy in the world. Yet people in Okinawa, a group of islands in southern Japan, enjoy even longer and healthier lives than the average Japanese do.

Life expectancy and death rates

World rank	Life Expectancy	Region	Death rates/100,000 people		
			CHD*	Cancer	Stroke
1	81.2	Okinawa	18	97	35
2	79.9	Japan	22	106	45
18	76.8	U.S.	100	132	28

Note: As of 1996 (the most recent figures available)
*Coronary heart disease

Okinawan diet

Scientists say Okinawans' diet is one of the key factors for their longevity. Here is the average diet of an elderly Okinawan compared with that of a typical elderly American compiled by a research group, the Okinawa Centenarian Study.

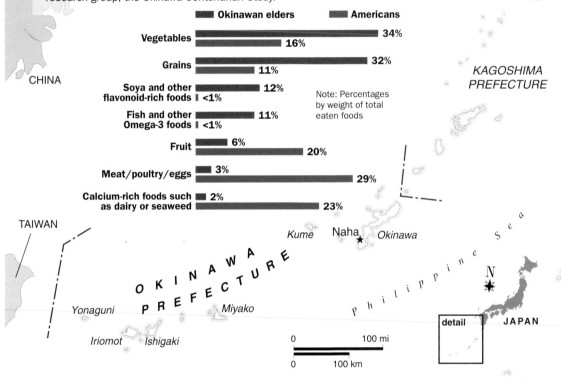

■ Okinawan elders ■ Americans

Vegetables	34% / 16%
Grains	32% / 11%
Soya and other flavonoid-rich foods	12% / <1%
Fish and other Omega-3 foods	11% / <1%
Fruit	6% / 20%
Meat/poultry/eggs	3% / 29%
Calcium-rich foods such as dairy or seaweed	2% / 23%

Note: Percentages by weight of total eaten foods

CHINA

KAGOSHIMA PREFECTURE

TAIWAN

Kume   Naha   Okinawa

OKINAWA PREFECTURE

Yonaguni   Miyako

Iriomot   Ishigaki

Philippine Sea

N

detail   JAPAN

0 — 100 mi
0 — 100 km

---

develop a skin cream when you're in your twenties, theoretically your skin will continue to look good as long as you use the cream. Unfortunately, if you were in your sixties when the product came on the market, you wouldn't be able to turn back the clock 40 years by using it,' says Dr. Doetsch. 'But preventing further skin ageing dead in its tracks is the next best thing.'

Elsewhere, researchers at Duke University in Durham, North Carolina, have found new clues as to why some people experience more rapid age-related memory loss than others. A team of researchers led by Dr. P. Murali Doraiswamy found

a link between nerve cell changes associated with ageing and a gene known as ApoE4. One in four of us carries ApoE4, which has already been linked to the early onset of Alzheimer's disease (onset is rare before the age of 60), as well as heart disease.

The scientists studied two groups of healthy men and women over the age of 55. One group carried the ApoE4 gene; the other didn't. All were tested for levels of N-acetylaspartate (NAA), a chemical inside the brain's nerve cells whose presence indicates that the cells are in good health. The study participants also took memory tests. When the measurements were taken again two years later,

> ## 'Some day, we may be able to develop a cocktail of different kinds of damage-reversing proteins, each of them good for enhancing the repair of a specific organ.'

the researchers found that everyone's NAA level had declined – a natural result of ageing – but that the decline was greater in people with the ApoE4 gene. The team hopes that further study will offer more clues and, eventually, treatments.

Eat less, live longer?

Not all potential anti-ageing strategies are high-tech. In fact, scientists have been able to extend the lives of animals – from protozoa to fruit flies to mice – merely by cutting back their food intake. Now researchers wonder whether this simple approach would work for primates, too. At one US centre in Baltimore, about 75 monkeys are currently on diets that contain all the necessary nutrients they need but only about two-thirds the calories they would normally consume. A parallel group of monkeys are allowed to eat as much as they want.

Scientists at the centre have been comparing the two groups as they mature and have detected some interesting early trends, including a lower incidence of heart disease, diabetes and cancer in the monkeys on lean rations. Warding off or delaying these diseases for as long as possible does, of course, extend the lifespan of the monkeys.

But this data is preliminary, and the researchers are quick to point out that it will be years before they know whether the same strategy will work in humans. To find out, the US-based National Institute on Aging is funding trials to study the impact of voluntary calorie restriction on people. Preliminary results will be available in a few years.

If you are not keen on cutting the amount of food you eat – even if it means living extra years – you are not alone. But imagine being able to reap the health benefits of calorie restriction without changing your diet. Scientists are looking at a chemical that may let you do just that. The chemical mimics the effects of a compound in the body called PPAR-delta, which is involved in the regulation of fat transport and insulin sensitivity.

To see if the chemical has any health benefits, Barbara Hansen, Ph.D., director of the Obesity and Diabetes Research Center at the University of Maryland, worked with six obese middle-aged male monkeys that had abnormally high levels of triglycerides (a type of fat) and abnormally low levels of HDL (good) cholesterol in their blood. In monkeys and people, these combined conditions are risk factors for heart disease. The monkeys were also insulin-resistant, an early sign of diabetes.

After four weeks on the chemical compound, the monkeys' HDL cholesterol levels were 79 per cent higher and their triglyceride concentrations were 56 per cent lower than they were at the beginning of the study. In addition, their sensitivity to insulin increased. Furthermore, there were no apparent negative side effects.

Researchers have begun to test the chemical in individuals who are at high risk of developing heart disease and diabetes. But it is not yet known whether PPAR-delta would extend the lifespan of healthy people who were not at particular risk of these diseases.

Exercise: the key to youthfulness

You do not have to go on a starvation diet or wait for a new drug or high-tech gene repairing technique in order to start lengthening your life straight away. In fact, rather like Dorothy in *The Wizard of Oz,* you have had the power all along – maybe not in the form of ruby slippers, but in something much more prosaic – exercise. Scientists

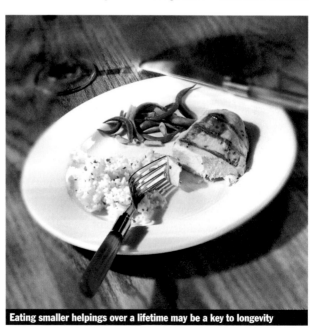

Eating smaller helpings over a lifetime may be a key to longevity

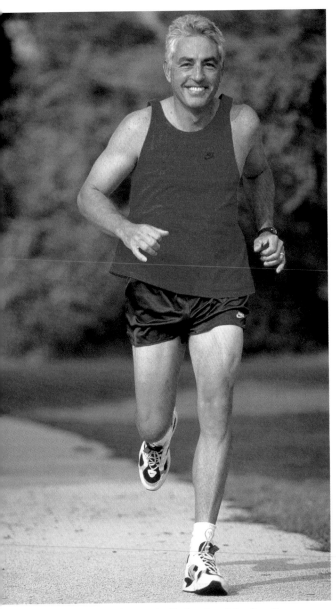

▲ Regular exercise may be the true fountain of youth. It can delay cell death that contributes to heart disease, help to keep arteries more pliable and boost your mood.

'Something as simple as walking can help to reverse part of the ageing process. You won't become 20 years old again, but you can certainly feel as if you are.'

are beginning to learn much more about how exercise slows down ageing. Below are two of the main ageing processes it combats.

■ **CELL SUICIDE** The heart is one of the first organs to show the effects of ageing. Now researchers at the University of Florida say that programmed cell death, known medically as apoptosis, is the reason. In apoptosis, a cell orders itself to stop functioning, shrinks, and ultimately dissolves. This process removes potentially dangerous cells, such as cancer cells, from the body but, as we age, it can also contribute to the death of cardiovascular cells.

In a study published in February 2002 in the *American Journal of Physiology*, Christiaan Leeuwenburgh, Ph.D. and a colleague at Florida University found that the hearts of older laboratory rats released greater amounts of a cell-death signal than did the hearts of younger animals. Dr. Leeuwenburgh blames damage caused by free radicals. But he and his colleague have early evidence to show that regular exercise can reduce the level of free radicals in laboratory rats. He believes it does the same for humans. 'If you exercise for an hour a day, you may produce more free radicals during that time because your body is under stress,' he explains, 'but for the remaining 23 hours your baseline level of free radical production will decrease.' And the key to living longer is to make fewer free radicals.

■ **ARTERY HARDENING** With age, the walls of our arteries tend to thicken, making it more difficult for the heart to pump blood. This causes high blood pressure, a risk factor for heart disease. A new drug called ALT-711 can reduce this hardening, according to a study conducted by the US National Institute on Aging. But drugs aren't the only answer. 'Something as simple as walking can help to reverse part of the ageing process,' says Dr. Kerrie Moreau Ph.D., who works in Human Cardiovascular Research Laboratory at Colorado University.

Moreau and her colleagues found that sedentary postmenopausal women who began walking at a moderate pace for 40 to 45 minutes a day five times a week could restore elasticity to their arteries. Previous work with male volunteers had produced similar results. When she announced her findings, in April 2002, Moreau said, 'You won't become 20 years old again, but you can certainly feel as if you are.'

Exercise has emotional as well as physical benefits, and it is never too late to reap them. Eva Kahana, Ph.D., is a research scientist based in Cleveland, Ohio. 'We studied people for nine years, beginning when they were about 75,' she says. Her research findings, published in a US journal, *Psychosomatic Medicine*, in summer 2002, provided evidence that those who took part in simple activities such as playing golf or walking scored considerably better, not only on physical criteria but on mental ones, too. 'We were surprised to discover that they were psychologically better off than those who were less active,' says Dr. Kahana. 'They were less depressed, had a greater sense of meaning in their life and more goals they wanted to achieve.'

The scientists involved in these projects say that too few doctors promote the benefits of exercise. It is widely known that moderate exercise can improve many chronic health conditions, from obesity to gallstones. It seems sensible, then, to take matters into our own hands – and just get out for a walk. As Dr. Kahana says: '… it's never too late to add life to your years. You may not be able to turn back the clock, but you can slow it down.'

NO TRUTH TO THE FOUNTAIN OF YOUTH

Few of us would get out our chequebooks if someone offered to sell us the Crown Jewels. But scientists believe that the public is far more gullible when it comes to buying products that supposedly delay ageing and add years to life.

In the US, a group of scientists involved in ageing research have published a paper warning people that no remedy on sale today 'has been shown to slow, stop, or reverse human ageing'. Although research is underway that may one day help scientists – and consumers – to slow down the ageing process, 'anyone purporting to offer an anti-ageing product today is either mistaken or lying'.

The article, signed by 51 scientists, was published in *Scientific American* in June 2002. It sets the record straight about the current state of research into human ageing. Here are some of the highlights:

■ **ANTIOXIDANTS** These chemicals, which neutralize damaging molecules called free radicals, occur naturally in the body and in many fruits and vegetables. And while there is no doubt that eating a diet rich in fruit and vegetables will benefit your health in a number of ways, antioxidant supplements cannot stop the clock. According to the article, 'there are a number of ongoing randomized clinical trials that address the possible role of supplements in a range of age-related conditions, the results of which will be reported in the coming years … but so far there is no scientific evidence to justify the claim that they have any effect on human ageing.'

■ **HORMONES** The levels of a number of hormones commonly decrease with age, including growth hormone, melatonin, testosterone, oestrogen and DHEA (dehydroepiandrosterone). DHEA is secreted by the adrenal glands and is converted into many other hormones involved in growth and strength. It may seem reasonable that replacing these hormones could reverse ageing. And several of them have indeed been shown to mitigate some of the physical effects of ageing. However, no hormone has been proved to slow down, stop or reverse the ageing process itself. And some hormone supplements have been proved to have harmful side effects.

■ **CALORIE RESTRICTION** Eating significantly less may extend the lives of people as it does in many other animal species, but no study has yet proved it.

■ **REPLACING BODY PARTS.** Some people have suggested that completely replacing body parts with more youthful components could increase longevity. But, say the scientists, while advances in cloning may make the replacement of tissues and organs possible, 'replacing and reprogramming the brain that defines who we are as individuals is, in our view, more the subject of science fiction than science fact.'

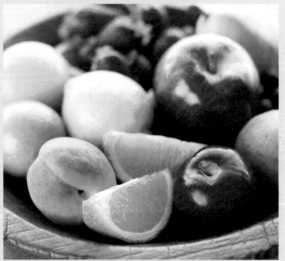

The antioxidants in fruit have many health benefits but antioxidant supplements do not appear to halt ageing.

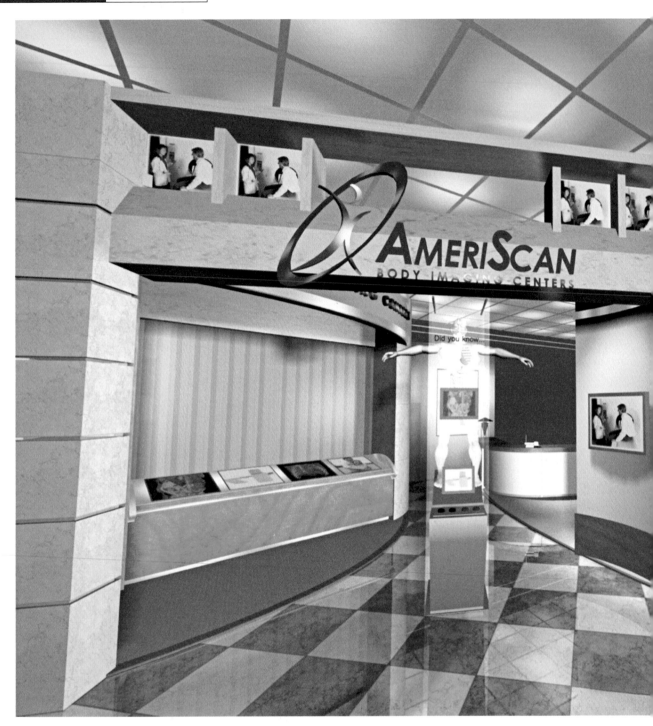

High street

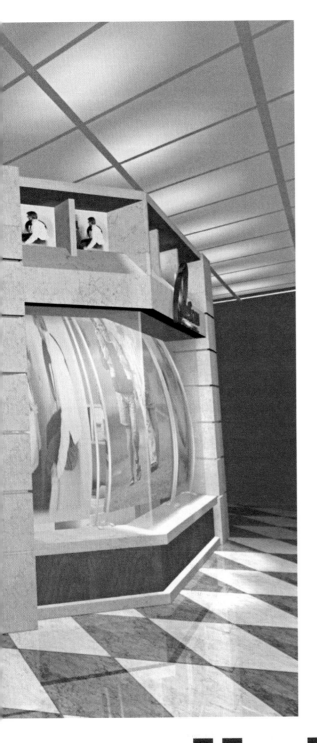

◄ The AmeriScan Body Imaging Center at the Chandler Fashion Square Mall in Chandler, Arizona.

medicine

A list for your next transatlantic shopping trip: jeans and trainers for the children, and, for you, a full-body CT scan? You won't need a doctor's referral or even symptoms – a fat chequebook is all that is required.

Heavily advertised in newspapers and on radio, smart walk-in centres offering these full-body diagnostic scans are springing up in affluent areas across the United States, luring consumers with the promise of detecting diseases such as cancer and heart disease long before any symptoms appear.

Because they are designed to attract healthy people, most of the centres are not in medical facilities but in shopping malls and other retail areas. Anyone with the price of admission (around £650) can get scanned for anything from suspicious growths to artery deposits to osteoporosis. Talk-show host Oprah Winfrey is among the many who have used these new diagnostic facilities.

Fantastic voyage

During the test, you lie still on a table that passes through a doughnut-shaped machine, called a spiral CT (computed tomography) scanner. An ultra-fast X-ray tube continuously rotates (or 'spirals') around you, generating up to a thousand or more cross-sectional images of your insides, from neck to pelvis. (Think of cutting up a cucumber into extremely thin slices in order to see inside.) Powerful computer software can stack these 'slices' in any plane, creating detailed 3-D images of the body that may reveal small tumours, aortic aneurysms, bone erosion, or calcified plaque in your arteries, for example. The entire procedure takes no longer than 15 minutes, including less than a minute of actual scanning.

Afterwards, you and a radiologist pore over the images, examining the inner recesses of your computerized body. For many, it can be almost a religious experience, says Dr. Harvey Eisenberg, full-body CT scan pioneer and founder of the HealthView Center for Preventive Medicine in Newport Beach, California.

Under a slogan that people in Britain might find a little too direct and slightly perturbing – 'You don't know what's inside until you look' – Dr. Eisenberg offers customers the possibility of uncovering early signs of heart, ovarian, endocrine, vascular and prostate disease, cancer, benign tumours, kidney stones and gallstones, osteoporosis, emphysema and aneurysms.

Says Dr. Eisenberg, 'We're in the middle of building a new technology whose goal is to replace the annual physical. Not the blood test, but pretty much the rest of it. What we think of as prevention today – the annual physical, chest X-rays, stress tests – doesn't work. We routinely see asymptomatic patients with masses in their bodies the size of grapefruits who have just passed their annual physicals. Or people who have advanced, life-threatening, coronary artery disease who have just had normal stress tests.'

Dr. Craig Bittner estimates that his four (and counting) AmeriScan body imaging centres in Arizona and California refer about 10 per cent of

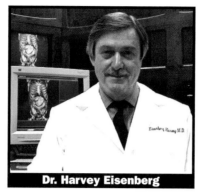

Dr. Harvey Eisenberg

'We're in the middle of building a new technology whose goal is to replace the annual physical. Not the blood test, but pretty much the rest of it.'

their customers for medical follow-up of apparently serious conditions. Dr. Eisenberg, whose centre scans up to 40 patients a day, refers about 80 per cent of his patients for follow-up. 'Emerging pathologies are almost always present,' he says. 'In 25,000 patients, I've seen maybe 10 that are completely normal.'

Proponents say that its potential to save lives by detecting disease is just one benefit of full-body CT scanning. The 'seeing is believing' quality of 3-D images that can show early signs of atherosclerosis, osteoporosis, or lung damage from cigarettes is a powerful incentive for people to make significant lifestyle changes, they say. 'While it's not as heroic as putting a balloon angioplasty in a woman having a heart attack, getting patients on board to be the captain of their health and helping them to make better health decisions is much better medicine,' says Dr. Bittner. Yet another benefit, scan proponents claim, is the potential for repeat scans every few years to assess the effects of such lifestyle changes and disease management therapies.

Radiation risks

Not everyone agrees that full-body scans are a boon to consumers. Critics pan the expensive tests as 'yuppie scans' that turn healthy people with no symptoms into angst-ridden patients who are often unnecessarily concerned about findings that will not, in the end, affect their health.

Although physicians can use a device in any way they think appropriate, the US Food and Drug Administration approved CT scanners to look only at specific organs, and only in people with suspected health problems. No US government agency or national health or medical organization has endorsed full-body CT scans – either for people with disease symptoms or for those without them. 'To date there is no evidence that total body CT screening is cost effective or is effective in prolonging life,' comments the American College of Radiology.

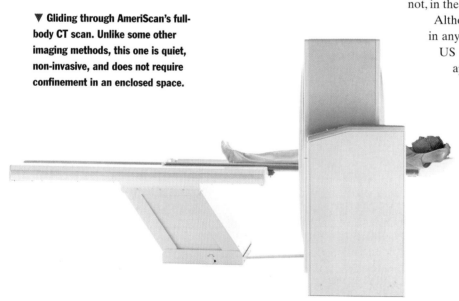

▼ Gliding through AmeriScan's full-body CT scan. Unlike some other imaging methods, this one is quiet, non-invasive, and does not require confinement in an enclosed space.

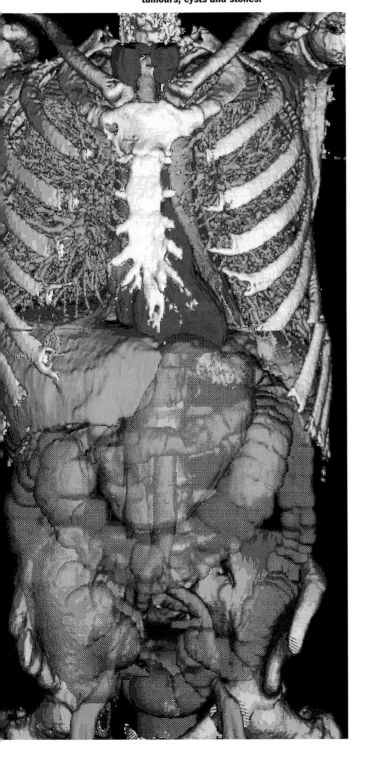

▼ The HealthView scan provides 3-D and cross-sectional views of your internal organs from neck to pelvis, revealing early evidence of disorders such as arterial plaque, tumours, cysts and stones.

One concern is that patients are unnecessarily exposed to radiation. At 1 to 2 rems (a measure of radiation that stands for 'roentgen equivalent man'), a full-body CT scan delivers an effective radiation dose 200 to 500 times greater than a simple chest X-ray, says Dr. Robert J. Stanley, president of the American Roentgen Ray Society. Contending that full-body scans are perfectly safe, though, Dr. Bittner notes that such doses are far less than those received annually by more than a million Americans in their chest area during heart angiograms. But critics have questioned the risks that would accrue with repeated follow-up scans.

Wild goose chases

Other worries include the risk of false-positives. These are scans that uncover, say, a questionable lump or growth that turns out to be harmless – but only after the patient has undergone further costly diagnostic testing. Dr. Yank D. Coble, president of the American Medical Association, is an endocrinologist in Jacksonville, Florida. Although he has scaled back his practice, over a recent 18 month period a dozen patients came to him after full-body CT scans detected what Dr. Coble termed lumpiness or nodules in their thyroids – conditions that are quite common. After further testing all the lumps or nodules proved benign.

Sometimes follow-up testing involves surgical procedures, all of which carry certain risks. For example, CT scans often cannot distinguish between benign and malignant lung nodules, and a biopsy may be required to tell the difference. Possible complications from lung biopsies include partial collapse of the lung, bleeding, infection,

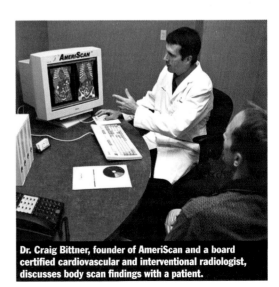

Dr. Craig Bittner, founder of AmeriScan and a board certified cardiovascular and interventional radiologist, discusses body scan findings with a patient.

Case histories

Are tests on demand good for you?

Is full-body CT scanning a fad for America's rich and its hypochondriacs, causing more panic than peace of mind? Or can it really help anyone to uncover a medical problem early enough to make a difference – or even save a life? Here are two stories that illustrate why the answers to such questions are not clear-cut.

For

FOR POLICE SERGEANT, SCANNING WAS JUST THE TICKET

Sergeant Bart Landsman of the Los Angeles Police Department didn't have a clue anything was wrong with him. In November 2000, however, he decided to have a full-body CT scan performed at the HealthView Center for Preventive Medicine in Newport Beach, California. His wife, Jacquelyn Landsman, an LAPD detective, had done so the year before. While most insurance policies don't cover such screens, Landsman had to pay only £120, and his LAPD health insurance covered the rest. So he figured, why not?

The radiologist reviewing Landsman's scans noticed an abnormality in his left kidney. Taking the radiologist's advice, Landsman spent the next 10 days visiting his family doctor and another radiologist. Their conclusion: Landsman, then 42, most likely had kidney cancer. The only way to be sure was to remove the organ. When the surgery was done on January 2, 2001, a lime-sized cancerous tumour was found inside Landsman's kidney.

Fortunately, says Landsman, the tumour still appeared to be encapsulated. 'I had an oncologist who came in and conferred with my radiologist,' says Landsman. 'They all say that with this kind of cancer, we wouldn't have found it until I had symptoms.'

Six weeks after his surgery, the 21-year LAPD veteran was back on the streets supervising patrolmen. 'I feel wonderful. I'm completely cured,' he says.

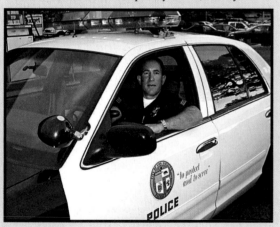

Against

EXPENSIVE LESSON: A SCAN, A SCARE, AND NEEDLESS SUFFERING

At 64, Dr. William Casarella, had no blood in his stools and no known polyps. But the chairman of radiology at Emory University School of Medicine in Atlanta did have a family history of colon cancer, so he scheduled a colonoscopy, the standard screening procedure.

However, the colonoscope could not get a full view of his colon. So he underwent a virtual colonoscopy, which uses computed tomography (CT) technology and is sometimes offered along with a full-body CT scan.

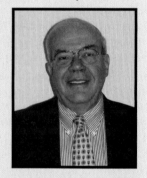

Though the colon was perfectly normal, the upper section of his CT scan revealed suspicious bodies in his liver and one kidney, and some non-calcified nodules in the base of the lungs – unlike calcified nodules that are usually considered harmless.

When a questionable lung nodule is found, doctors often suggest repeated scans at six-month intervals for two to three years to see if the nodule changes or grows. But Dr. Casarella opted to have more tests done immediately. This led to a complete CT scan of the chest; a CT scan of the kidneys enhanced with intravenous dye; a liver biopsy; and, finally, video-assisted thoracoscopic surgery to biopsy his lungs, which resulted in four days of hospitalization.

'There's a lot of pain,' says Dr. Casarella. 'You feel pretty terrible for four or five days, and it takes four to six weeks before you feel good enough to be fully active.' Five months later, he still felt numbness and occasional pain in his chest. His total bill was $47,000 (almost £30,000) – all to determine that he had a benign kidney cyst and, in his lungs and liver, healed histoplasmosis scars caused by a very common fungus.

'I don't think the country can afford to do this kind of work-up on every patient with a positive lung scan,' says the doctor. 'You just wind up converting a lot of normal people into patients.'

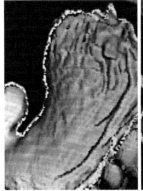 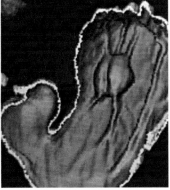

▲ The difference between normal stomach tissue (left) and an early tumour (right) can show up even before any symptoms arise.

pain, discomfort, nerve damage and even death. Dr. Stephen Swensen, chairman of radiology at the Mayo Clinic and a world expert in pulmonary radiology, has noted that the lung biopsy fatality rate was 4 per cent in a study conducted in Southern California community hospitals.

The risk of false-positive readings is heightened by the failure of full-body CT centres to use intravenous dye. When a diagnostic CT scan is used on people with symptoms, this dye is often injected into the body to illuminate inner structures that are otherwise hard to see on X-ray film. The dye helps radiologists differentiate between abnormalities that matter and those that don't. The CT centres don't use the dye because there is a risk of an allergic reaction to it. Hospitals are willing to use the dye because, in patients with symptoms, the benefits outweigh the risks.

Even when a full-body CT scan produces a clean bill of health, critics worry that this could give consumers a false sense of security – in effect, carte blanche to live as they please, without regard to their health. Yet they may have a disease the scan missed or a problem such as diabetes that won't show up on any scan.

All about arteries

But the potential of more focused CT screenings, at least for at-risk patients, does intrigue many researchers. One of the hottest areas of interest is the use of CT scans to screen people for coronary artery disease.

Electron beam CT (or EBCT), which is often offered as part of a full-body CT scan, examines artery walls

Even when a full-body CT scan produces a clean bill of health, critics worry that this could give consumers a false sense of security...

for calcium deposits. Theoretically, the greater the calcification, the greater the risk of coronary artery disease. (Oprah Winfrey had an EBCT scan at Dr. Eisenberg's centre in the autumn of 2000, which revealed minor calcium deposits in her arteries.)

Doctors debate the ultimate value of EBCT scans. Some data indicate that the scans are no better at predicting coronary artery disease than standard risk assessment criteria such as blood pressure, cholesterol levels, smoking history and age. And high calcium scores don't always mean a higher risk of heart attack. While calcium deposits do indicate atherosclerosis, or artery narrowing, it is unclear how likely these deposits are (as opposed to soft, noncalcified plaques) to rupture and cause a significant artery blockage that could lead to a heart attack.

Nevertheless, EBCT could eventually become valuable for screening people who, based on such standard criteria as cholesterol levels, are

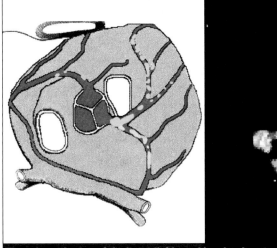

The schematic view of the heart (left) provides visual context for an electron beam CT scan image (right), which reveals the precise location of calcified plaque deposits in a coronary artery. Such a scan might prompt life-saving intervention.

traditionally considered to be at intermediate risk of heart disease, says cardiologist Dr. Sidney C. Smith Jr., chief medical officer of the American Heart Association. Dr. Smith says that if EBCT identifies such people as being at higher risk than previously thought, they could benefit from intensive prevention efforts. These could include medication and diet to lower cholesterol and blood-thinning therapies such as daily aspirin to help prevent dangerous blood clots from forming.

Meanwhile the research continues in the USA. The American National Heart, Lung, and Blood Institute recently launched a large, long-term study to determine, in part, whether CT scans are actually better than other methods at predicting who is most likely to develop heart disease.

Looking for lung cancer

Another area of keen interest is the use of spiral CT to detect lung cancer. In 1999, the British medical journal *The Lancet* published findings touting the benefits of CT over conventional chest X-rays in detecting small lung cancers.

Smokers started begging for the scans, which unquestionably offer better resolution than chest X-rays. But does this earlier detection help patients

RESEARCH ROUND-UP

Blood tests on demand

Want to check your thyroid function, test your cholesterol or even find out if you have AIDS? In the USA you can do this simply by walking into one of a growing number of direct-to-consumer diagnostic labs. In Britain, too, an increasing number of tests can be ordered by mail or via a web site, or bought in stores such as Boots.

In America tests include screening for specific conditions such as gout or pregnancy as well as comprehensive blood and urine profiles that include tests for blood, heart, kidney, liver and thyroid functions, diabetes, osteoporosis and prostate cancer. To get them, customers can walk into a retail store or order them over the phone or internet, then have blood taken at a collection site, which might be in an office complex or even a hospital. (Healthcheck USA has more than 3,000 affiliated collection sites. Quest Diagnostics maintains more than 1,300 collection sites, which include several QuestDirect retail stores.) The results are often available within 24 hours, via a confidential web site, fax or mail. There's one catch, about half of all states require that a doctor request diagnostic tests. Certain labs skirt this issue by hiring physicians to sign the requisitions, usually without seeing the patient.

Some people use such services with their doctor's blessing. Dr. Christopher Kopecky, a cardiologist in San Antonio, recommends Healthcheck USA to both his poor, uninsured heart patients and to those whose insurance won't cover as many tests as he'd like.

But the College of American Pathologists and the American Medical Association does question the ability of lay people to select the most appropriate tests or interpret them correctly. 'Perfectly normal people might lie above or below so-called "normal" blood test ranges, and some abnormal results might

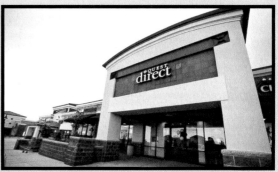

A Quest Diagnostics facility at the local mall.

lie within the "normal" range,' cautions Dr. Yank D. Coble, president of the American Medical Association. 'People can be artificially reassured and at times alarmed about results that are not really meaningful.'

Dr. Kopecky recommends that patients send a copy of test results to their doctor. Healthcheck USA will also indicate on the customer's lab report that a doctor should be consulted if results are above or below certain norms. If the results are deemed critical or 'panic' values, the lab organizations or affiliated physicians call the customer to urge him or her to see a doctor immediately.

Because of the wide availability of NHS services, far fewer people buy private diagnostic tests in Britain, although pregnancy testing kits are sold in most chemists and Boots offer a small range of home kits to test cholesterol, allergies and for blood group identification. While home kits are regulated under the EC In Vitro Diagnostic Medical Device Directive, there are no mandatory regulations for the private British laboratories now offering allergy and even DNA testing, although the Royal College of Pathologists and the Association of Clinical Pathologists have established a Clinical Pathology Accreditation scheme, to which most NHS laboratories belong.

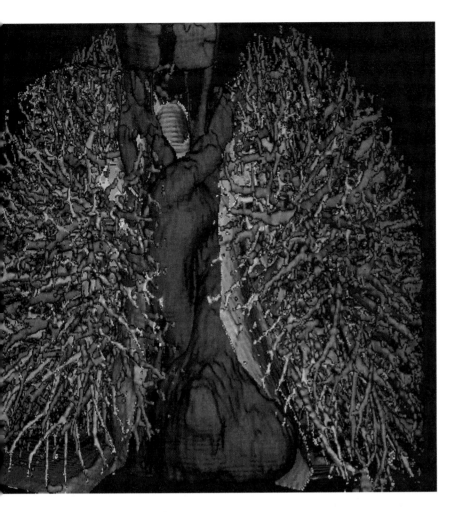

◀ A spiral CT scan shows with startling clarity the bronchioles, or tiny tubes, of healthy lungs, with the heart in the middle.

comprehensive health screening test there is. Not only can it find disease early, but it's also the first to screen for such diseases as kidney cancer.'

Dr. Bittner resents the medical profession's 'paternalistic attitude that people aren't intelligent enough' to make decisions about their health. 'We're not saying, don't go to see a doctor. We're saying, let us help you and your doctor be better informed.'

Counters Dr. Stanley, a co-editor of an authoritative CT textbook: 'I strongly believe CT is a modern miracle of diagnosis that has vastly improved the management of disease. But you can really wreak havoc on the general public by scanning everyone who is asymptomatic and finding all these little, inconsequential bumps.' Indeed, suspicious but ambiguous findings might only lead to riskier, more invasive, more expensive tests, which may or may not prove useful. In the USA, opinion is clearly divided but patients are advised to consult their doctor before having a scan and to make sure he receives a copy of the findings.

live longer – or does it simply alert them earlier to a fatal disease? Lung cancer cells may spread (metastasize) when the lesions are 1mm to 2mm in diameter, before even CT screens can detect them. Since 1951, when the link between smoking and lung cancer was first clearly established, more than 350,000 patients have been studied. 'None of these studies has shown that you have a decreased chance of dying from lung cancer by detecting it early with either chest X-ray or CT,' says Dr. Swensen. But the research continues. America's National Cancer Institute is currently studying CT to see if it can detect lung cancers early enough to save lives.

Meanwhile false-positives generated by spiral CT lung scans are common. After three years of annual screening, a Mayo Clinic study of 1,520 smokers found abnormalities that required more tests or biopsies in 80 per cent of participants. Of those, says Dr. Swensen, 99 per cent were benign.

Conceding that full-body CT scans result in false-positives and false-negatives, Dr. Bittner says, 'It's not a perfect test, but it's the single most

THE SITUATION IN BRITAIN

In Britain, full-body CT scans are not generally available on demand without a doctor's referral although private patients can choose to have general health check-ups involving a whole battery of other diagnostic tests. Both BUPA and the Portland Hospital (one of eight in Britain run by the Hospital Corporation of America) feel that full-body scans may pose an unnecessary risk to patients who have no clinical reason to undergo them.

But Peter Fermoy, communications manager of the Independent Healthcare Association, which represents 95 per cent of private British hospitals, says the scans are available on request but are not marketed. 'Patients are becoming increasingly empowered to make decisions for themselves. But I feel that if patients want these diagnostic tests, they should first seek their GP's advice.'

The world is

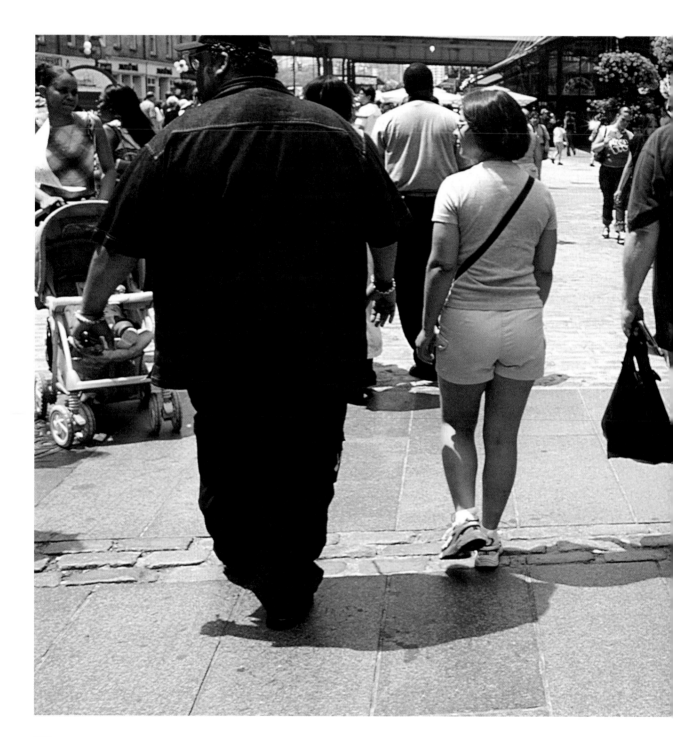

getting fatter

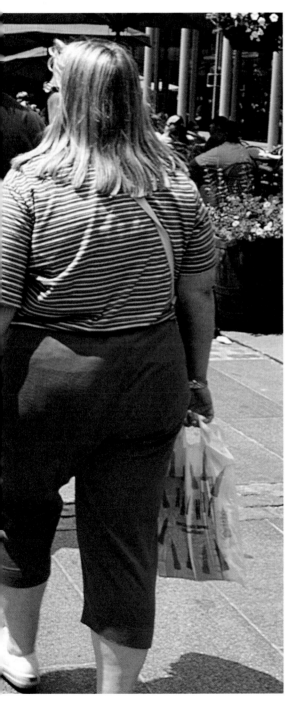

Fat is becoming a major medical problem in the developed Western world. And the extent of the problem is beginning to stretch even farther. For instance, one study found that more than a third of city-dwelling women in India weighed significantly more than was healthy. Many countries now record 20 per cent of their populations as clinically obese, and more than half the UK population is overweight to some degree.

Obesity is growing at such a rate among the young that parents could outlive their children. Too many live on fast food diets and take too little exercise. 'These young people are storing up for themselves enormous ill health for the future', says Andrew Prentice, professor of international nutrition at the London School of Hygiene and Tropical Medicine.

Seriously obese children can expect to lose some nine years of their lives through conditions that were far less common in their parents' generation, such as diabetes, stroke and coronary heart disease.

The problem is even worse in the USA. There, a government study on obesity, published in September 2001, reported that more than 60 per cent of American adults were

◀ **About one in five Britons is clinically obese and half the population seriously overweight – and the numbers are rising.**

overweight and almost 30 per cent were classified as obese. This is a huge leap from 20 years ago, when the rates were about 45 per cent overweight and 15 per cent obese. Doctors say you are overweight if your body mass index (BMI) is 25 or higher; you are obese if your score is over 30. To calculate your own body mass index, see the box on page 63.

'The recent increase in girth ... may undermine much of the progress that has been made in the last century in terms of health and longevity,' says Professor Prentice. Dr. David Satcher, the US government's Surgeon General, agrees, warning that those ever-expanding waistlines are not merely an issue of vanity. As many as 300,000 Americans are dying each year from illnesses caused or worsened by obesity. In fact, Dr. Satcher predicts that obesity may soon displace smoking as the chief cause of preventable deaths in the USA.

Obesity has led to an epidemic of Type 2 diabetes, as well as an increase in the number of people suffering from heart disease, cancer, arthritis and breathing problems. Diabetes alone can lead to blindness, kidney failure, nerve damage and heart disease. It is the leading cause of amputations in the US. And the problem is getting

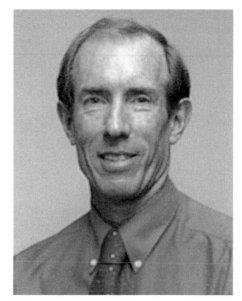

▲ Andrew Prentice, professor of international nutrition at the London School of Hygiene and Tropical Medicine.

worse. One in ten British children is now classed as overweight and 2.6 per cent are obese. This means that the ill health effects of those excess pounds start early. An American study published in March 2002 found that in one group of obese children, 25 per cent had already developed high blood sugar, putting them at increased risk of diabetes.

A tax on fattening foods?

The huge cost to the healthcare systems in both the UK and the USA has led to the suggestion of taxing soft drinks and fast foods – fizzy drinks are one of the main high-calorie culprits. In fact the Californian state legislature already has a draft bill for levying a tax on soft drinks to generate money to fight obesity in the young. If the bill is passed, the culprits will soon be helping to pay for the damage they cause. Other US states are now considering banning drinks and confectionery machines from schools, and New York has passed laws banning the sale of foods that have 'minimal nutritional value' until after the lunch break.

An editorial published in the British publication *The Lancet* suggested further radical solutions, including subsidies for nutritious foods and an advertising ban on junk foods targeted at children.

Obesity on the rise in Europe

Throughout Europe obesity has reached epidemic proportions. At least 135 million EU citizens are affected, according to the latest figures from the International Obesity TaskForce. The chart shows percentages of overweight and obese people in 14 EU countries.

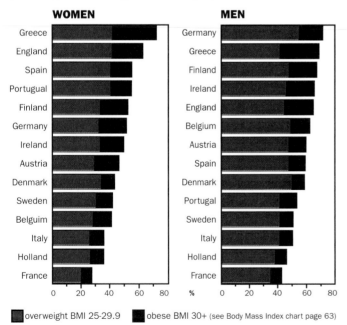

Researchers are finding that, in some people, the body fights especially hard to maintain its stores of fat.

Why is it so easy to get fat?

For years, doctors told their patients that losing weight was merely a matter of willpower. They shook their heads and said if you weren't losing weight, then you just didn't know how to say no. But now, experts acknowledge that shedding pounds is a lot more complex than simply resisting the lure of the chocolate digestives in the cupboard. Genetics appears to play a larger role than once thought. And researchers are finding that, in some people, the body fights especially hard to maintain its stores of fat.

The problem is that we are battling with a weight regulation system, evolved over hundreds of thousands of years, designed to keep us well covered, no matter how scarce food becomes. Early man had to be able to endure long periods of famine. And as the species evolved, those with more efficient metabolisms survived to procreate.

In 1991, a search for clues to some of the mysteries about genetics, environment, and obesity led a US health researcher, Eric Ravussin Ph.D, deep into Mexico's Sierra Madre mountain range. Dr. Ravussin was looking for a group of Pima Indians whose ancestors had settled in this isolated, rugged land some 500 years earlier. For decades doctors had been perplexed by the high rates of obesity, high cholesterol and diabetes in Pima Indians living in the Phoenix, Arizona, area. Almost 50 per cent of the tribe is diabetic – the highest rate in the world. The chance to examine the Mexican Pimas could help to settle the burning question – are obesity and diabetes the result of genetics or environment?

Dr. Ravussin and his colleagues have now been studying the Mexican Pimas for more than a decade. Their conclusion: both nature and nurture play a significant role. In an environment that requires a lot of manual labour to produce food, the Pimas tend to be leaner and have a much lower rate of diabetes than those who have ready access to high-calorie foods. But even in this environment, the Pimas still have a high risk of diabetes compared to other groups. About 7 per cent of the Mexican Pimas have diabetes, compared to 3 per cent of their neighbours.

'What we have learned is that the Pimas have a huge genetic liability in terms of obesity,' says Dr. Ravussin. 'It's probably an asset in periods of famine, but a very big liability in times of feast.'

Bigger helpings: size does matter

No doubt one reason for our expanding waistlines is the advent of the 'kingsize' or 'whopper' syndrome. In the past 30 years, some so-called 'single' portions have expanded hugely. Look at the new larger-size single servings that are now available:

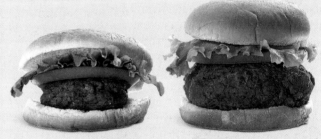

	1970s	NOW
Fast-food burger	25g (1oz) (standard burger)	175g (6oz) (double burger)
Cola drink	300ml (½ pint) (standard can)	600ml (1 pint) (large single-serving in restaurants and cinemas)
Chips (French fries)	115g (4oz) (medium portion)	200g (7oz) (supersize portion)
Yoghurt	150g (5½oz) (standard size)	200g (7oz) (large standard size)
Muffin	50g (1¾oz) (standard size)	100g (3½oz) (standard size)
Crisps	28g (1oz) (single-serving bag)	50g (1¾oz) (large single-serving bag)
Mars bar	65g (2¼oz) (regular bar)	100g (3½oz) (King-size bar)

The efficient metabolism theory

Research on the Pimas led scientists to wonder if there might be a set of genes – 'thrifty genes' – that were linked to a more efficient metabolism and a propensity to lay down large stores of fat. The idea is that some of us are born with low-fuel metabolisms: a little goes a long way. Other, more fortunate, people – fortunate, that is, during times of plenty – have gas-guzzling metabolisms that burn up fuel, keeping the body slim.

Although no one has found the exact bits of DNA responsible for obesity, plenty of evidence supports the thrifty gene hypothesis. For example, researchers at Columbia University have found that if you compare the metabolisms of two 12 stone people, one of whom weighed 20 stone in the past

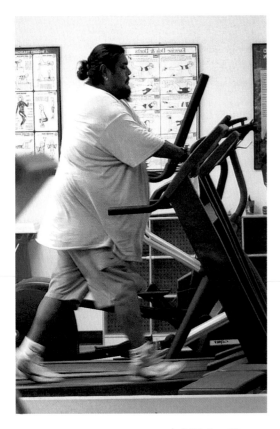

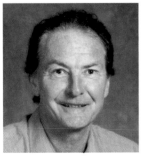

▲ A 27-stone Pima man works out at the Gila River Indian Reservation in Sacaton, Arizona, which has one of the highest rates of obesity in the world, according to Eric Ravusssin, Ph.D. (left).

and the other whose weight has been stable, you'll find that the once-heavy person needs 200 to 300 fewer calories per day to survive.

But thrifty genes and metabolism may not tell the whole story. Ask yourself how easily you can say no to a slab of gooey chocolate cake? Part of the answer could be locked deep in your DNA, according to researchers from the University of Maryland in Baltimore. Their study, published in June 2002, suggests that eating habits leading to obesity may be predetermined at least in part by genes. They looked at 624 adults from 28 Pennsylvania Amish families. (Genetics researchers favour Amish families because their gene pool is isolated and well documented by genealogical records.)

Each participant filled out a questionnaire about three factors related to eating. One was hunger. A second was restraint – a measure of whether people say no if they think eating another goody might make them fat. The third was disinhibition – how hard it was to say no to second helpings of a favourite food that they had already started eating. The researchers found that the answers given by overweight people correlated with obesity, and that high scores tended to run in families. When the researchers scanned the human genome, they could link the eating behaviours with segments of certain chromosomes. The next step is to find the exact genes linked to restraint and disinhibition.

A new way of looking at fat

Why some of us get fat is only one aspect of obesity that is being studied. Scientists are also gaining new information about fat itself, and the damage it can cause. It seems that fat is much more complicated than we once thought.

For years, researchers thought of fat simply as a tissue designed to store energy. But within the past year or so, they've come to see fat – known clinically as adipose tissue – as a hormone-producing organ, in much the same physiological group as the ovaries or the thyroid gland.

'Fat cells are essentially a gland,' says Dr. Louis Aronne, clinical associate professor of medicine at Weill-Cornell Medical College and director of the Comprehensive Weight Control Program in New York City. 'They produce a lot of different hormones. And the bigger the fat cell, the more hormones it produces.'

Bloated fat cells secrete more harmful hormones than their leaner counterparts, Dr. Aronne says. The main ones are known as plasminogen activator inhibitors, which make the

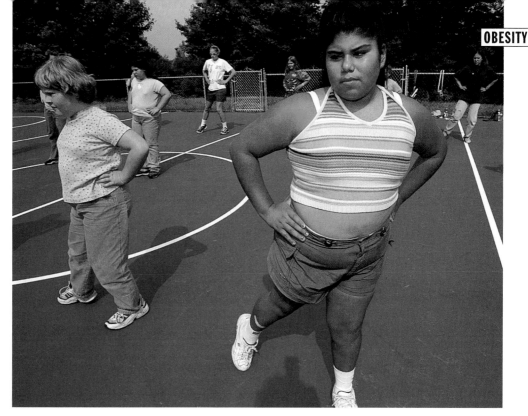

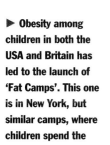

▶ Obesity among children in both the USA and Britain has led to the launch of 'Fat Camps'. This one is in New York, but similar camps, where children spend the school holidays getting fit, exist from Bradford to Brighton.

Bloated fat cells secrete more harmful hormones than their leaner counterparts.

blood clot more easily – triggering heart attacks and strokes, and tumour necrosis factor-alpha (or TNF), which is associated with inflammation. In women, fat cells also produce oestrogen. This may explain the higher rates of reproductive cancers in obese women. And the hormone leptin, which increases with weight gain, has been associated with an increased risk of blood clots, says Dr. Aronne.

What can we do?

For better or for worse, most of us in the Western world now live in an age of plenty. Delicious food is abundant, and physical exercise has become a voluntary luxury rather than a necessity. Still, it is clear that plenty of people want to be thinner. How can they go about it?

Many doctors now view obesity as a chronic medical problem, like diabetes or high blood pressure. To lose weight and keep it off, they acknowledge the fact that some people will need the help of structured programmes. Some will need personal coaches who will be responsible for monitoring progress and offering support. Some will need medication, just as they would for high

blood pressure, and many may need to stay on them for life. Others will opt for the drastic measure of stomach-shrinking surgery (see box on page 65).

For one American woman, Barbara Izykowski, the structured-programme approach did the trick. Barbara is 56 years old and 5ft 5in tall. For most of her life, she has been on a diet. And, for most of her life, she has been overweight. 'I tried Weight Watchers,' she says. 'I tried liquid diets. I tried pills.' But when she tipped the scales at 19 stone 4lb (122.5kg) she knew she had to try something else. So she volunteered to take part in a research study into exercise and weight-loss being run by scientists at the University of Pennsylvania.

To take part in the study, she had to agree to exercise four times a week and limit her calories. 'They gave us little books to look up the calorie count for everything we ate,' Barbara remembers. 'I was so angry to begin with. You had to look up everything you put into your mouth.'

The exercise was difficult, too. 'I had to start slowly,' she says. 'Before I started the study, I was lucky if I could walk from the house to the car. So I wasn't happy with that either.'

But today, after two years of limited calories and regular exercise – she walks for 50 minutes four days a week – Barbara Izykowski has lost 6st 9lb (43kg) and sees the exercise regime and calorie counting as a lifelong commitment. She remembers with joy the day a saleswoman told her to leave the

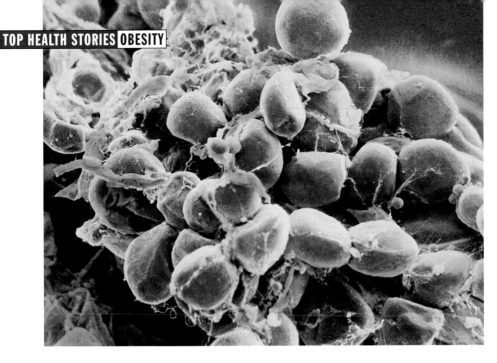

◀ Dietary fat that is not metabolized immediately is stored in fat cells such as these (shown in yellow).

'outsize' dress section in a local department store and look among the regular sizes: 'She told me I didn't need size 24 or 28 any more. I realized I could finally start shopping in the "misses" department.'

Medicines to dissolve weight

When Mary Beth Syrnick's weight suddenly ballooned, she became quite worried. She knew she had a strong family history of high blood pressure and stroke. She feared that the extra weight would take years off her life. But the lure of biscuits and chips was intense. 'It wasn't so much a feeling of hunger as it was a craving,' she says. 'All day I would graze – on junk food especially.'

Mary Beth, who lives in Philadelphia in the USA, went to see her doctor. He thought she might need some extra help. Along with a regular exercise routine and a diet plan that included keeping a food diary, he prescribed Meridia. This is a weight-loss drug that curbs appetite. It was approved by the US Government in 1997.

Mary Beth lost weight fast, and with the help of the diet drug has kept off most of the weight. 'It helps with the cravings,' she says. 'When I wasn't taking the medication I'd just eat and eat and eat before I would eventually feel full. If I weren't on the medication, I'm sure I would put the weight back on in no time.'

In the UK, a drug called Orlistat is available on prescription, but its use is strictly controlled. Medically described as a pancreatic lipase inhibitor, it reduces the body's absorption of dietary fat by as much as one-third. The drug works by tying up the enzyme that helps the body break down fat,

explains Dr. Thomas Wadden, of the University of Pennsylvania's School of Medicine. Some of the weight loss probably occurs as a result of individuals cutting their fat intake voluntarily because of what happens if they eat too much fat: if someone taking Orlistat eats more than 20g of fat, they suffer with flatulence and offensive-smelling diarrhoea. 'Of course, if you eat a healthy diet, you won't have to worry about those gastrointestinal symptoms,' says Dr. Wadden. Orlistat cannot be prescribed for longer than two years because there has not been enough research into its long-term effects beyond this period. There is also a risk that someone coming off the drug may gradually regain the weight they have lost.

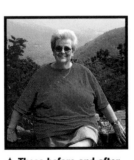

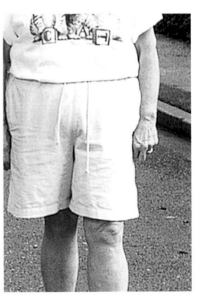

▲ These before-and-after photographs show how a well-planned diet and exercise routine helped Barbara Izykowski to lose 6st 11lb (43kg).

Alternatively, there are weight-loss aids. One example is a herbal extract called Metabolife. This is sold over-the-counter in the USA; anyone else can buy it via the Internet. Many people can take this herbal concoction safely, says Dr. David Heber Ph.D., professor of medicine and director of the Centre for Human Nutrition at the University of California. Metabolife contains caffeine and a substance called ephedra. 'There's good data in Europe showing that ephedra, aspirin and caffeine work well together,' Dr. Heber says. Still, he warns against taking herbal remedies without medical supervision. In certain people, these substances can cause serious side effects, such as cardiac arrhythmia (irregular heartbeat). So it is important to consult your GP before taking any over-the-counter weight-loss product.

Medical treatment for obesity is not recommended for children. It is possible that the drugs used could have adverse effects on puberty or on later eating behaviour.

Drug treatments in the pipeline

Research scientists are looking at 200 possible anti-obesity formulations for future development. Not all of them will make it onto the market, but any new weapons in the fight against fat will be welcome. Two promising drugs currently undergoing clinical trials work by altering the body's weight-regulating system. One, known as Axokine, is in its final phase of testing in the USA before it can be submitted for Government approval. It is not available anywhere else yet.

Axokine was originally developed as a treatment for a neurological disorder. When it was tested in patients, the results were disappointing. But researchers noticed an interesting thing: patients on the drug lost a lot of weight. This was not necessarily surprising, because the patients were terminally ill. But when the researchers took

Scientists are looking at 200 possible anti-obesity formulations for future development. Not all of them will make it onto the market, but any new weapons in the fight against fat will be welcome.

Are you overweight or obese?

The Body Mass Index (BMI) is used to determine whether a person is at a healthy weight, overweight, or obese. BMI has some limitations, in that it can overestimate body fat in people who are very muscular and it can underestimate body fat in people who have lost muscle mass, such as many elderly.

Calculating your BMI   Body Mass Index (BMI) $= \dfrac{\text{Weight (pounds)}}{\text{Height (inches)}^2} \times 703$

Body Mass Index (BMI) chart

Key   ☐ Healthy weight (Below 25)   ☐ Overweight (25-29)   ▨ Obese (30+)

Weight in pounds

Height	120	130	140	150	160	170	180	190	200	210	220	230	240	250
4'6	29	31	34	36	39	41	43	46	48	51	53	56	58	60
4'8	27	29	31	34	36	38	40	43	45	47	49	52	54	56
4'10	25	27	29	31	34	36	38	40	42	44	46	48	50	52
5'0	23	25	27	29	31	33	35	37	39	41	43	45	47	49
5'2	22	24	26	27	29	31	33	35	37	38	40	42	44	46
5'4	21	22	24	26	28	29	31	33	34	36	38	40	41	43
5'6	19	21	23	24	26	27	29	31	32	34	36	37	39	40
5'8	18	20	21	23	24	26	27	29	30	32	34	35	37	38
5'10	17	19	20	22	23	24	26	27	29	30	32	33	35	36
6'0	16	18	19	20	22	23	24	26	27	28	30	31	33	34
6'2	15	17	18	19	21	22	23	24	26	27	28	30	31	32
6'4	15	16	17	18	20	21	22	23	24	26	27	28	29	30
6'6	14	15	16	17	19	20	21	22	23	24	25	27	28	29
6'8	13	14	15	17	18	19	20	21	22	23	24	25	26	28

NOTE: Chart is for adults aged 20 and older.

OBESITY LINKED TO KIDNEY CANCER

In September 2002, Cancer Research UK announced that kidney cancer in women has increased by 22 per cent over the past decade. Cigarette smoking is a major risk factor for the disease. But Dr. Nick James, a kidney cancer specialist at the Queen Elizabeth Hospital, Birmingham, says, 'being overweight causes changes in hormones in the body, particularly for women, and it could be this hormone imbalance that increases the risk of kidney cancer'. Fat cells produce excess amounts of the female hormone oestrogen which speeds cell division. The faster cells duplicate, the greater the chance of something going wrong and a cancer cell being formed.

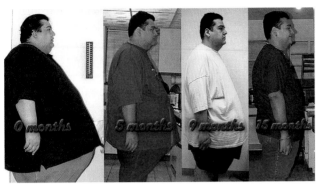

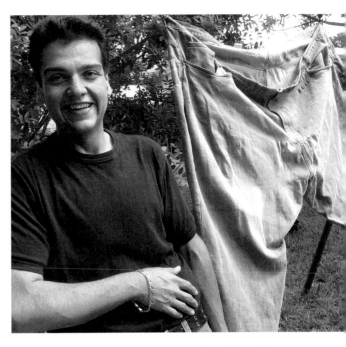

▲ Andy Schlesinger of North Miami Beach, Florida, is seen in a progression of photos as he lost some 36 stone in the two years after he underwent stomach-reducing surgery. Now, weighing just a little over 14 stone, he stands victoriously next to the trousers he once wore.

a closer look at how the drug worked, they discovered that it stimulated the brain's hypothalamus in a way very similar to the weight-regulating hormone leptin.

Trials in obese patients have been promising. 'An interesting thing about this drug is that people don't regain the weight right after stopping it,' says Dr. Louis Aronne of New York City. However, the drug has one major drawback – it has to be injected.

Another fat-fighting medication blocks substances that occur naturally in the body called cannabinoids. As the name suggests, these very closely resemble the active ingredient in marijuana. Researchers wondered whether – since marijuana gives you what is popularly known as the 'munchies' – an anticannabinoid drug might suppress the appetite. In a study published in the journal *Nature* in 2001, mice genetically engineered to be deficient in cannabinoid receptors ate 40 per cent less than normal mice. In a separate experiment, obese rats genetically modified to have low levels of leptin – the hormone that leads to feelings of fullness – produced higher amounts of cannabinoids than occur naturally. When the rats were injected with leptin, their cannabinoid levels dropped.

Fat hormones regulate metabolism

Several years ago, when scientists discovered leptin, they thought they had a magic bullet for obesity. Leptin is a hormone released by fat cells. The larger fat cells get, the more leptin they release. Normally, when the brain gets a surge of leptin, it concludes that the body has a safe store of fat, and it sends out a message to dampen the appetite. So researchers concluded that all they needed to do was give overweight people more leptin. Surely this would kill appetite and cause weight loss.

But when they tried it, the experiments were a dismal failure. It emerged that obese people produce large amounts of leptin naturally. And adding more doesn't seem to help them lose weight.

But there is a happy ending. A recent study showed that additional leptin may help to keep the weight off in people who have already managed to shed excess pounds through other methods. A small pilot study, published in the US *Journal of Clinical Endocrinology and Metabolism* in May 2002, concluded that leptin injections could help to maintain weight loss by regulating metabolism.

The researchers observed that the body goes into 'survival mode' when people try to lose weight. Their metabolism slows right down, their thyroid production diminishes, and their leptin levels plummet. The body tries to conserve energy and becomes more fuel-efficient as it becomes thinner,

The researchers observed that the body goes into 'survival mode' when people try to lose weight. Their metabolism slows right down.

WHEN ALL ELSE FAILS: SURGERY

Increasingly, obese Americans are turning to stomach-shrinking surgery to help shed stubborn pounds. In 2002, there were nearly 62,000 such operations, compared to 36,000 five years ago, according to Georgeann Mallory, a specialist in the field.

To help patients resist the temptation of calorie-laden foods, doctors choose one of several procedures that limit the amount of food the stomach can hold. The most common is called a gastric bypass. In this surgery a pouch is constructed out of the top of the stomach, and then the contents of this pouch are rerouted directly to the intestines. The pouch initially can hold only about 25g (1oz) of food.

'Eventually, as the pouch stretches, it will get to the point where you can eat a small meal of about 115g (4oz),' says Mallory. 'That's about the size of a Weight Watchers meal.'

Because the stomach is smaller, the patient feels full sooner. Furthermore, the outlet from the new pouch is small, so it doesn't empty as fast. 'Your food stays trapped in there longer, and you feel full longer. You also have to really chew your food well so that it can fit through that small opening,' explains Mallory.

The surgery is reversible. The part of the stomach cut off from the pouch can be reattached. 'But that's not common,' Mallory says. 'You'd just gain the weight back.'

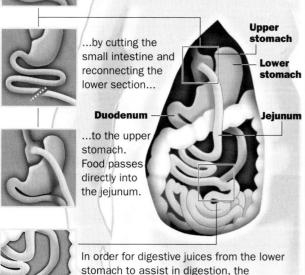

A Roux-en-Y gastric bypass – one of four stomach-shrinking surgical operations

The stomach is separated into two parts. The upper part forms a small egg-sized pouch. The lower stomach and first portion of the small intestine are bypassed...

...by cutting the small intestine and reconnecting the lower section...

Upper stomach

Lower stomach

Duodenum

Jejunum

...to the upper stomach. Food passes directly into the jejunum.

In order for digestive juices from the lower stomach to assist in digestion, the duodendum is reconnected to the lower section of the small intestine.

burning up fewer calories during the day, even when it does the same amount of exercise as before – a phenomenon that will be recognized by all too many frustrated dieters.

'Nature wants you fatter, not skinnier,' explains Dr. Rudolf Leibel, the study's co-author and a professor and head of the division of molecular genetics at Columbia University in New York City. 'There's a lot of biology set up to defend body fat.'

Dr. Leibel and his colleagues studied the effects of weight loss and maintenance in four people. The team found that they could return someone's metabolism and thyroid levels to normal if they simply boosted the amount of leptin in that person's blood to pre-weight-loss levels. However, far more research is needed before leptin injections become a standard treatment.

A little weight loss goes a long way

Whatever your approach to losing weight, there's very hopeful news on one front. A study published in February 2002 in the *New England Journal of Medicine* found that small lifestyle changes – including moderate weight loss – can greatly reduce the chances of developing diabetes, even among people prone to the condition.

In the study, researchers followed more than 3,000 overweight patients who were deemed to be at high risk for diabetes. The patients were randomly assigned to receive a placebo (dummy pill), take an oral medication (the diabetes drug Glucophage) to lower their blood sugar, or to take part in a programme of diet and exercise – at least two-and-a-half hours a week. Ultimately, diet and exercise proved to be far more effective than medication at preventing diabetes. The drug cut the risk of developing diabetes by an impressive 31 per cent, but the lifestyle modifications cut the risk by a whopping 58 per cent.

'People didn't need to lose 7 stone (45kg) to lower their risk of diabetes,' says study co-author Dr. David M. Nathan, a professor of medicine at the Harvard Medical School. 'Some only lost 15lb (7kg), and that was enough to prevent diabetes.'

Finally, for those who say it is pointless to lose weight if you're destined to regain it, there's now evidence to the contrary. In spite of the fact that many of the patients in the study regained some of the weight they lost after three or four years, their risk of diabetes was still significantly lower than those who had lost no weight at all. It seems that it's better to have lost and regained than never to have lost weight at all.

The organ shortage: pigs to the rescue?

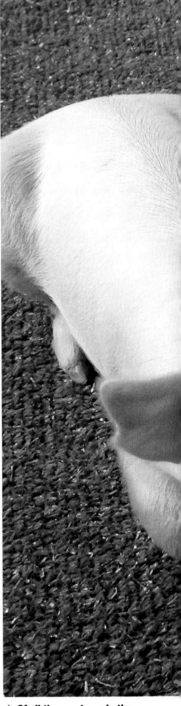

▲ Of all the creatures in the animal kingdom, it turns out that pigs are the best candidates to serve as organ donors to humans.

L ife is a long waiting game for the thousands of British patients who need a kidney, liver, heart, or heart and lung transplant. Demand has spiralled in the last decade; in 1991, for instance, 4113 people needed a new kidney, but by 2000 the figure was 6284. On average someone in the UK dies every day because the organ they need is not available.

Could xenotransplantation – transplanting a cell, tissue or organ from another species – be part of the solution? Some scientists believe so. Among them are pioneering researchers at PPL Therapeutics, the Edinburgh-based biopharmaceutical company, and Dr. David Sachs, a professor at Harvard Medical School who heads the Transplantation Biology Research Center at Massachusetts General Hospital, in Boston.

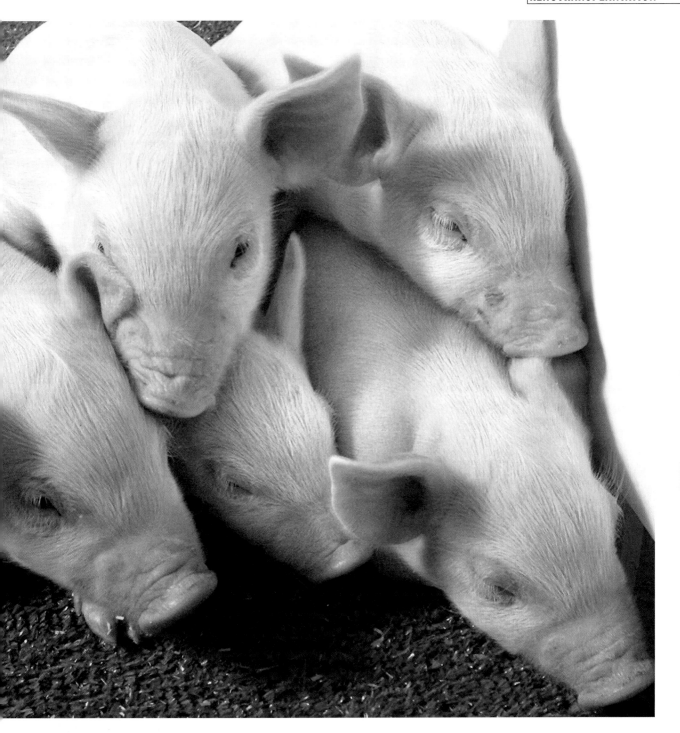

A priceless litter

In January 2002, colleagues of Dr. Sachs at Immerge Bio-Therapeutics in Charlestown, Massachusetts, and at the University of Missouri in Columbia, reported a break-through. Writing in the journal *Science*, the researchers described a litter of genetically altered pigs born in September 2001. The pigs, cloned from cells taken from the colony of miniature swine Dr. Sachs has bred for

nearly 25 years, had one copy of a specific gene 'knocked out' of their DNA, potentially making their organs more compatible with those of humans. The same month PPL announced that they too had produced a Christmas litter of similar 'knock-out' pigs.

These pigs are important because they remove one of the biggest stumbling-blocks in pig-to-human transplants: sugar molecules that sit on the surface of the transplanted pig organ's cells. These sugar molecules are known as galactose-alpha (1-3-galactose). During evolution, humans and primates, such as monkeys and apes, lost the enzyme that makes this molecule. Today, our immune system recognizes the sugar as foreign and produces antibodies that attack it, leading to rejection of the transplant and, ultimately, organ failure. Dr. Sachs and his team can initially suppress and eliminate these antibodies, but they always return.

The 'knockout' pigs are missing one copy of the gene that is responsible for manufacturing this enzyme. The next step for Immerge Therapeutics is to breed those otherwise-normal piglets to produce males and females with just one copy of the gene, and then breed those offspring, to produce a litter in which one out of four piglets will lack both copies of the gene. PPL have already achieved this by another route, and in July 2002 announced the birth of four healthy 'double knock-out' pigs at their US subsidiary in Virginia.

'This advance brings us closer to the promise of a potential solution to the world-wide shortage of organs and cells for transplantation,' says David Ayares, chief operating officer and vice-president of research at PPL Therapeutics Inc.

Organs and cells from the newly-developed pigs will now be tested in studies at the Thomas E. Starzl Transplant Institute at the University of Pittsburgh. But as scientists move closer to the possibility of animal-to-human transplants, practical and ethical concerns are being aired.

Genetically altering pigs for humanity

PPL Therapeutics, the Edinburgh-based company that worked with the Roslin Institute to clone Dolly the sheep, has also developed a technique to clone genetically altered pigs whose organs the human body is less likely to reject.

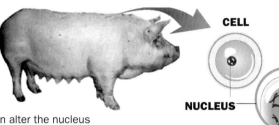

A cell is collected from a pig.

CELL

NUCLEUS

Scientists then alter the nucleus to inactivate the alpha 1-3 galactosyl transferase gene, which adds a particular sugar group to the pig's cell that the human body would reject as foreign.

CHROMOSOME

DNA STRAND

The altered nucleus is inserted into an egg cell whose original nucleus has been removed.

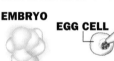

EMBRYO

EGG CELL

DNA HELIX

ALTERED NUCLEUS

The egg is allowed to divide for a few days until it becomes an embryo. Several embryos are implanted into a surrogate mother pig who carries them to term and delivers 'knock-out' offspring. A 'knock-out' is an animal produced with the specific gene inactivated or knocked out.

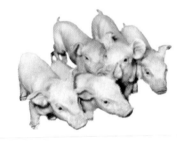

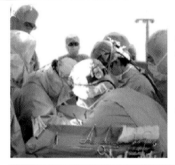

The hope is that organs and cells taken from these knock-out pigs can be transplanted into humans without rejection.

Pigs are the preferred species for xenotransplantation (transplants from animal to man) on scientific and ethical grounds.

Questions of ethics

One of the concerns centres on the risk of transferring pig retroviruses into humans. Retroviruses are a special kind of virus that become integrated into the DNA of host cells, taking over the cell. The human immunodeficiency virus (HIV), which causes AIDS, is a human retrovirus. The porcine endogenous retrovirus (PERV) in pigs is similar to retroviruses present in all human cells

and has the potential to infect humans. Although their transfer to humans is a valid concern, Dr Sachs points out that 'to date, there is no evidence that pig retroviruses have caused human disease'.

One US study tracked nearly 160 cases involving human patients who had received transplants of – or had otherwise been exposed to – pig tissues or cells. (As yet, no such work has been done in the UK.) These people included stroke survivors and patients with Parkinson's disease who had neural swine cells implanted, and those whose livers had failed and were connected to an external pig liver which filtered their blood while they were waiting for a human liver transplant. No evidence of viral transmission was found, even years later. Additionally, tissue culture from Dr. Sachs' specially bred miniature swine, inbred for so long that they're similar to identical twins, appears not to contain the pig virus that infects human cells.

But Chris Rudge, medical director of UK Transplant, the NHS organization which coordinates transplantation services across the UK, says that 'very real concerns' remain about the risks of transferring infections from pigs, although he hails the work as an 'exciting development'.

Animal rights activists have also protested against the use of pigs as unwitting donors for organ transplants. Pigs are the likeliest animal to be used for xenotransplantation because, next to non-human primates (which are either endangered or too small to provide suitable organs), pigs are the most abundantly available species and have the greatest physiological similarity to humans. Since millions of pigs are slaughtered every year for food anyway, notes Dr. Sachs, 'it seems unlikely that there will

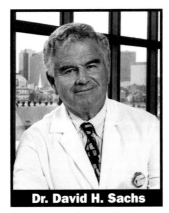
Dr. David H. Sachs

'When you have that kind of potential [life-saving] benefit, it makes sense to me to keep going forward with the research.'

be widespread ethical reservations about using them as a source of life-saving organs'. Or as Dr. Robert Lanza, vice-president of medical and scientific development at Advanced Cell Technology in Worcester, Massachusetts, puts it, 'If it is acceptable to kill pigs to make sausages, surely it must be acceptable to kill them to save lives.'

And therein lies the most important reason for this kind of research, says Dr. Sachs. 'We know patients' lives depend on it,' he says. 'So when you have that kind of potential benefit, it makes sense to me to keep going forward with the research to see if we can do something for all these people in such dire need, and try to balance that potential benefit against the possible risks, and other drawbacks.'

No time to wait

In Britain, however, clinical trials of xenotransplantation are 'likely to be a number of years away,' according to Chris Rudge. Meanwhile, the number of organs from cadavers is declining as medical science saves more lives, but demand is increasing and people are being actively encouraged to donate living organs for transplantation.

In 2001, the number of living organ donors increased to about 32 per cent of all donors – a figure that has been steadily increasing in recent years, according to UK

SURGEONS WARM TO PORTABLE ORGAN SYSTEM

As the number of people waiting for organ transplants continues to grow, scientists are looking for a way to make more organs available. They may have found it with a device called POPS (Portable Organ Preservation System). The experimental machine can keep organs alive and functional for hours or days, and potentially for an unlimited amount of time.

'This could transform the way transplants are performed,' says Dr. David Cronin, assistant professor of surgery at the University of Colorado, who is working with biotech company TransMedics of Woburn, Massachusetts, to develop the device.

Currently, solid organs for transplant, such as hearts, kidneys and lungs, are removed from donors and immediately placed on ice, severely limiting the time during which they are viable. The process damages even the best organs and renders some marginal organs unsuitable for transplant. Also, while the organ is on ice it can't be tested for proper functioning.

To solve the problem, POPS pumps a warm, blood-based, oxygenated nutrient solution through the organ in rhythmic pulses, in the same manner in which the heart pumps blood. 'This not only avoids the damage that comes from being in a cold, non-oxygenated environment,' says Dr. Cronin, 'but we can test the organ and see if it's functioning properly before we transplant it into the recipient. If it doesn't work, we can either repair it or discard it.' So far, POPS has been successfully tested on more than 500 animal organs. Chicago researchers also tested it on a human heart, a couple of kidneys and a liver that was deemed unsuitable for transplant. It worked so well with the kidneys, says Dr. Cronin, that the organs actually began to produce urine. The process also dramatically improved the status of the liver to the point where it might have been usable as a transplant after all.

TransMedics are awaiting approval to begin clinical trials in humans in the UK and the USA very soon.

Transplant. But with a transplant waiting list exceeding 5000, more are urgently required. Among the suggestions aired, in 2002 consultations that will pave the way for new UK laws relating to human organs and tissue, was the proposal that donors should receive some form of compensation. In fact, hospital trusts are permitted to offer donors some compensation, says Maxine Walter, UK Transplant's media and public relations officer, but are not legally required to do so, which creates disparities.

The most common organ transplants from living donors are kidneys, which are usually very successful (humans need only one healthy kidney to survive), and livers because liver tissue has the capacity to regenerate.

The case for living kidney donations got a boost in April 2002 from data presented by US researchers from Johns Hopkins University in Maryland. The researchers showed they could transplant organs between any two people, regardless of blood type or antibodies resulting from a previous transplant, if they filtered the kidney recipient's blood of antibodies that would normally reject a donor kidney.

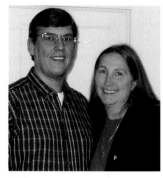

▲ Cheryl McCullough has never regretted donating a part of her liver to husband, Randy.

Living liver transplants are a more difficult area because the surgery required to cut out part of a liver is so intense and long – about 18 hours. Only 58 living-donor liver transplants have been performed in the UK since 1992, many of them at King's College Hospital in London, which has the largest liver transplant programme in Europe and was the first programme to perform living related liver transplantation in children.

Living liver transplants are always 'lobe transplants', that use just a small part of the liver. (The King's programme has also pioneered a new surgical technique which means that a donated cadaveric liver can be divided to save two or even three children's lives.)

Despite the complex surgery, no living liver donor deaths have been recorded in the UK. But in the USA, where 1000 living liver transplants have been performed in the past decade, a few have died as a result of the procedure, either from the surgery itself or from post-surgical complications. One study found that 71 per cent of donors complained of mild, ongoing abdominal symptoms. The death of one healthy liver donor – allegedly due to inadequate postsurgical care – made front-page news in New York in January 2002.

Persuading the public to donate organs to save lives can be an uphill struggle – particularly if there is any risk attached. But some people have a very clear incentive. Cheryl McCullough of Green Bank, West Virginia, donated part of her liver to her fiancé (now husband) two years ago. 'When it was all said and done, the bottom line was I had a choice,' she says. 'A choice I have never regretted making and would do all over again in the blink of an eye. Everyone is motivated by something – money, power, nice possessions, and the like. For me, to know I had truly made a difference in someone's life – that was my compensation.'

As Maxine Walter of UK Transplant says, 'That's our key message. Transplants do save lives. As a result of increasingly sophisticated surgical skills, more people can now benefit from a transplant – ironically at a time when the supply of organs is dwindling. Living donors are particularly important because their organs can provide the most successful type of transplant.'

THE ORGAN WAITING GAME

UK ACTIVE TRANSPLANT WAITING LIST AT 30 SEPTEMBER 2002

Organ	Patients Waiting for Transplant
Kidney	4945
Liver	184
Heart	91
Lung	269
Kidney & pancreas	90
Pancreas	20
Heart & lung	80
Total waiting	5679
Total at 30 September 2001	5498

NUMBER OF TRANSPLANTS PERFORMED IN THE UK IN 2001

Organ	Transplants
Kidney alone (358 were living donors)	1691
Liver	675
Heart	166
Lung (single and double)	93
Kidney & pancreas	41
Pancreas	6
Kidney & heart, kidney & liver	11
Heart & lung	32
Heart & liver, liver & heart-lung	2

PATIENT PROFILE

Islet cells transplanted, she tosses her insulin needles

Merry Brunson, a diabetic, didn't need a whole new pancreas – just the pancreatic cells called islet cells that produce insulin. The cells, currently derived from donor pancreases but potentially available from pigs as well, may one day change the future for diabetics.

For 30 years, Merry, of Greeley, Colorado, gave herself injections three times a day, trying to keep her Type 1 diabetes under control. She followed a strict diet – giving up foods she loved, like ice cream – and checked her blood sugar levels several times a day.

By the time she was in her late 30s, however, all the conscientious self-care in the world had stopped working. Merry began experiencing dangerous episodes of low blood sugar that left her woozy and disoriented. There were nights her husband found her convulsing in her sleep from low blood sugar, and days when her two young children had to call the emergency services because she'd passed out.

'It was getting to the end, where I knew I had to do something for myself,' says the 41-year-old finance officer. She opted for the latest technology – an implantable insulin pump, which regulated her insulin and helped to maintain a more even blood sugar level – but it still wasn't enough.

Then Merry read an article about researchers in Canada who had succeeded in transplanting insulin-producing islet cells into people with Type 1 diabetes. She went online to find out more and learned that researchers at the University of Miami were beginning islet cell transplants. In spring 2001 she signed on and the following Memorial Day weekend, at the end of May, she underwent the brief procedure.

Islet cell transplantation is not new. In the past 25 years or so, more than 300 people around the world have undergone such transplants. (Leicester General Hospital hopes to begin the UK's first programme this year.) But few of the procedures, if any, worked for long, because the immunosuppressant drugs patients needed to keep their bodies from rejecting the transplanted cells harmed the islet cells themselves. Then Canadian scientists at the University of Alberta, in Edmonton, developed a novel, steroid-free combination of three anti-rejection drugs that appear to prevent rejection and halt autoimmune destruction of the islets. Traditional anti-rejection drugs contain steroids, which can cause serious side effects.

After the successful Canadian islet cell transplants in 2000, the National Institutes of Health launched a multi-centre clinical trial in the United States.

To perform the transplant, doctors inserted a catheter through Merry's upper rib cage into the portal vein, which leads to the liver, and infused hundreds of thousands of donor islet cells (from a cadaver) through the thin tube. Merry remained awake during the procedure and left the hospital the following morning. A couple of weeks later, she returned for a second transplant.

The results, she says, have been nothing short of miraculous. No need for insulin. No finger pricks (although she still checks her blood sugar periodically because she simply can't believe she's cured). And all the ice cream she could want. 'Sometimes I have to think, Is this really real?'

Early results appear to indicate that her recovery is perfectly real. By mid-2002, about 80 people had undergone the experimental procedure as part of a clinical trial sponsored by the Immune Tolerance Network, an international collaborative research effort. In December 2001, Miami researchers announced that eight of the ten patients who had received the islet cell transplant there (including Merry) were free

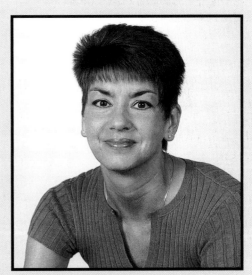

Following Islet cell transplantation Merry has resumed a normal life, all but cured of diabetes.

of the need for insulin injections, and the remaining two would no longer need injections after undergoing the second infusion.

The transplant is still experimental, and donor islet cells are scarce. Each patient receives cells from at least two pancreases, relatively few of which are donated each year. The organ shortage is one of the main reasons researchers are looking for ways to use cells from animals, such as pigs, in humans.

Bioterror: science fights back

Imagine an explosion ripping through the heart of London, leaving in its wake a deadly dust of radioactive isotopes or anthrax spores. Or what might happen if fanatics released nerve gas on the city's underground system – just as the Japanese terrorists did in Tokyo in March 1995. For some people, biological warfare has already become a reality – notably the Kurdish population in the later stages of the Iran-Iraq war.

Fears that bioterrorism might strike here have prompted the government to buy millions of doses of smallpox vaccine and to brief the nation's doctors on how to deal with a deliberate release of anthrax. It has even been suggested that NHS Direct might be used to detect outbreaks of such killer diseases. And, behind the scenes in Britain and the USA, scientists are renewing their efforts to discover ways to protect ordinary people against the threat of biological weapons including anthrax, smallpox, Ebola virus and other pathogens as well.

▶ Members of the US Marine Corps Chemical-Biological Incident Response Force demonstrate anthrax clean-up techniques at a news conference in October 2001.

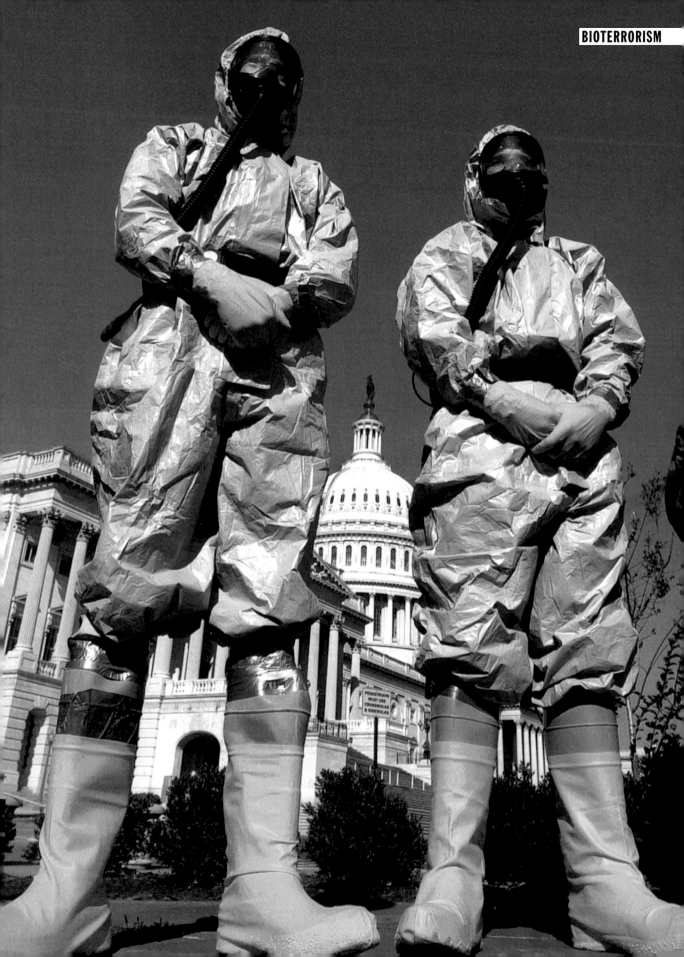

In the quest to find both drug treatments for the infected and vaccines to protect the uninfected masses, inspiration has come from some fascinating places – even outer space.

ET-inspired research

Oddly enough, technology developed for the Search for Extraterrestrial Intelligence (SETI) project may have accelerated the discovery of a cure for people infected with anthrax.

In 1999, space scientists in the United States launched a novel programme that links the home computers of some 5 million volunteer computer buffs. Software for the SETI@home programme runs in the 'background' of those computers, using their untapped processing power to sift through

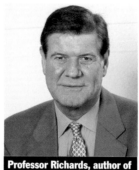

Professor Richards, author of the 'Son of SETI' programme.

more than a billion radio telescope signals for any signs of intelligent life existing in outer space.

Professor Graham Richards, chairman of the chemistry department at Oxford University, realized that the same 'desktop grid computing' could be used to fight anthrax. His task: to sift through 3.5 billion molecules to identify those which might block the formation of the deadly toxin produced by anthrax.

Starting in February 2002, the programme Prof. Richards calls 'Son of SETI' used 1.4 million volunteers' computers to whittle down that

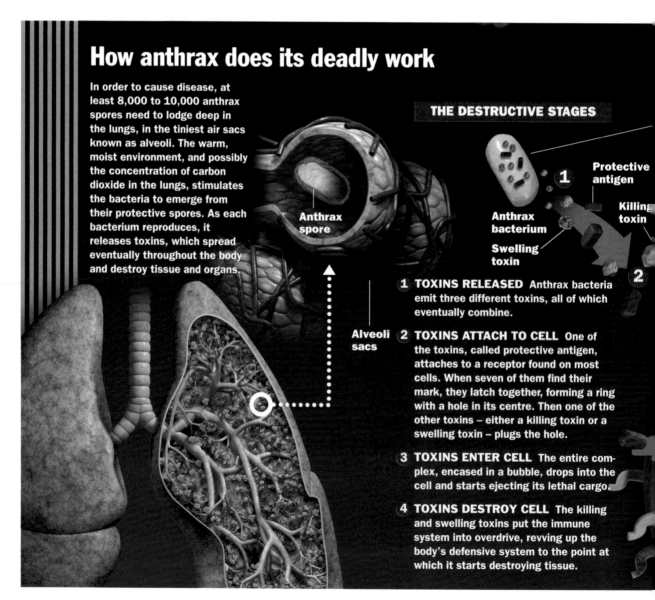

How anthrax does its deadly work

In order to cause disease, at least 8,000 to 10,000 anthrax spores need to lodge deep in the lungs, in the tiniest air sacs known as alveoli. The warm, moist environment, and possibly the concentration of carbon dioxide in the lungs, stimulates the bacteria to emerge from their protective spores. As each bacterium reproduces, it releases toxins, which spread eventually throughout the body and destroy tissue and organs.

Anthrax spore

Alveoli sacs

THE DESTRUCTIVE STAGES

1 **Protective antigen**

Anthrax bacterium

Swelling toxin

Killing toxin

2

1 TOXINS RELEASED Anthrax bacteria emit three different toxins, all of which eventually combine.

2 TOXINS ATTACH TO CELL One of the toxins, called protective antigen, attaches to a receptor found on most cells. When seven of them find their mark, they latch together, forming a ring with a hole in its centre. Then one of the other toxins – either a killing toxin or a swelling toxin – plugs the hole.

3 TOXINS ENTER CELL The entire complex, encased in a bubble, drops into the cell and starts ejecting its lethal cargo.

4 TOXINS DESTROY CELL The killing and swelling toxins put the immune system into overdrive, revving up the body's defensive system to the point at which it starts destroying tissue.

In just 24 days, the worldwide network had run calculations that otherwise would have taken 20 years.

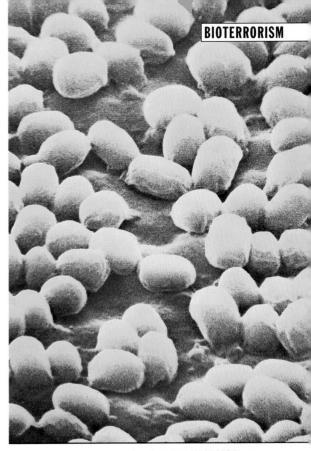

huge list of molecules to 12,000 likely contenders. In just 24 days, the worldwide network had run calculations that otherwise would have taken 20 years. The results were turned over to the US and British governments, who will use them to help develop a drug that targets one of anthrax's three poisonous proteins.

Duelling with a toxic trio

To understand how one of those potential drugs might disable anthrax, it is useful to know how the insidious anthrax bacterium works.

For decades, anthrax has been viewed as a potential biological weapon. So scientists had already made progress in unravelling its mysteries years before the anthrax-laced letters appeared in American government offices and media outlets in 2001. Thanks to that head start, by January 2002 – just three months after the letter attacks – researchers had worked out how anthrax wreaks havoc in the body.

Anthrax usually spreads through amazingly resilient, microscopic spores – each one less than one-twentieth the diameter of a human hair. Once a spore is inhaled or sneaks in through broken skin, it will germinate into active bacteria that flood the bloodstream with toxins. Through a cunning biological hijacking scheme, the toxins can enter cells and turn off the cells' natural internal defence against bacterial invasion.

'The anthrax toxin consists of three proteins,' says Prof. Richards. 'Individually they're not toxic. But the three come together to form the lethal toxin.'

Here's how: The first protein, called protective antigen, gathers in clusters to form a ring that serves as an entrance into cells. The protein's name is actually a misnomer; originally the protein was thought to have protective properties, but in fact it acts more like a Stealth bomber to deliver the other two proteins – known as lethal factor and oedema factor – into the cell.

Lethal factor destroys immune cells from the inside. In January 2002 oedema factor – originally named for the swelling it causes – was discovered to play an even more sinister role. It disables a messenger molecule in the host cell and begins sending out its own signals that quickly block the body's natural immune response to the invader, allowing that invader to spread.

Now that this mechanism is understood, it's theoretically possible to develop an antitoxin that would stop the progression of the disease while antibiotics wipe out the bacteria that caused it. 'There are very elegant ways of blocking the effects of the various anthrax toxins,' says Dr. Anthony Fauci, director of the National Institute of Allergy

▲ ANTHRAX SPORES can survive for years and are resistant to extremes of heat, cold, and dryness. The bacteria within become activated as they germinate inside their host.

WHEN IT CAN BE STOPPED

CIPRO and other antibiotics kill bacteria by interfering with an enzyme that the bugs need to create their DNA.

ANTITOXINS do not yet exist against anthrax, but scientists are working on compounds that would soak up the toxins before they could bind to cells.

Cell receptor

Macrophage cell

Macrophage enzymes

and Infectious Diseases at the National Institutes of Health (NIH) in the USA. 'That's a direction that's being actively pursued.'

The computer project run by Prof. Richards screened molecules for substances that could block the site where the lethal factor and oedema factor proteins enter cells. Identifying such molecules would guide the development of drugs that could treat anthrax in much the same way that protease inhibitors work against HIV.

Building a better anthrax vaccine

Drugs to inhibit the anthrax toxin are only one approach being pursued. Scientists are also racing to produce a new anthrax vaccine, because the existing one has limitations. It's recommended only for people over the age of 18 who have robust immune systems and a high likelihood of coming into contact with anthrax spores. Such candidates include military personnel and certain lab workers. Another problem with the current vaccine is that it doesn't confer full protection quickly enough; it requires a series of six separate injections given over 18 months, plus a yearly booster.

'We need to develop a second generation of anthrax vaccine,' Dr. Fauci says. 'That's very much at the top of our current priorities.' The most promising research involves a vaccine developed by the NIH and the US Department of Defense. It uses a genetically engineered version of anthrax's protective antigen protein to provide immunity against the real thing. That new vaccine should be ready for testing on humans by mid-2003, Dr. Fauci says.

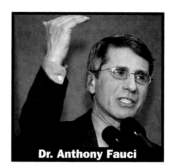

Dr. Anthony Fauci

'I think it would be at least a little naive to think there isn't the possibility that some of that material got into the hands of people who would use it in a nefarious way.'

In Britain, researchers have also developed a vaccine based on the protective antigen protein. It may offer protection in just two doses through a nasal spray. Laboratory mice gained immunity to anthrax after they were given the vaccine by nasal spray, injection, or both.

Meanwhile, researchers at the Howard Hughes Medical Institute in Chevy Chase, Maryland, discovered an anthrax-resistant gene in mice that safeguards the mice even after they've been exposed to anthrax. A form of the gene is known to exist in humans, but it's not known whether it offers similar protection. Although the gene's discovery is an encouraging step, says Dr. Fauci, the key question is whether scientists can develop a drug that mimics the gene to block anthrax in humans.

Smallpox: a large threat?

Anthrax dominated the headlines after the letter attacks, but another potential biological threat has since overshadowed it.

The eradication of smallpox was perhaps the greatest medical success story of the past century. The last recorded outbreak in the general population occurred in Somalia in 1977; in 1980 the World Health Organization triumphantly declared that smallpox had been wiped out. So why are we worried about it now, more than two decades later? Because official stocks of the virus still exist in labs in Atlanta and Moscow. And because the Soviet Union, years after signing an international bioweapons treaty, produced tons of the virus to use in cluster bombs and intercontinental missiles.

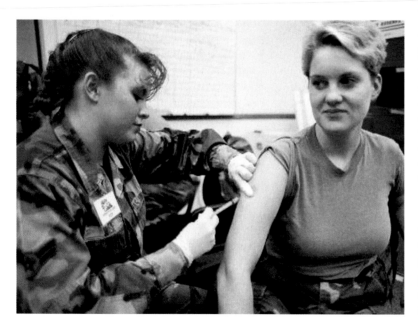

◀ The current anthrax vaccine is recommended for military personnel, but not for the general public. Scientists are developing a newer, safer vaccine for everyone.

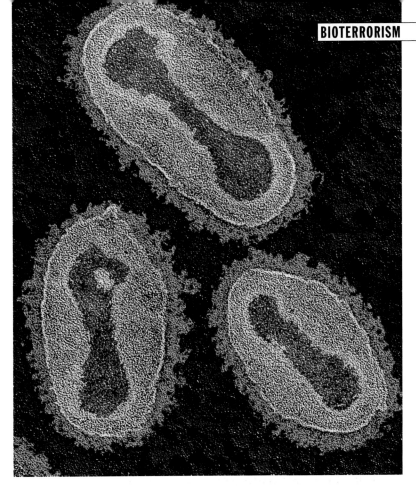

'I think it would be at least a little naive to think there isn't the possibility that some of that material got into the hands of people who would use it in a nefarious way,' Dr. Fauci says.

Even before the anthrax attacks, US health officials had become concerned that there were only 15 million doses of smallpox vaccine available for Americans. But they discovered that each dose could be diluted five times and still retain its potency, so the USA instantly had 75 million doses to hand. After September 11 2001, more were ordered – to bring the US stockpile to around 300 million doses by the end of 2002 – enough to vaccinate everybody in the United States,' Dr. Fauci says, though no decision to do so has yet been made.

In Britain, some 16 million doses were ordered in April 2002, and further supplies are being sought. However, in late 2002 the Government said that vaccination in advance of any possible terrorist attack would only be offered to an as yet unspecified number of health workers and other key personnel because of the smallpox vaccine's inherent dangers.

The current vaccine uses *Vaccinia* virus, which spurs production of antibodies that also protect against smallpox. This vaccine made it possible to wipe out smallpox (and those who have been vaccinated will still have some immunity). But it does have shortcomings. Based on use of the vaccine worldwide, researchers have estimated that vaccinating everyone in Britain could result in at least 300 serious illnesses and 60 deaths.

The vaccine causes one to two deaths for every million people vaccinated and comes with an array of rare but serious side effects, ranging from skin lesions and eczema to encephalitis – a potentially fatal inflammation of the brain. As no cases of smallpox have been reported since the 1970s, is that an acceptable price to pay? Perhaps not.

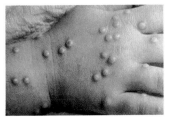

▲ Above, the smallpox virus as seen through an electron microscope. Infection (right) causes fever, exhaustion and pustular rash. The virus is transmitted via inhaled airborne droplets.

Researchers estimate that vaccinating everyone in Britain [against smallpox] could result in at least 300 serious illnesses and 60 deaths.

The solution, Dr. Fauci says, is to develop a new, safer vaccine. 'If in fact we got that – and we are putting a lot of effort into getting that – then there would be very little doubt that you would vaccinate everybody,' Dr. Fauci says. 'By doing that, you would completely eliminate the threat of smallpox.'

While developing a new vaccine to prevent smallpox infection is the top priority, researchers are also working on antiviral drugs that would stop the virus from replicating once a person is infected. The most promising is an existing drug called cidofovir, used to treat eye infections caused by cytomegalovirus, a complication in some people with HIV. Researchers initially found that the drug was highly effective in blocking a virus very similar to smallpox when injected into animals, including primates. But because any outbreak of smallpox is likely to create a public health crisis, health officials want something that can be handed out in pill form, rather than having people line up for shots.

So far, studies in animals and in the laboratory show that the oral form 'actually is even more potent than the intravenous one,' Dr. Fauci says. But because of the time it takes to test drugs for safety, particularly using animal trials, it will probably be at least a year – and probably two years or more – before an oral drug is available, he adds.

DIAGNOSIS: BIOTERRORISM

When terrorists strike – with bombs, guns or even airplanes turned into missiles – the attack is immediate and obvious. But with bioterrorism, it could be days before we know that killer germs have been unleashed among us. Smallpox, for example, incubates for 7 to 17 days before the first symptoms appear. The first signs of the inhalation form of anthrax that killed five people in the USA in 2001 are virtually indistinguishable from the flu.

So, in addition to finding vaccines and drug treatments to deal with these threats, researchers are focusing on ways to identify an outbreak faster. Here are a few ways they are doing this in America:

■ To diagnose anthrax infection, scientists are developing molecular probes to detect subtle changes in the blood that occur even before the anthrax spore germinates and begins spewing toxins into the bloodstream. The blood culture test used in the USA in October 2001 requires 24 to 72 hours to get a result. The new test would provide results within minutes.

■ A computerized system is being built to analyse US sales data of common drugs such as cough syrup or aspirin. A sudden, unexplained rise in sales could be a first alert of a biological attack.

■ A web site funded by the US Agency for Healthcare Research and Quality has been expanded to help medical professionals to learn to respond quickly to a bioterrorist attack. The site can be found at www.bioterrorism.uab.edu.

■ A handheld device is being developed for use in the field to scan genes from blood samples for signs that a person has been exposed to a potentially lethal agent.

■ A device is being developed to analyse the DNA from a swab test (fluid samples taken from the nose or mouth) to identify patterns that would indicate exposure to a bioterror agent.

■ In a project funded by the US Department of Defense, bees are being trained to recognize the scent of biological or chemical agents.

Progress is being made towards better testing of smallpox vaccines and treatments. In June 2002, microbiologists at the Centers for Disease Control and Prevention in the USA were able to infect monkeys with smallpox in a way that created symptoms similar to those that humans experience. The idea is to create an animal model of the disease for testing purposes – without putting human volunteers at risk. Previous attempts to infect monkeys with smallpox produced only mild symptoms.

Ebola: closer to a cure

Perhaps the most terrifying of all the bioterror threats is the Ebola virus, a deadly disease that has plagued certain parts of Africa over the past few decades. One of the infectious diseases categorized as a viral haemorrhagic fever, nightmarish Ebola induces a plethora of gory symptoms – including uncontrolled bleeding out of the body's orifices— and kills up to 90 per cent of infected people within a week after their first symptoms appear. There is no known cure, but scientists are on the case and have made major breakthroughs in recent years.

First, researchers at the NIH developed a vaccine that prevents Ebola infection in monkeys. The vaccine is expected to undergo phase 1 trials in humans in the USA before the end of 2002. But, at best, it will be two years or more before a vaccine is available. NIH researchers have also identified the type of protein that causes bleeding in Ebola victims, and they are trying to develop an inhibitor that will block it.

And in the spring of 2002, scientists at the US Army Medical Research Institute of Infectious Diseases at Fort Detrick, Maryland, reported an astounding discovery that may hold the key to vanquishing Ebola. While the scientists were experimenting with Ebola DNA, they found that harmless, Ebola-like particles were assembling themselves from proteins within culture cells. The particles are barely distinguishable from Ebola particles – even to the most highly trained eye. Because of the striking similarity, it's possible that the harmless particles could be used to trick the body's immune system into producing antibodies that would effectively fight off an Ebola infection.

Bioterror research pays off doubly

A cure for anthrax. A new smallpox vaccine. An Ebola vaccine. Authorities warn that future biological attacks are likely and we will need tools like these to defend ourselves. But even if such predictions prove wrong, research into vaccines and drugs

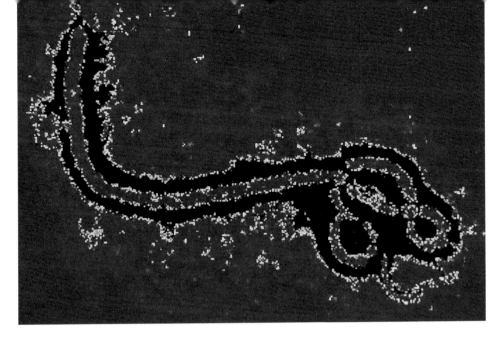

◄ A colour-enhanced transmission electron microscope image of the Ebola Zaire Virus. The tiny microbe is devastatingly powerful, ultimately causing every major organ system of the body to fail within weeks of infection.

to combat these killer microbes 'will pay off in much larger ways against the infectious diseases that we see every day,' says Bill Frist, the Tennessee Republican who is the only physician in the US Senate. Many of the discoveries made, he pointed out, could be directly applicable to victims of more common infectious diseases. Though far less prevalent than heart disease, stroke or cancer, lower respiratory infections, tuberculosis and measles are still among the top ten killers in the developed world. And HIV/AIDS has yet to find a cure.

When the World Health Organization (WHO) proclaimed victory over smallpox back in 1980, the international scientific community seemed confident that the world would soon be free from the threat of virtually all major infectious diseases. 'The fact that we were able to eradicate smallpox – a disease which killed a half billion people – led to complacency that was reflected throughout our scientific and academic culture in the United States,' says Senator Frist.

WHO has now warned that the world dangerously overestimated its ability to control disease, and that just a handful – AIDS, TB, measles, malaria, diarrhoeal diseases and acute respiratory infections – are a major threat to world prosperity.

In January 2002, England's chief medical officer, Sir Liam Donaldson, outlining a new strategy for combating infectious disease,

warned of the 'global threat' they posed, and also noted that: 'Since the early 1970s at least 30 previously unknown infectious diseases have become prominent, for which there is no fully effective treatment.' And, say US researchers, another two dozen that were once considered banished for good have re-emerged.

Which makes today's research all the more vital. That work must involve, 'not just developing an Ebola vaccine, but really understanding the virus,' says Senator Frist, 'so that you'll be prepared in the short term for Ebola and can apply that knowledge more generically to other viruses in the future.'

WHAT DOES IT MEAN TO YOU?

Here are just a few of the ways that scientific research may make us more secure against bioterror attacks:

■ The current anthrax vaccine is only for people over the age of 18 and takes too long – six doses given over 18 months – to provide full protection. Recent breakthroughs may lead to a vaccine and drug treatments that would be safe, fast and effective for everyone.

■ In October 2002, chief medical officer Sir Liam Donaldson said that Britain would vaccinate key personnel in advance. And, in the event of an attack, the strategy would be to 'ring fence' an outbreak, by rushing in stocks of vaccine and immunizing all contacts of those showing signs of the disease. But, given the potential side effects, development of an improved vaccine could save lives and spare many from serious illness.

■ Currently, there is no vaccine or treatment for Ebola virus, which carries a fatality rate of up to 90 per cent. But scientists are getting nearer to discovering ways to protect the public from dreaded Ebola.

■ The quest for cures for potential bioterror agents is likely to have spin-off benefits in the fight against other infectious diseases, such as AIDS and tuberculosis.

ALSO IN THE NEWS

Here's an update on three ongoing health stories: cloning, stem cells and personalized medicine

Cloned kitten grabs headlines, but deeper problems emerge

With the birth of 'cc' (short for 'carbon copy'), the world's first cloned cat, on December 22, 2001, the issue of cloning hit the front pages once again. The breakthrough, which was announced in February 2002 in the journal *Nature,* marked the fourth species successfully cloned by Texas A&M University, in the United States – watch out for dogs and horses coming next. Perhaps unsurprisingly, though, the emotional appeal of a kitten excited far more attention than the pigs, goats and cattle that the university had previously worked with. And that same emotional connection unleashed another round of debate, both on the ethics of cloning itself and on the particular ethics of cloning a cat, when thousands of domestic felines are destroyed each day because they don't have homes.

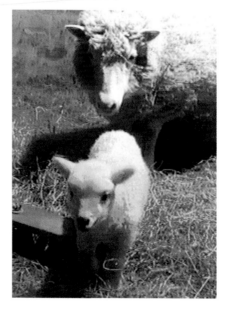

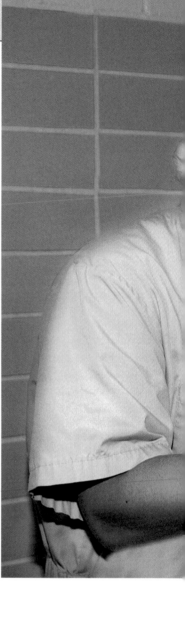

◄ Dolly the sheep, the first mammal to be successfully cloned from an adult cell, is shown here with her first lamb, Bonnie, whose birth proved that Dolly – despite being a clone – is able to breed normally and produce healthy offspring.

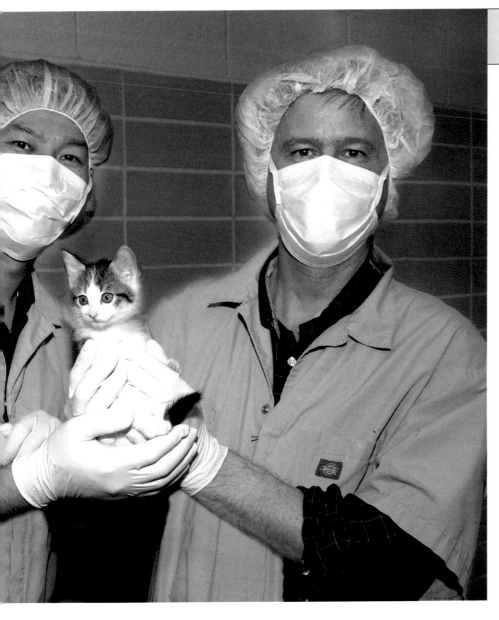

◀ Tai Young (left) and Mark Westhusin (right) successfully cloned the first cat with the birth of 'cc', pictured here at seven weeks old.

is that in mice, where the most cloning research has been conducted, clones have a 30 per cent shorter lifespan than their natural cousins and experience major problems with their livers and lungs.

The cloning express, however, speeds on. In October 2002, the Italian gynaecologist, Severino Antinori, claimed that the first cloned human was about to be born. This isn't science fiction: the techniques are straightforward, but 'genetic defects,' Joyce Harper, a lecturer in human genetics and embryology at University College, London, remarks, 'put everyone off. Every animal that has been cloned has had something wrong'. Work in Britain – such as that of Ian

But given the health problems associated with cloned animals, the debate is premature, according to Dr. Rudolf Jaenisch, of the Whitehead Institute in Cambridge, Massachusetts. Dr. Jaenisch is one of the founders of transgenic science, in which new genes (often human ones) are added to an organism, such as a mouse, to create animal models of human diseases for the purposes of study.

Dolly, the sheep who started the current cloning frenzy, is suffering from arthritis that may be related to genetic defects from cloning. Researchers at the University of Cincinnati College of Medicine reported in March 2002 that mice they cloned are becoming obese despite eating a normal diet. Maybe more troubling, Dr. Jaenisch notes,

Wilmut, the Scottish creator of Dolly the sheep – is focused on cloning human tissue for therapeutic purposes.

Even if reproductive animal cloning does become commonplace, don't imagine that when Fido or Fluffy dies, you can simply order another pet just like them, because the chances are they won't look exactly the same. 'Cc's' coat, for example is different from its genetic mother's, partly because its fur is patterned. During embryonic development, the genes that code fur colour are randomly turned 'on' and 'off' in millions of cells, creating a new, unpredictable pattern. The new pet might not behave the same as the old one did, either. Traits, such as a friendly disposition, are not necessarily reproducible by cloning.

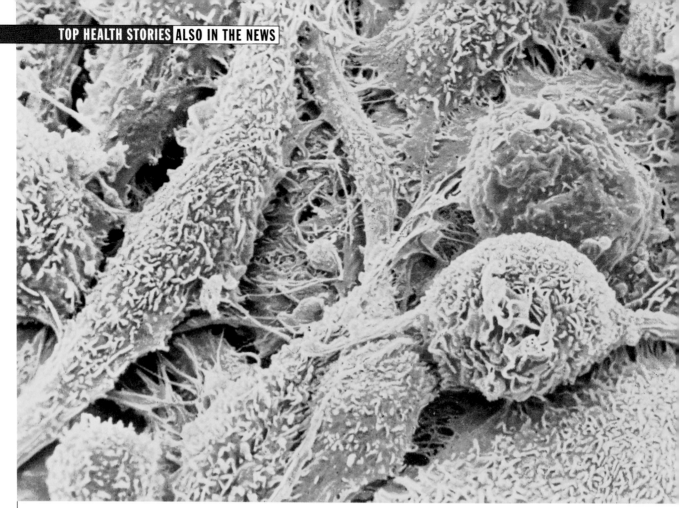

▲ Embryonic stem cells can potentially be used to produce any other type of cell in the body.

Stem cell bank to open for business in Hertfordshire

Scientists in the UK are leading the way in the field of stem cell technology and the science of therapeutic cloning. But the plans to establish Europe's first stem cell bank in Britain, announced in early September 2002, hit the headlines as much for their ethical implications as for their scientific significance.

The laws governing such research are more liberal – although nonetheless strictly controlled – in Britain than the rest of the world, allowing scientists to forge ahead with the potential use of human stem cells in the treatment of conditions such as Parkinson's disease and diabetes. Health minister, Lord Hunt of King's Heath, praised the go-ahead for the European cell bank in *The Independent*, saying that it 'will ensure that the UK retains its international position in this exciting field, which promises to bring a revolution in health care'.

Stem cells, or 'mother' cells, can develop into a range of different types of cell, giving them the potential to repair damaged tissue or organs in the body. In January 2002, genetic scientists at Advanced Cell Technology in Worcester, Massachusetts, said they had used cells from cloned cow embryos to grow kidney-like organs. When implanted into adult cows, the organs actually worked, and weren't rejected by the animals. This important news

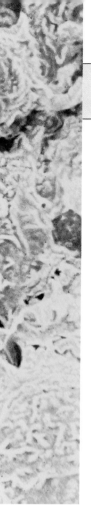

suggests that, one day, healthy cells cloned from a human being could be used to grow new organs that will not be rejected by the person's immune system.

In April 2002, a paper in the journal *Cell* described the use of therapeutic stem cell cloning to treat an immune deficiency disease in mice. The scientists – Dr. George Daley, Ph.D., of the Whitehead Institute in Cambridge, Massachusetts, and his colleagues – first cloned the animals, then harvested stem cells from the embryos and repaired the genetic defect in these cells. Then they placed the cells back into the mice, where they partially restored normal immune function: the first time researchers had shown that cells grown in a culture could be introduced into an animal to treat a disease.

The new European stem cell bank, which hopes to be in operation within a year, would hold stocks of stem cells taken from embryos and adults, making them available to the research community and, ultimately, for medical treatment. Any scientists conducting stem cell research will also be obliged to deposit samples of any cell lines created in the bank.

The ProLife Alliance opposes the bank and all activities that involve harvesting stem cells from foetus or embryo, fearing that the process will lead to the large-scale destruction of human embryos. They argue that stem cells derived from adult tissues will work just as well, quoting reports of the successful use of adult stem cells derived from bone marrow. But in early 2002, a team led by Professor Austin Smith, at Edinburgh University, discovered that adult stem cells appear to fuse with the cells of damaged tissue, rather than actually 'morphing' into a new type of cell in order to replicate fresh, healthy tissue, limiting their therapeutic benefits. The earlier in life stem cells are collected, scientists believe, the greater their potential adaptability.

Drug treatments get personal

Could slight variations in a gene that controls an enzyme in your liver influence how you react to medicines? With the unravelling of the human genome, the days of one-size-fits-all drugs may be coming to an end.

The so-called 'poor metabolizer' gene variation in the liver was first identified by scientists from the Imperial Cancer Research Fund in the early 1990s. LGC, the UK's leading genetic testing organization, took on the rights to research and work with the gene and, in June 2002, sub-licensed them to Orchid BioSciences in the United States. Here, they are developing a panel of DNA tests that could quickly determine how well a patient will absorb around 300 of the most commonly prescribed drugs – and, therefore, how well they will react to the treatment, so that the dose can be tailored to the patient.

Genes not only affect how much of a drug is metabolized by the body, they also help to determine which drugs will work. In March 2002, researchers at the Mayo Clinic in Rochester, Minnesota identified 14 genes that indicate that a woman's tumour is most likely to respond to the standard chemotherapy drugs for ovarian cancer. A test based on this finding could be used to spare thousands of women each year from undergoing treatments with drugs that probably won't help them at all. Ultimately, perhaps, testing kits could be held in doctors' surgeries to enable your GP to identify which of a choice of medicines will work best for you. The Mayo Clinic has even more sophisticated plans for an electronic database to eventually house not only the medical records but also the complete genome of all of its patients. If successful, the database, a hugely expensive collaboration with IBM, will provide clues to how each patient's genetic makeup might influence the success of various treatments, and could make it easier to diagnose rare diseases.

Meanwhile, in Britain, genetic researchers are investigating the links between genes and human behaviour. With the help of funding from Cancer Research UK, the Health Behaviour Unit, based at University College, London, is proposing a system of personalized testing for smoking-related diseases. They also plan to compare the genetic tendency of someone to smoke with their success or failure in programmes aimed at helping them to kick the habit.

PART 2

GENERAL HEALTH

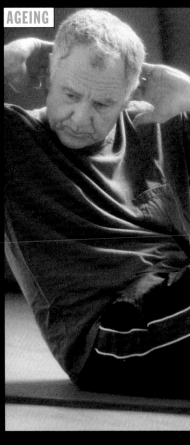

AGEING

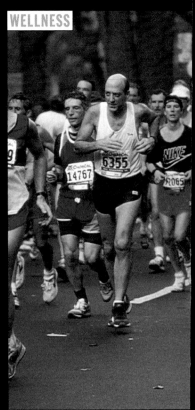

WELLNESS

Whether you're an infant, a centenarian or somewhere in between, medical scientists are hard at work to bring you a longer, healthier life. In the Ageing chapter, you'll find cutting-edge revelations about Alzheimer's disease and new ways to turn back the clock. In Children's Health, read about a natural treatment for hyperactivity and laser surgery that takes the fear and risk out of inserting grommets. If you're already healthy and want to stay that way, turn to Wellness to find out what to drink on long flights, what not to do when you have a sore throat and how to lower your cholesterol by eating more often.

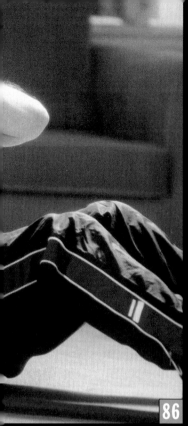

86

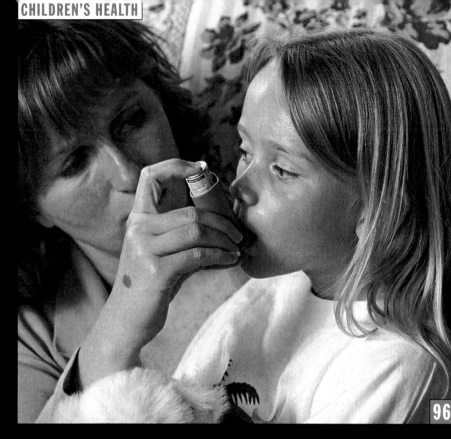

96

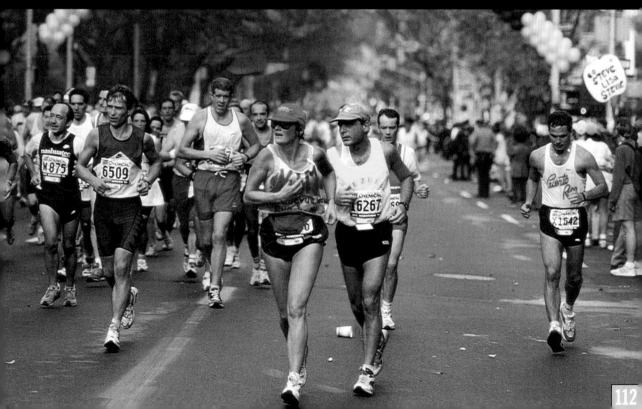

AGEING

With the oldest baby boomers pushing 60, it's feared that dementias, including Alzheimer's disease, could affect 1.5 million British people by 2050. But medical science is fighting back. In the past year, no fewer than three possible new treatments have emerged. Two are familiar for their role in combating other diseases: the cholesterol-lowering drugs called statins and the B vitamin folate. The other is a new drug that cripples a rogue protein associated with the brain-draining disease.

And there's further good news for healthy ageing: research tells us that if you're middle-aged and unfit, you can get back into the shape you were 30 years ago with a mere six weeks of moderate exercise. Concerned about your memory? Scientists have found that it's not lost, just untapped. Finally, a combination of two common supplements has been shown to rejuvenate ageing cells, preventing the energy drain often associated with getting older.

Progress in prevention

Lower your cholesterol to save your brain

Back in the year 2000, medical investigators began to suspect some kind of connection between commonly prescribed cholesterol-lowering medications and a reduced risk of brain-wasting Alzheimer's disease. Research results announced in 2002 delivered a clear message: subjects who used the cholesterol-lowering drugs known as statins were as much as 79 per cent less likely to develop Alzheimer's. The statin defence now looks so promising that clinical trials are under way in Europe and North America to test the drugs' mettle against this cruel degenerative disease.

In the largest of the several recent studies, Boston University researchers reviewed the medical records of more than 800 families at 15 different medical centres. The researchers looked at people who developed Alzheimer's and their siblings who didn't. The results? More than four times as many people who remained free of the disease had used statins. That revealing difference was valid regardless of the presence of the gene variant ApoE4, which is known to increase the risk for Alzheimer's.

How it works Researchers don't know how statins protect against Alzheimer's. Is it the same way they protect against heart disease – by lowering levels of the dangerous LDL type of cholesterol? It could be, since experts strongly suspect a connection between Alzheimer's and vascular disorders such as high blood pressure and stroke, which can be caused by elevated cholesterol levels.

One explanation may be that, by inhibiting the liver's cholesterol production, statins reduce the number of brain-damaging 'micro-infarcts', tiny brain lesions caused by blockages throughout small arteries in the brain, which are known to be associated with a history of transient ischaemic attacks, or mini-strokes. Micro-infarcts have already been linked with certain types of dementia, and they may play a role in Alzheimer's as well.

But researchers aren't ruling out the possibility that something else besides statins' cholesterol-lowering power is responsible for these benefits. The drugs could also slow the formation of amyloid deposits, the clumps of proteins that cause brain tissue degeneration. Or they could suppress the brain inflammation associated with Alzheimer's. Nobody knows – yet.

Availability Doctors have been prescribing cholesterol-lowering statins since 1987, under such brand names as Lipitor or Pravastatin among others. However, before the drugs can be prescribed expressly for treating or preventing Alzheimer's, they'll have to prove themselves in large studies. To date, the research has been mostly observational – that is, based on analyses of past medical records. The new studies, which will take years to complete, are controlled clinical trials in which the researchers follow the progress of study participants to determine whether use of statins affects their development of Alzheimer's.

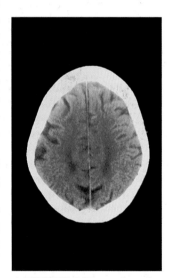

▲ **DEMENTIA A** CT scan shows the death of cerebral tissue – marked by deep ingrowths in the brain – as a result of multi-infarct dementia.

Progress in prevention

Could one vitamin beat Alzheimer's?

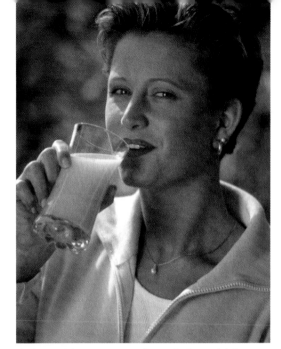

Researchers have come up with the most solid evidence yet that high levels of a simple amino acid in the blood will increase the risk of developing Alzheimer's disease. The suspect substance – homocysteine – is a normal by-product of metabolism. Scientists already know that people with Alzheimer's (and heart disease too) have high homocysteine levels. But a study published in February 2002, in the *New England Journal of Medicine* showed evidence that high concentrations of homocysteine in healthy adults may lead to Alzheimer's.

▲ Orange juice, oranges and grapefruit are rich in folate, a B vitamin that lowers homocysteine levels. Green leafy vegetables are excellent sources too.

That means a reversible risk factor may exist for Alzheimer's disease, and the solution could be as simple as ensuring an adequate intake of the B vitamin folate (folic acid), which is known to reduce homocysteine levels in the blood. Experts stop short of recommending taking supplements of folate for Alzheimer's prevention, because there is no direct proof that supplements can stave off the disease. But, says Boston University Medical Center's Dr. Joseph Loscalzo, Ph.D., 'It's intriguing to contemplate the possibility that consumption of these vitamins might help to prevent the development of Alzheimer's disease and other dementia.'

How they know Starting in 1976, investigators followed the progress of more than 1,000 older men and women who did not have Alzheimer's disease or any other type of dementia. By the year 2000, 111 of them suffered from dementia, with 83 of those cases diagnosed as Alzheimer's. But the key finding was this: those with high homocysteine levels were twice as likely to develop Alzheimer's disease within eight years.

That significant connection should encourage people to be sure to consume enough folate through their diet or by taking supplements. But researchers want to know more. Do elevated homocysteine concentrations actually cause Alzheimer's? Or are they merely a result of some other component of the disease process? Does folate supplementation reduce Alzheimer's risk? In the USA large nationwide studies to answer those questions have begun.

Take action

Super sources of folate

The B vitamin folate can help to drive down homocysteine levels and possibly reduce the risk for Alzheimer's. Folate is available in B complex vitamin supplements, folic acid supplements or these naturally folate-rich foods:

1 GREEN LEAFY VEGETABLES spinach, kale, watercress, cabbage, rocket, chard
2 OTHER GREEN VEGETABLES Brussels sprouts, broccoli, asparagus
3 PULSES lentils, chickpeas, black-eyed peas, kidney beans, borlotti beans
4 ORANGES AND ORANGE JUICE
5 LIVER
6 BREWER'S YEAST
7 WHEATGERM

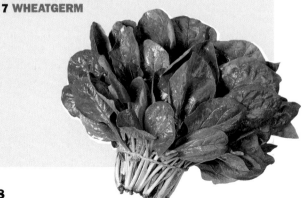

Is there a cure in curry?

Elderly villagers in India almost never suffer from Alzheimer's disease, and their favourite spice may have something to do with it. Researchers suspect that curcumin, the compound in the spice turmeric that turns curry yellow, has properties that discourage amyloid deposits, which may cause brain impairment. Neurologists at the University of California, Los Angeles, explored that hypothesis by engineering amyloid-laden rats and putting some of them on a high curcumin diet. Sure enough, the curry-fed rats showed less amyloid accumulation than the others and did better on memory tests. If further studies on humans confirm curcumin's protective effect, it will come as no surprise in much of India, where turmeric is a centuries-old traditional medicine.

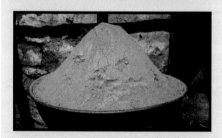

Common vaccines may fend off Alzheimer's

While the quest for an Alzheimer's vaccine continues, you may already be protected by other vaccinations you've had. Canadian investigators examined the records of several thousand men over age 65 who had been participating for five years or more in a study of dementia. They found that the men who'd had tetanus or diphtheria shots were 59 per cent less likely to develop Alzheimer's disease. Polio vaccinations reduced risk by 40 per cent, and even flu shots appeared to have a protective effect. The possibility that vaccinations against infectious diseases may carry an added anti-Alzheimer's bonus is consistent with the theory that infectious agents, along with a compromised immune system, could contribute to the development of Alzheimer's disease.

Drug development

New drug may prevent brain deposits linked with Alzheimer's disease

A promising new drug that could combat Alzheimer's disease has emerged. It stops the formation of amyloid, a starch-like protein linked to Alzheimer's, and so prevents waxy amyloid deposits from building up in brain tissue. As the deposits are prime suspects in the devastating mental impairment of Alzheimer's, discouraging their formation could stop the disease.

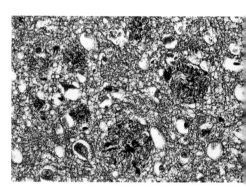

▲ In Alzheimer's disease, waxy amyloid protein accumulates in the brain to form hard, insoluble plaques.

British researchers who synthesized the drug, called CPHPC, did some impressive detective work. They analysed roughly 100,000 compounds to find a candidate that could be chemically modified to act on the target protein. After they showed that the winning compound could work on mice, the investigators tested CPHPC on 19 people who did not have Alzheimer's but who did have amyloid deposits in organs such as the kidney and liver. The results, published in the British science journal *Nature* in May 2002, showed that, after nine months of daily doses of CPHPC, the targeted protein was essentially gone from the bloodstream of the study subjects.

How it works The guilty substance is called serum amyloid protein (SAP). Its crime is aiding and abetting amyloid build-up by sticking to amyloid molecules, helping them clump together. CPHPC stops the action of SAP with a one-two punch. By binding to SAP, it leaves no way for the protein to bind to the amyloid molecules. In addition, it can bind to two SAP molecules at once, creating a sort of double SAP that gets the attention of defender cells in the liver, which attack it. Since the body wants to maintain its usual supply of SAP in the bloodstream, it raids amyloid deposits in tissue for SAP, robbing the dangerous deposits of the mortar that holds them together.

Availability CPHPC is tantalizingly promising as an Alzheimer's treatment, but testing is still in early stages. Although the drug has been shown to cripple SAP, researchers still must prove that amyloid deposits break down as a result. More important, the work to date has dealt with amyloids in general, not with brain amyloid deposits specifically. Finally, it's never been shown that amyloid deposits in brain tissue actually cause Alzheimer's; they may simply be a symptom of the disease. The answers could come in a few years from new clinical studies in which researchers will test the drug on people who already have Alzheimer's disease.

Key discovery

Workouts turn back the clock

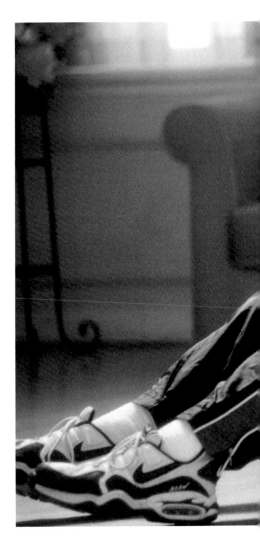

If you were to run into five men you knew 30 years ago at college, you wouldn't be surprised to see that they were out of shape and had gained a bit of weight. Which was exactly what researchers from Dallas discovered when they revisited five now-middle-aged men who had taken part in a physical conditioning study back in 1966. But they also found something much more exciting: after just six weeks on a programme of regular, moderate exercise, those five men recovered their fitness levels of three decades earlier.

The message is an exciting one for maturing baby boomers – and their parents. Simply put, it's not too late to get back into shape. 'This study clearly provides evidence that even an older person who has failed to maintain fitness over time can benefit from an exercise programme,' says Dr. Benjamin Levine, a specialist in internal medicine who worked on the study. 'Starting an exercise programme when you are older can combat the effects of ageing.'

How they found out The five men were subjects in the landmark Dallas Bed Rest and Training Study. That study demonstrated something we take for granted today: regular exercise can restore the fundamental levels of physical fitness that being a couch potato takes away. In 1966, the researchers found this out by putting 20-year-old subjects in bed for eight weeks before running them through an eight-week endurance training programme. Throughout, they measured aerobic capacity (the body's ability to use oxygen to perform endurance exercise). That capacity declined with bed rest and improved with exercise.

The follow-up study, carried out in 1996 and published in September 2001, resulted in two very encouraging findings. First, the impact of 30 years of ageing on aerobic capacity was in fact less drastic than the original eight weeks of bed rest. Second, when the men, now in their fifties, completed their six weeks of steadily progressing endurance exercise, their aerobic capacity proved to be much the same as it had been 30 years earlier. What about that extra body fat? No improvement at all. But the reason is clear: the men were not asked to alter their diet.

> **When the men, now in their fifties, completed their six weeks of steadily progressing endurance exercise, their aerobic capacity proved to be much the same as it had been 30 years earlier.**

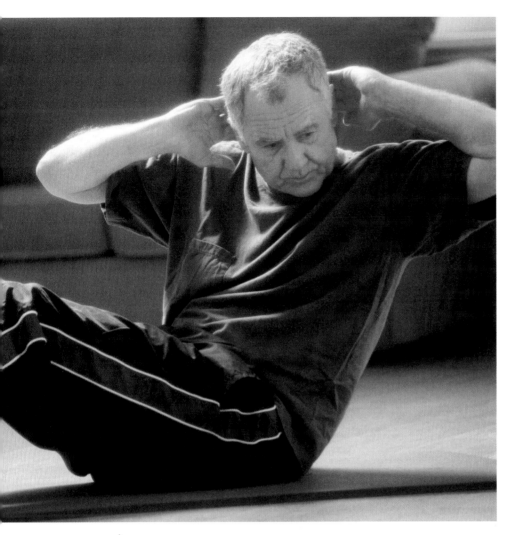

◄ Good news for ageing baby boomers: adopting a regular endurance training programme can quickly restore your aerobic fitness to what it was decades earlier, even after years of inactivity.

Take action

Walk away from the effects of ageing

The latest research shows you can recapture the fitness of your youth with moderate endurance exercise. Here's how to follow in the path of the Texas study subjects who recovered their full aerobic capacity in just six weeks, after three decades of ageing.

■ EMPHASIZE ENDURANCE Your goal is to increase aerobic capacity, which requires steady, extended (20 minutes or more) efforts like walking or jogging, rather than shorter bursts like sprinting or lifting weights.

■ PICK YOUR EXERCISE The subjects chose walking, jogging and cycling on a stationary bike. Other endurance options include swimming, rowing machines, and cross-country ski machines.

■ DO IT OFTEN The test subjects were required to exercise four or five times a week.

■ WORK YOUR WAY UP Start out at a comfortable pace and try to work a little longer each time.

■ FIND THE RIGHT INTENSITY Exercise intensity is measured by your heart rate as you exercise. The study subjects kept it between 70 and 80 per cent of their maximum heart rate (220 minus your age). They used a wristwatch-style heart rate monitor – a good investment.

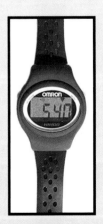

■ REACH FOR YOUR PEAK The subjects showed improvement by working their way up to four or five 45 to 60 minute sessions per week by the sixth week. (It may take you longer to get there. Proceed at a pace that's comfortable.)

■ STICK WITH IT The study leaders credit the men's success to their tenacity. They didn't slack off or sustain any injuries. They just kept at it.

Key discovery

Eat less, live longer

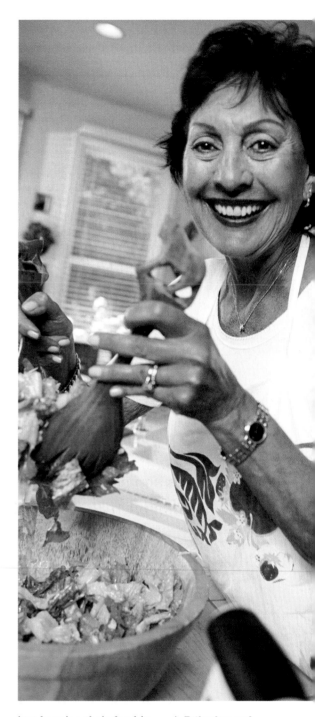

▲ Eating less and eating healthily may be the keys to adding years to your life and life to your years.

Think you eat more than you should? New anti-ageing discoveries may provide some extra motivation – beyond simply losing weight – to give your spoon and fork a rest. After putting mice on very low-calorie diets, investigators from the University of California at Riverside found that just a few weeks of such a diet slowed the ageing process and even reversed some of its consequences.

Science has known since the 1930s that caloric restriction – that is, eating much less than usual – delays ageing and extends the lifespan of laboratory animals. But scientists always assumed that those results were a cumulative effect of an entire lifetime of skimpy meals. Now it looks as if the anti-ageing benefits of caloric restriction kick in almost immediately. That means that middle-aged or older people may still be able to reap the rewards even after a lifetime of gluttony.

How it works The Californian research team cut the calorie intake of some very old mice by 20 per cent for two weeks and then by 20 per cent more for two additional weeks. They were then able to measure the effect on ageing by observing which genes were turned on (expressed) as a result of the caloric restriction. They found that gene expression associated with such ageing factors as inflammation and cellular stress was reversed – just as it was for old mice that had been on lean rations all their lives.

The animal studies are encouraging, but whether caloric restriction could be recommended as an anti-ageing strategy for humans remains to be seen. The National Institutes of Health is sponsoring a study of humans that may provide some answers. One danger for individuals who try caloric restriction on their own would be malnutrition, which would more than offset any benefits. And since so many people in the developed world have difficulty just keeping their food intake down to the generally recommended levels, it's hard to imagine a mass conversion to crash-dieting among the middle-aged.

A more likely benefit of this research would be the development of a drug that mimics the anti-ageing effects of caloric restriction. (See related article on page 40.)

ALSO IN THE NEWS

A possible solution to appetite loss

Appetite tends to shrink with age, even in healthy, active people. But too great an appetite loss is a common and serious problem for the elderly, leading to dangerous weight loss and malnutrition. The cause of this 'anorexia of ageing' remains unknown, but in late 2001 a team of Australian researchers pinned down the role of a key hormone, cholecystokinin (CCK), which is known to act as an appetite suppressant. It is also known to be more plentiful in the bloodstream of older persons. The researchers discovered that CCK affected older adults more powerfully than younger ones. They confirmed this by offering meals on three occasions to 12 healthy older subjects between 67 and 83 years of age, as well as to 12 younger people between 18 and 33. Everyone was given a pre-meal intravenous infusion of either CCK or an inert substance, and the older people who received CCK ate much less than the younger ones. This suggests that a drug to inhibit CCK's strong action in older adults could fight severe loss of appetite in the elderly.

Time to forget ginkgo?

The popular herb ginkgo biloba has been touted as a memory enhancer for years, and a few studies – some of them involving Alzheimer's patients – have indicated that it works. But a new, well-designed study of 230 healthy people over age 60 found no benefit. Half were given ginkgo supplements (40mg three times a day, as per the herb supplier's instructions) and the other half received dummy pills (placebos). After six weeks, tests that measured memory, learning, concentration and attention revealed no difference between the groups. (The product was advertised as producing benefits within four weeks.) The study was conducted by researchers at Williams College in Williamstown, Massachusetts and The Memory Clinic in Bennington, Vermont, and the results were published in the August 2002 issue of the *Journal of the American Medical Association*. It did not address people who already have memory problems, whom ginkgo may still help, or any potential benefits of taking ginkgo over the long term.

Beat flu and also avoid a stroke?

Have you had your flu shot this year? If you're over 65, it's free on the NHS and well worth having. New research from France shows for the first time that older people who were vaccinated against influenza were also much less likely to suffer a stroke. This was determined by comparing the flu vaccine histories of 90 recent stroke survivors over

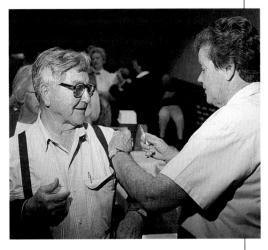

age 60 with the histories of people who had not had strokes. A much higher percentage (56.1) of the stroke-free group had been vaccinated in each of the five previous years than the stroke sufferers (41.1 per cent), indicating that the shots were protective. The researchers believe that their immune-boosting effect reduces the likelihood of all types of infection, not just influenza. Infections increase the risk of stroke and heart attack in older people, probably because they destabilize the plaque build-up on artery walls. But the benefits were not evident in people over the age of 75, perhaps because other stroke risk factors, such as high blood pressure, are so pronounced at that age that they eclipse the vaccine's protective effect.

Key discovery

The memory power of older people isn't lost; it's just untapped

Neurologists have been telling us for years that we can slow down age-related memory loss by stimulating our brains with regular mental challenges. Now they've got photographic evidence and it indicates that older adults have all the brainpower required for good short-term memory. They just need to use it better.

By using MRI (magnetic resonance imaging) to scan brain activity while study subjects tried to memorize words, American researchers at Washington University in St. Louis found that older adults (in their mid-seventies) were less likely than younger ones to use certain regions of the brain's 'memory centre'. That's an encouraging finding

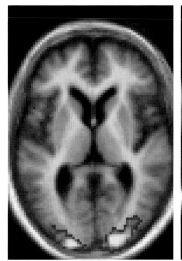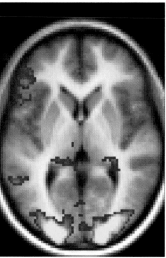

▲ **BRAIN SCANS REVEAL** how regions involved in memory can be coaxed into action. In the image on the left, the blue pointer shows an absence of activity in one area of the 'memory centre' as an older adult attempts recall using normal memory strategies. But the image on the right shows activity in these regions when the volunteer was offered memory support strategies.

for people who are tired of 20 minute car-key searches and embarrassing pauses to remember names. Why is it encouraging? Because it offers the first solid evidence that the memory loss that often accompanies normal ageing is not the result of lost capacity, but rather of a tendency to tap into the wrong part of the brain for memorizing. And that's good news, because that tendency is not irreversible and can be overcome with practice.

The researchers weren't looking at people with the severe mental impairment of dementia but healthy adults who were typical candidates for the far less serious age-related decline in short-term memory sometimes called benign senescent forgetfulness. When those men and women

attempted to memorize a string of words, the MRIs detected little activity in the left prefrontal cortex memory centre. But when they were asked to think more deeply about the words – for example, by designating each noun as either concrete or abstract – the memory centre lit up and they were more likely to remember the word later.

The researchers, who published their results in the US journal *Neuron* in February 2002, conclude that older adults can learn to tap into their memory capacity with the help of cognitive training which emphasizes memory techniques such as associating words with images or other words. The findings also show that the ageing brain is still quite capable of functioning at a very high level.

Take action

Flexing your memory muscles

Your memory gets better when you challenge your mind to think in new ways. Here are five pursuits that may improve your ability to tap into your brain's memory centre.

1 Learn to read music and play a musical instrument.
2 Take up a new career or an absorbing hobby.
3 Learn a foreign language.
4 Follow current events and put them in context.
5 Read and then discuss what you read.

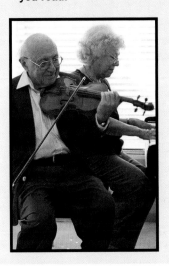

Evidence ... indicates that older adults have all the brainpower required for good short-term memory. They just need to use it better.

Key discovery

Two supplements may boost energy... and the brain

Browse the supplement section of your local health food store and you'll find two nutritional supplements hailed as anti-ageing wonder drugs that actually seem to offset time's vigour-draining effects. When researchers at the University of California at Berkeley and Oregon State University fed alpha-lipoic acid (ALA) and acetyl-L-carnitine to aged rats for a month, the animals did better on memory tests, had more energy and showed improved cellular functioning.

'With the two supplements together, these old rats got up and did the Macarena,' says Bruce Ames, Ph.D., professor of molecular and cell biology at UC Berkeley, who published the study results in the February 2002 issue of the *Proceedings of the National Academy of Sciences*. 'The brain looks better. They are full of energy. Everything we looked at looks more like a young animal.' Dr. Ames and colleagues have founded a company called Juvenon to market the anti-ageing supplement combination they discovered.

How it works The researchers think the rejuvenation effect takes place in the mitochondria, the cell's power centres. Deterioration of mitochondria is a key factor in ageing. ALA is produced naturally in the mitochondria, where it acts as an antioxidant, wiping out damaging by-products of metabolism called free radicals. ALA is one of the few antioxidants capable of entering the mitochondria from the outside, so introducing more of it substantially reduces the age-promoting effects of free radicals.

Acetyl-L-carnitine, another of the body's proteins, brings a different kind of action to the rejuvenation party. When present in the large quantities that a supplement delivers, it boosts the age-diminished performance of a key mitochondrial enzyme responsible for fuel-burning. Result: more energy.

Availability The research so far shows that ALA and acetyl-L-carnitine rejuvenate rats in the short term. Whether they rejuvenate humans in the short or long term is the subject of new clinical trials under way. The supplements are widely available in UK health stores and should be taken in tandem to benefit from their anti-ageing effects, say the researchers. The formula used in the studies is marketed in the USA as Juvenon; each tablet contains 200mg of ALA and 500mg of acetyl-L-carnitine and the recommended dose is two or three tablets a day with food.

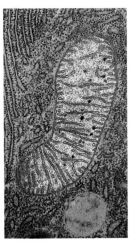

▲ The mitochondrion – seen here in orange, greatly magnified – is the power centre of the cell. In ageing, deterioration of mitochondria is a key factor, which Juvenon may be able to combat.

CHILDREN'S HEALTH

If there's one thing paediatricians have learned over the years, it's that children are not simply little adults. They have their own unique metabolism and physiology, and they're not always as fragile as you might think. For instance, new research finds that infants as young as two months have an immune system capable of handling up to 10,000 vaccines. They also have strong minds of their own, as one doctor learned during the first-ever scientific study of toilet training.

Researchers are also beginning to tackle the increasingly high incidence of obesity among children. From infant feeding to childhood exercise, they're looking for ways to keep children slim – and healthy. A further benefit to exercise may be better control of attention deficit hyperactivity disorder. Finally, learn what thumb sucking really does to your child's teeth, the significance of your child's asthma symptoms, and the latest on chronic ear infections.

Alternative answers

Hyperactivity – could more exercise help?

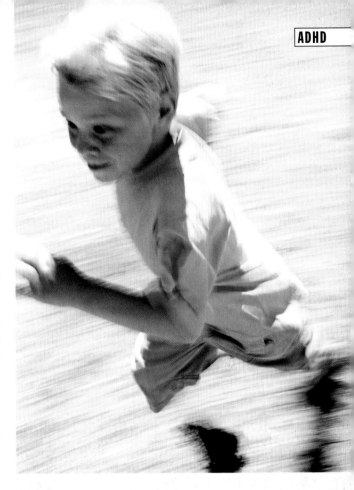

I f your child has attention deficit hyperactivity disorder (ADHD), the gym or sports ground may provide a better solution than taking medicine. Research from the University of Georgia in the USA, published in February 2002, suggests that vigorous exercise may be just as effective as medication in managing the behavioural factors involved in ADHD.

Around 5 per cent of all school-aged children in the UK are thought to have ADHD to some degree. These children are easily distracted, interrupt or intrude on others, and have difficulties waiting their turn or sitting still. One per cent suffer from a severe form of the disorder and some are prescribed long-term medication.

► BURNING OFF all that excess energy with brisk exercise may be a natural alternative to medication for children with ADHD.

The University of Georgia researchers looked at 18 children, aged 8 to 12, with ADHD. They took them off their medication the day before the study began, then assigned them either to intense treadmill walking or rest, and compared their responses to a control group that did neither – and had no medication. While boys improved more with exercise than girls, the researchers believe that the results were promising enough for exercise to be studied further as a tool for managing ADHD.

The results came as no surprise to Stephen C. Putnam, M.Ed., author of *Nature's Ritalin for the Marathon Mind: Nurturing Your ADHD Child with Exercise* (Upper Access, 2001). Putnam says that exercise influences neurotransmitters (chemicals that transmit nerve impulses) in the brain, and that helps to moderate ADHD. 'Stimulants like Ritalin increase the amount of dopamine, a neurochemical that affects motivation and hyperactivity as well as our ability to focus,' he says. Aerobic exercise also stimulates production of the 'feel-good' chemicals dopamine, serotonin and endorphins. Not all exercise is good,however.

'Exercise that's too easy might not do enough', Putnam says. 'Exercise that's too intense can produce fatigue, irritability, and inattention.' So if you decide to try this route with your ADHD child, talk to your doctor first.

RESEARCH ROUND-UP

Snoring and ADHD linked

When children are small and they become whiny and overstimulated, their parents apologize, saying they are 'overtired'. Well, they are right. A study from the University of Michigan finds that children who snore often are twice as likely as other children to have attention and hyperactivity problems. This is because snoring interrupts sleep and therefore leaves children tired. In boys under the age of eight, habitual snorers were three times more likely than non-snorers to be hyperactive. The study authors don't know why, but suggest that 'children who are sleepy may be more likely to shift their attention frequently and create stimulation to keep themselves awake'. In other words, they fidget a lot. If your child snores and has excessive daytime sleepiness, talk to your GP, says study author Dr. Ronald Chervin, associate professor of neurology.

Restless nights can lead to restless days.

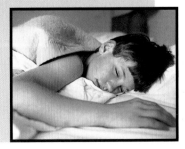

Key finding

Asthma linked to clean living?

Draught-proofed, double-glazed, super-clean houses may be contributing to increasing rates of asthma in children. The provocative theory – with studies to support it – was voiced as experts from around the world gathered at a major global conference on asthma in New York in September 2002.

'Our clean living ways perhaps might be leading to this global rise in asthma and allergies,' said Dr. Andy Liu, who runs a children's asthma clinic in Denver, Colorado in the USA, which has also seen a spiralling increase in cases.

The National Asthma Campaign's statistics show that 5.1 million people in the UK are currently being treated for the condition: that's one child in eight and one in every thirteen adults. Asthma has become a nationwide epidemic and is now our most common childhood illness. In the USA, over the past 20 years the number of people with asthma has risen by 154 per cent – interestingly precisely the same rate of increase in weekly asthma episodes reported in the UK over the same period.

Most people think that asthma is caused by air pollution such as diesel fumes, greenhouse gases and other dirt in our environment. But it may be caused by just the opposite. Recent research shows that the cleaner the environment, the more cases of childhood asthma. It's all to do with our immune systems.

It seems that children who avoid the repeated coughs, colds and snuffles of infancy have immune systems that overreact to dust or other allergy triggers – with asthma as the result. But in poor countries, where children are often ill, cases of childhood asthma are rare. In communist East Germany, for example, asthma rates were low, but since the Berlin Wall coming down and unification, the country has become less polluted and its people healthier – and asthma rates have rocketed.

Other studies appear to back the theory that too much cleanliness is bad for you. It has been shown, for instance, that children growing up with dogs in the house have less asthma. The same applies to those who grow up on farms.

What does this mean for families in Britain? Well, for one thing, it should help to alleviate the guilt felt by the thousands of mothers who go to work and leave their children to be cared for by childminders or in nurseries.

'Children in day care settings who have illnesses early on seem to be more resistant to asthma as they get older,' says Bill Davis, a New York doctor. This is because their immune systems have tackled all manner of infections and become stronger and more resilient in the process.

Nevertheless, asthmatic symptoms must be treated as soon as they appear. If your child wheezes or has a persistent cough, keep track of when the symptoms are most apparent and the frequency of attacks, and make an appointment to see your doctor.

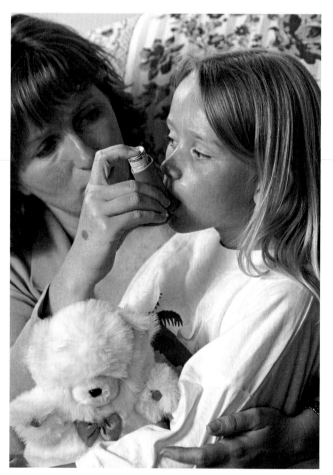

◄ **CHILDHOOD ASTHMA spells lost school days for as many as half of those with the disorder, according to UK health statistics.**

Surgical solution

Brain tumour zapped by radioactive bullet

Paediatric neurosurgeon Andrew Reisner, of Atlanta, Georgia in the USA will never forget the Sunday he was called to the hospital to examine one-year-old McEllery Badio. The otherwise healthy toddler was twitching with convulsions, and a magnetic resonance imaging (MRI) scan showed he had a brain tumour. Emergency surgery revealed a horror: of the 50 different types of brain tumour that can occur in children, McEllery had the very worst – atypical teratoid tumour, an extremely rare, extremely deadly cancer.

'Untreated, these children die within a month of diagnosis,' says Dr. Reisner. Even with treatment, the cancer is so aggressive that death is almost certain.

Dr. Reisner removed the tumour and gave the toddler chemotherapy, but four months later the tumour returned. Another operation, another round of chemo – and still, four months later, the same stubborn cancer. Radiation, the one treatment that might have helped McEllery, was dangerous in such a young child. Then one of Dr. Reisner's colleagues had an idea. Why not try a new device called GliaSite, one of only three new treatments approved for brain tumours in the past 20 years?

GliaSite is a balloon catheter that delivers internal radiation directly to malignant brain tumours, treating the target area while minimizing radiation exposure to healthy tissue. It's like a bullet of radioactivity. At the time, in late 2001, the technique had been tried on just 200 adults and no children. McEllery would be the first.

So doctors operated for the third time, placing the balloon in the cavity formerly occupied by the tumour and filling it with a radioactive liquid. The toddler spent five days in isolation to minimize the risk of exposing other people to radiation. He also wore a lead-lined cap so his parents could hold him without risking contamination. Then there was a fourth operation to remove the balloon, followed by another agonizing five-month wait. And the results? By April 2002, there was no sign of cancer.

GliaSite is a device Dr. Reisner would rather never have to use. But now that he knows it works, he's glad to have it in his arsenal. Treatment usually takes less than a week, as opposed to the six weeks or so for standard external beam radiation therapy. Will it be used in the UK? Kirk Mundy of Proxima Therapeutics, GliaSite's American manufacturer, says that the technique has been approved in Europe and will be available in Germany and Italy by the end of this year. However, because it is so costly, its introduction in Britain will depend on funding.

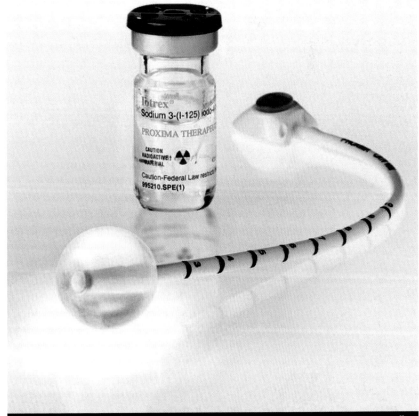

The GliaSite system allows radiation to be delivered directly to areas likely to contain cancer cells.

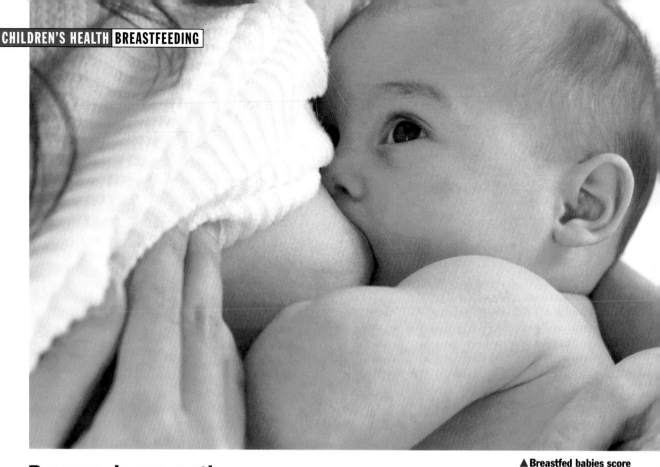

Progress in prevention

British media imagery discourages women from breastfeeding

▲ Breastfed babies score an average of 3.2 points higher on IQ tests when they reach school age. And mothers who breastfeed have a lower incidence of breast and ovarian cancer and osteoporosis.

As any new mother who's given birth in a hospital knows, formula companies make themselves known right from day one. From the souvenir blue and pink baby name cards in the cribs to the educational booklets and bounty bags you take home, formula manufacturing sponsorship tends to be involved. Not an ideal springboard from which to push breastfeeding.

Researchers from Brunel University say that breast and bottle feeding are portrayed very differently in the UK media – whether on television or in print. According to an article published in the *British Medical Journal*, the team claims that the media could be partly to blame for the reluctance of so many women to breastfeed their babies, despite numerous public health campaigns to try to persuade them that breast is best.

It is known that breastfeeding protects babies from various infections, and allergies such as asthma and eczema. And mothers too enjoy some protection from breast, uterine and ovarian cancer.

Nevertheless, bottle feeding is shown on television and in newspapers more often than breastfeeding and tends to be presented as the more straightforward option. In March 1999, the Brunel researchers analysed some 200 television and newspaper references and found that bottle feeding was associated with 'ordinary' families, whereas breastfeeding was linked with wealthier middle-class women or celebrities like Victoria Beckham.

When the researchers looked at the portrayal of mums and babies on television, they observed 170 visual references to formula feeding across all programmes against just one scene – on Channel 4's 'Brookside' – of a woman breastfeeding. Breastfeeding problems, such as sore nipples and the practical and emotional difficulties of leaving a baby, were mentioned 27 times across all programmes, while there there was just one reference to the problems of bottle feeding.

'Breastfeeding is associated with the most health benefits and yet it is the form of feeding that is not portrayed in a positive light,' observed researcher Dr Lesley Henderson. She added that the media was a powerful tool for changing public attitudes and behaviour, and more could be done to promote breastfeeding.

In television drama, 'breastfeeding is almost used as a shorthand to portray middle-class women,' says Dr. Henderson. 'This could make some women less likely to think that breastfeeding is something that they should try.'

It seems that her conclusions carry some weight. Despite the Government's commitment to policies designed to boost breastfeeding, its campaigns to promote this method of feeding are failing to reach disadvantaged women. And the number of women breastfeeding in the UK remains low. Between 40 and 60 per cent of mothers currently breastfeed – and many for less than three months, the minimum period recommended by health experts – with mothers on the lowest incomes and in the lowest social classes being those least likely to breastfeed.

But, as a spokesperson from the National Childbirth Trust observed, 'Not only is breastmilk by far the best food for baby but it is also free – so what better choice for "ordinary" families?'

RESEARCH ROUND-UP

Soya formula does not affect sex organs

After decades of infants being fed soya formula, a large study published in the *Journal of the American Medical Association* finds no negative long-term effects of soya on the reproductive system of males or females. This was initially a concern, says lead researcher Dr. Brian Strom, of the University of Pennsylvania School of Medicine, because soya contains some natural phyto-oestrogens, oestrogen-like substances that can have feminizing effects, particularly during infancy. So Dr. Strom and his colleagues contacted about 800 adults who, as infants, had participated in feeding studies at the University of Iowa (248 had been fed with a soya-based formula). The only significant difference they found was that women who had been fed soya formula bled for slightly longer when they menstruated and had slightly more menstrual discomfort. Another study in the *Proceedings of the National Academy of Sciences* in May 2002 warned that genestein, one form of phyto-oestrogen, may weaken babies' immune systems. However, the study was conducted only in mice, and so is very preliminary.

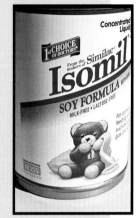

PATIENT PROFILE

Success, after a night-time lesson

Martha Davis always planned to breastfeed her first baby, but had it not been for a patient nurse and a middle-of-the-night breastfeeding session, she would have given up before she even left the hospital.

Martha, 34, gave birth to her son, Mandela, in late March 2002 at Boston Medical Center in the USA. By the second day of her hospital stay, she was frustrated and discouraged by her attempts to breastfeed, certain she couldn't do it.

'I thought it would be easy. I thought I would just put him on there and he would know what to do,' she recalls. She didn't know that babies and their mums often need some help to breastfeed properly. The nurse sat with her for hours that night, showing her how to hold the baby in the best position, how to get him to latch on, and how to keep him awake while he fed.

Interviewed two weeks after leaving the hospital, Martha said she and Mandela were doing fine. She loved breastfeeding and hoped to continue for at least six months, even after she returned to her job as a medical technician. 'There's a comfort in knowing I can feed him and he's totally satisfied,' she said.

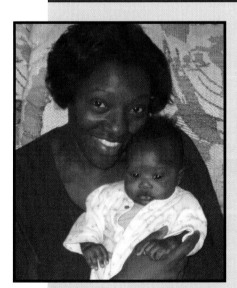

A happy Martha and Mandela Davis

Key discovery
The effects of bullying linger on

Did you breathe a sigh of relief when the bully in your daughter's class moved away? Did you think she could put the teasing, taunting, pinching and hair-pulling behind her? Well, think again. A study published in the *British Medical Journal* found that a history of being bullied is linked to future anxiety or depression – especially in adolescent girls.

In this study of 2,680 Australian high school students who completed questionnaires, 51 per cent said that they had been bullied at the age of 14–15. The same year, 18 per cent of those who had been bullied reported symptoms of anxiety or depression, while the following year, 7 per cent reported such symptoms, all related to the incidents of past bullying. In fact, in 30 per cent of the students who had been bullied and who were depressed, bullying was given as the main reason for their depression. Girls were more likely than boys to complain of depression and anxiety.

The researchers, from the Centre for Adolescent Health, Royal Children's Hospital, in Victoria, Australia, suggest that reducing the incidence of bullying in schools may also reduce anxiety and depression among school children. Their findings were published in September 2001.

Related, not a cause It's important to note that the study did not find that bullying was a direct cause of the anxiety or depression – just that they were related, says bullying expert Nancy J. Cunningham, Ph.D., who directs the Center for Safe Urban School Communities at the University of Louisville in the USA.

'The processes of developing clinical depression and anxiety are complex, with multiple risk factors that are both biological and environmental,' she says. 'We can probably say that an adolescent at risk for depression or anxiety will have a harder time handling bullying than a more resilient child. So bullying can exacerbate the anxiety or depression.'

In her own research on bullying, Dr. Cunningham found that children who identify themselves as either bullies or victims (or both – some youngsters fall into both groups) see themselves as less resilient and the school environment as less supportive. These children will need help to succeed at school, both socially and academically.

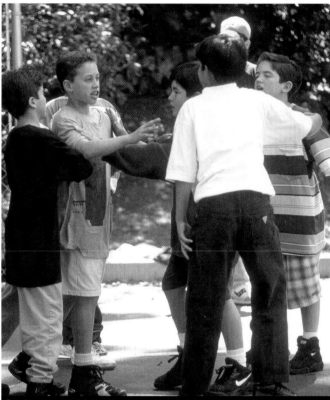

Cruelty some might dismiss as mere horseplay can have lasting repercussions

Take action

Stop bullying in its tracks
US expert on bullying, Nancy J. Cunningham, Ph.D., suggests the following tactics to parents whose children are regularly bullied:

■ **COMMUNICATE WITH YOUR CHILD** Know what is going on at school and within your child's peer group.

■ **LOOK OUT FOR PROBLEMS** That means anxiety, depression, emotional withdrawal, a fear of going to school, avoiding school and truancy. If your child is depressed or suicidal, get professional help.

■ **EDUCATE YOUR CHILD** Let your child know that the bullying is the problem – the victim is not.

■ **FIND PEACEFUL SOLUTIONS** Discourage your child from dealing with the problem by bullying others. Also, help your child to develop assertive strategies for getting away from the bully.

■ **TEACH YOUR CHILD** Help your child to develop social skills and encourage his or her friendships with other children.

■ **ASK THE SCHOOL FOR HELP** Your child's school should have policies and procedures in place to deal with bullying. It should also have a philosophy that aims for a school climate of caring and respect.

Key discovery

Sucking a dummy or thumb is fine for first two years

For years, parents have guiltily watched their infants happily sucking away on rubber dummies (now sold as 'soothers') or on their own thumbs. The guilt comes from warnings they'd had from their parents that this habit would inevitably lead to braces later on. But a recent study should, to some extent, set parents' minds at ease.

While long-term sucking on a soother or thumb can cause dental problems, children can safely suck away for up to two years without causing serious damage, says John J. Warren, assistant professor at the University of Iowa College of Dentistry in the USA.

What the study found Dr. Warren and his colleagues followed 372 children from birth to age 5, questioning their parents every few months about how much the children sucked on soothers or thumbs. Then, when the children reached 5, the dentists took impressions of their teeth and looked for abnormalities.

Dental development differed depending on whether the child sucked a soother or thumb, says Dr. Warren. With a soother, children tend to suck so hard that their cheek muscles tighten. This prevents the upper jaw from expanding sideways as it should, making it narrower and pushing the teeth together. Additionally, having the soother in a child's mouth for so long pushes the tongue down into the lower teeth more, driving them apart. 'So you end up with a cross bite, where the lower teeth stick out to the side more than the upper teeth, the opposite of how it should be,' he says.

With thumb sucking, the pressure of the thumb against the teeth causes damage. 'That forces the upper front teeth out and the lower front teeth in,' Dr. Warren says.

Still, Dr. Warren doesn't discourage parents from letting their babies suck on soothers or thumbs. 'An infant up to 12 months of age really needs some comforting that a soother or thumb can provide,' he says. But beyond then it could become a problem. So get rid of the soother and discourage thumb sucking by the time the child is 2. And, since it's easier to hide a soother than a thumb, consider handing your newborn a soother right from the start.'

Otherwise, warns Dr. Warren, you might end up with a child like some of his patients – youngsters of 8, 9, 10, or even older who still suck their thumbs.

'An infant up to 12 months of age really needs some comforting that a soother or thumb can provide.'

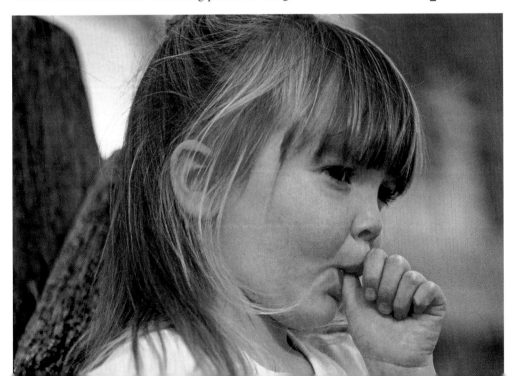

◄ Four out of five children give up thumb-sucking on their own before the habit has done any long-term harm to their teeth.

Progress in prevention

New bacteria could mean fewer fillings

How many of us as children had our sweets strictly rationed – with dire warnings that too much sugar would rot our teeth? Thanks to Jeffrey Hillman, Ph.D., children – and mums – of the future may not have to worry any more.

A University of Florida researcher, Dr. Hillman spent 25 years creating a new strain of *Streptococcus mutans,* a naturally occurring bacterium that breaks down food sugars, resulting in the formation of lactic acid. Over time, the acid destroys tooth enamel, causing cavities. Studies suggest that *S. mutans* causes 85 per cent of tooth decay. But Dr. Hillman's strain disarms this enemy.

How it works By removing the gene responsible for producing the lactic acid, Dr. Hillman has created a kinder, gentler *S. mutans,* one that still digests sugars, but without creating the tooth-etching acid. No acid, no cavities. The strain worked on rats even when the rodents were fed high-sugar diets.

Availability Dr. Hillman and OraGen, the company licensed to market any products arising from the new strain, hope to receive permission from the US Food and Drug Administration to begin testing in humans during 2002. In the early 1980s, however, an early strain of the bacterium was applied to three men in Dr. Hillman's lab. That strain is still the only *S. mutans* in their mouths, proving it has staying power. In case this is a bug you don't want in your mouth, rest assured – the bacterium was not passed on to the men's wives or children, indicating that it probably can't be spread by kissing. The group was too small to permit a test of the bacterium's effect on cavities.

Dr. Hillman hopes the new *S. mutans* will some day eradicate most tooth decay. He envisages inoculating infants when their teeth first appear, giving a lifetime of protection. But don't throw away that toothbrush yet. 'Good dental hygiene will always be necessary because of plaque build-up,' says Dr. Hillman. And to freshen morning breath.

> **Dr. Hillman envisages inoculating infants when their teeth first appear, conferring a lifetime of protection [against tooth decay].**

RESEARCH ROUND-UP

British children benefit from anti-cavity remedy

Over the past ten years, millions of UK children have benefited from the use of dental sealants – plastic coatings which dentists bond into the groove of the chewing surface of a tooth to help prevent the formation or spread of tooth decay. According to statistics from the Dental Practice Board (DPB), which records all NHS dental procedures, almost 1.9m sealant restorations were performed in 2001–2002 at a cost of more than £14m, compared with just over 7,000 at a cost of £46,814 ten years earlier. This procedure is free from NHS dentists for children with dental caries and can also be performed as a preventive measure on a private basis, which would not be recorded by the DPB. In the USA, there is particular concern that poorer children are not receiving the treatment. One recent survey showed that while 33 per cent of the children studied had dental caries, only 23 per cent received sealants under State-funded health programmes. A Spanish study, published in 2002, that had followed 607 young children with and without fissure sealants for 4½ years, concluded that the treatment should be offered to all schoolchildren to reduce the risk of dental caries.

Surgical solution
Grommets the easy way

It is 2am and you are awakened by your screaming toddler, who's running a high temperature and tugging on her ear. You know the score; your daughter has an ear infection, and in the morning you'll go to the surgery for a prescription for that pink medicine that makes it go away. Your child has Otitis media, or middle ear infection. By the time children reach their third birthday, two out of three will have had at least one ear infection.

But for thousands of children each year, Otitis media occurs so often that even the pink medicine (amoxicillin) isn't enough. Generally, these children's Eustachian tubes, which connect the middle ear to the back of the throat, haven't developed properly, allowing pressure and fluid to build. This condition is known as persistent glue ear. To release the pressure, surgeons often insert tiny tubes or grommets into the child's eardrum. This allows mucous fluid to drain down the Eustachian tube and into the back of the throat. The operation is not performed as widely in the UK today as it was 20 or so years ago.

In the UK, grommets are inserted into the eardrum in hospital under general anaesthetic. But a new procedure is being used in America. Family doctors are performing grommet insertion in their own practice offices using laser surgery and a local anaesthetic. This takes away much of the fear, as well as the risk of general anaesthetic, says Dr. Gordon Siegel, assistant clinical professor at Northwestern University Medical School, one of the pioneers of the laser procedure. It also cuts the cost.

In January 2002, the largest study so far on surgery-based grommet insertion concluded it was a 'safe and effective alternative to grommet insertion in the operating theatre'. That does not mean that the procedure isn't still somewhat traumatic for the parent and child, comments Dr. Siegel.

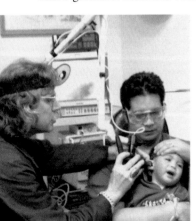

◀ **Dr. Siegel performs grommet insertion under local anaesthetic in his office.**

Otitis media: middle ear infection

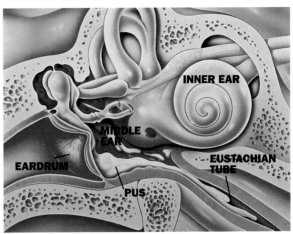

INNER EAR

MIDDLE EAR

EARDRUM

EUSTACHIAN TUBE

PUS

Infection of the middle ear – between the eardrum and the delicate structures of the inner ear – may lead to blockage of the Eustachian tube, so that pus and mucus build up and cause pain.

'The children are screaming because they don't like to be held down, but we know we're not hurting them,' he says.

He numbs the ear with an anaesthetic, then makes a small hole in the eardrum with the laser. 'They feel a little pop, there's a bit of warmth, then a sudden pressure change,' he says. Then, using a microscope to guide him, he inserts the grommets.

Dr. Siegel has performed thousands of these insertions in his Chicago surgery since perfecting the technique a few years ago. Families come to Dr. Siegel from all over the country. That's because, at the moment, only about 100 doctors in the United States offer the procedure, largely because the laser equipment is so expensive.

RESEARCH ROUND-UP
Weaning parents off antibiotics

Doctors know that most ear infections will clear up on their own. But some GPs find it hard to resist a parent who insists on antibiotics to treat a screaming child. Now doctors at Cincinnati Children's Hospital in the USA have worked out a way of dealing with those problem parents. They supplied parents with pain medication for children's ear infections and a 'safety net' prescription for antibiotics – to be filled only if the child's condition didn't improve in 48 hours. Of the 153 families that participated in the study, just 47 filled the prescription and resorted to the antibiotics. Seventy per cent got by just on the pain medicine – either children's ibuprofen or ear drops, or a combination of the two. And sixty per cent said that they would be willing to treat future ear infections without antibiotics, just using painkillers.

Progress in prevention
Screening programmes for newborn babies

I n the UK, all newborn babies are screened for several conditions. Remember that Guthrie heel-prick test that doubtless provoked a little scream? Those drops of blood collected on a card were tested for phenylketonuria or PKU, an inherited disorder that affects one baby in 16,000. If caught early, PKU can be treated effectively with diet. The National Health Service plans to use the Guthrie Bloodspot card to test babies nationally for cystic fibrosis, too – at present, just 20 per cent of the country is covered by neonatal screening for CF. Some health authorities also screen for hypothyroidism, though again, coverage around the UK is patchy.

The NHS is also introducing a linked antenatal and newborn screening programme for two blood disorders, sickle cell disease and thalassaemia. This should start happening in 2004.

Newborn screening is high on the agenda in the USA. In January 2002, the March of Dimes – an American children's charity dedicated to saving babies' lives – launched a campaign to alert policy makers and doctors to the importance of newborn screening. They observed that, rather like in the UK, it's the luck of the draw as to whether you live in an area where babies are screened for certain conditions or not.

Women in Massachusetts and Maine are fortunate – their babies are screened for nine metabolic diseases for which the March of Dimes recommends infants be tested. These can be devastating or deadly if not caught early. If an abnormality is found, the baby should begin treatment immediately – usually with a special diet, or else with supplemental doses of the hormone, vitamin, or enzyme he or she is missing.

A new screening test has been developed that makes it possible to check for as many as 40 conditions using only five drops of blood and one analytical procedure. The March of Dimes says that there's no excuse for not testing all newborns. A blood specimen should be taken from every newborn prior to release from the hospital. Some of the tests (such as the one for PKU) may not give accurate results, however, if they are done too soon after birth.

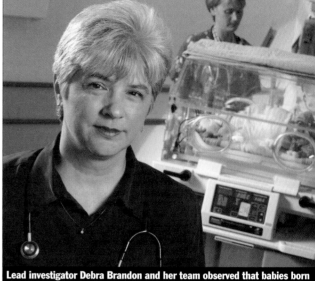

Lead investigator Debra Brandon and her team observed that babies born before 31 weeks fare better when exposed to cycled levels of light.

Key discovery
Give night and day to early babies

S ome newborn intensive care units are rather like a theatre just before the curtain goes up. Lights are dimmed and sounds are muted to protect these fragile babies. But a study published in the American *Journal of Pediatrics* in February 2002 found that this may not be the right approach.

Earlier research had proved that continuous bright light can restrict the growth and development of pre-term infants. But in this recent study, the babies were exposed to varying levels of light, which were regulated to mimic day and night.

According to research leader Debra Brandon, Ph.D., R.N., the cycled light accelerated the babies' growth rates, perhaps because it helped to establish their natural circadian rhythms – hormonal cycles that create the pattern of sleep and wakefulness – and therefore helped them to sleep better. 'If infants sleep better, they should grow better,' she says. Additionally, infants secrete certain gastro-intestinal enzymes that are related to circadian rhythm. Improving that rhythm may help them to digest their food and use the calories properly.

ALSO IN THE NEWS

Soccer mums, beware

Many soccer mums wince when their kids head the ball, envisioning concussions and declining SAT scores. But what many may not realize is that the size of the ball itself carries a significant risk for injury, particularly if young players use adult-sized balls. That's the finding of a British study, published in December 2001, that tracked all children and young adults who passed through a fracture clinic over 17 months. Among the 1,920 young patients seen, 28 goalies sustained 29 wrist fractures trying to 'make a save'. In nearly three out of four incidents, an adult (size 5) ball had been used. This ball can weigh nearly half a kilo (and be kicked at speeds of up to 25 miles per hour). Goalkeepers take the full force on their hands. Although smaller balls (size 4 for those aged 8 to 11, size 3 for younger children) are recommended in the United Kingdom and the United States, they are not often used.

Kids suffer computer vision syndrome

Forget telling your kids to move back from the television. It's the computer that may be damaging their eyes. A study by researchers at the University of California at Berkeley found that as many as 30 per cent of American children who use a computer place undue stress on their eyes and may need special computer eyewear. The results, announced in March 2002, also found a strong connection between children spending many hours at a computer and premature nearsightedness. Children are particularly at risk for computer vision syndrome (CVS) because they work on computers for hours with few breaks, are likely to ignore eye problems adults would notice, and use computers arranged for adult-sized users, which can lead to an inopportune viewing angle. The most common symptoms of CVS include eyestrain or eye fatigue, dry eyes, burning eyes, light sensitivity, blurred vision, headaches, and pain in the shoulders, neck, or back. 'It's important to pay attention to children's workstations and try to accommodate the area to the child,' concludes lead researcher Pia Hoenig, chief of the binocular vision clinic.

Cold prevention: send kids to nursery

Mothers who work outside the home now have another weapon in their arsenal to counter the criticism from stay-at-home mums. Their children, at least the ones who attend large nurseries, are likely to have fewer colds when they begin primary school, according to Dr. Thomas M. Ball, associate professor of clinical paediatrics at the University of Arizona, whose research was published in the *Archives of Pediatric and Adolescent Medicine* in February 2002. Studying more than 1,000 children, Dr. Ball and associates found that, while at age 2 the children in large day-care nurseries (with more than five unrelated children) had more colds than those cared for at home, by the time they started school they had fewer colds. 'This study gives credence to the hypothesis that acquired immunity obtained in day-care protects a child from colds later in life', Dr. Ball says.

Getting a handle on bike safety

So, you succeeded in getting your children to wear helmets when they are riding their bikes. But before breathing a sigh of relief, be sure to check out their handlebars. In 30 years of studying abdominal injuries in 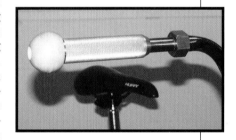 children, a team of US researchers found that the main cause of injury resulted from handlebars, mainly when children hit something and toppled over them. So bioengineers at the Children's Hospital of Philadelphia designed a safer model. Unveiled in late 2001, it's fitted with a spring and damping system (like the spring in a pogo stick) that absorbs up to half the force transmitted through the handlebars upon impact. The engineers hope to commercialize the device, which should add only a few pounds to the cost of a bike.

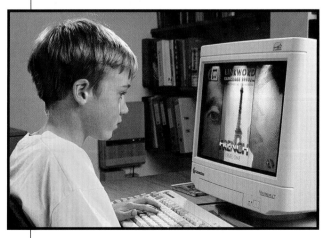

Key discovery

'Baby fat' gets new significance

When friends talk to a new parent, the 'Is he sleeping through the night?' question is second only to 'How much weight has he gained?' Now, parents might want to pay particular attention to their answer to that latter query. A report in the February 2002 issue of the US journal *Pediatrics* finds that rapid weight gain during the first four months of life could be linked to obesity later in childhood.

The study examined 19,000 children born between 1959 and 1965. Researchers found that if babies gained just an extra 3½ ounces (100g) per month, they were about 30 per cent more likely to be overweight by the time they were 7 years old. Starting with a birthweight of 7lb, that baby would weigh 14lb by four months, compared to the 13lb average weight of babies who ate less.

'Babies double their birthweight during the first four to six months, so this may be a period for the establishment of weight regulation,' suggests Dr. Nicolas Stettler, a paediatric nutrition specialist at the Children's Hospital of Philadelphia and the lead researcher for the report.

One theory is that these early months are when the biological mechanism that regulates obesity develops. Another is that it's fate – that is, early weight gain reflects a child's genetic predisposition to be fat. Or maybe it's just that parents who stuff their *babies* with too much food are just as likely to stuff their *children* with too much food. The timing of the study may also be signficant. When these children were born, in the early 1960s, babies were often fed solid food much earlier than they are today.

The researchers certainly don't recommend putting your newborn on a diet. But they do suggest we may need to take another look at how we feed infants. If the association is confirmed by other studies, researchers note, it may lead to new approaches to preventing childhood obesity.

A review of 32,200 Scottish three-year-olds published in *The Lancet* in June 2002 discovered that obesity was significantly less common in those that had been breastfed.

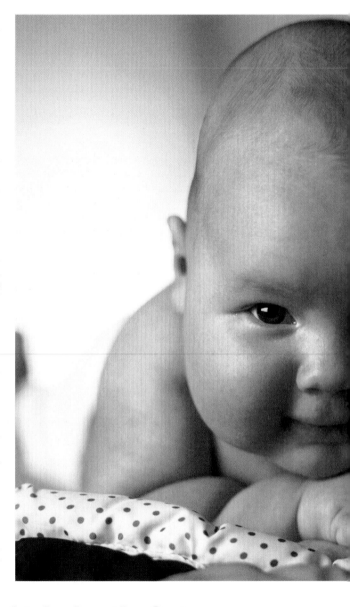

'Babies double their birthweight during the first 4 to 6 months, so this may be a period for the establishment of weight regulation.'

RESEARCH ROUND-UP

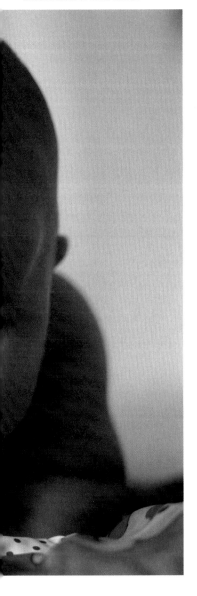

▼ ONE WAY to prevent infant obesity, suggests Dr. Nicholas Stettler, is to heed the American Academy of Pediatrics' advice to breastfeed exclusively for six months, followed by gradual introduction of solid foods.

What's next? Health clubs for newborns?

Being carried, strapped into a chair, or ferried around all day in a pushchair does little to prepare a baby for a lifetime of regular exercise. That's the thinking behind the first-ever activity guidelines released in the USA in February 2002 for infants and toddlers. Developed by the National Association for Sport and Physical Education, they suggest, for example, that babies should not remain in car seats and other devices that restrict movement for long periods of time, and toddlers and preschoolers shouldn't be immobile for more than an hour, unless sleeping. Child obesity is a serious problem in the USA, and now in Britain too. According to the British Heart Foundation, the number of obese six-year-olds has doubled and the number of obese 15-year-olds has trebled in ten years. Yet the time that is allocated to sport in primary school has roughly halved in the past five years.

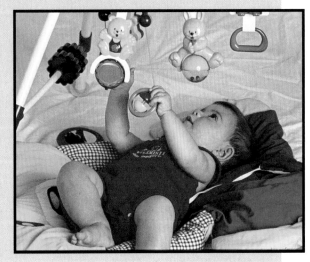

Tiny babies face big problems

For years, medical professionals knew that very tiny (low-birthweight) babies had a higher risk of various medical problems, including blindness, cerebral palsy and learning disabilities. Now a study finds that learning disabilities and low academic performance may persist even into young adulthood. The study, published in the USA in the *New England Journal of Medicine,* is the largest, most comprehensive follow-up to date of the first group of very-low-birthweight infants who survived because of advances in newborn care technology that began in the 1970s. The researchers followed 242 of these children, who weighed an average of 2.5lb when they were born. Fewer had graduated from high school and more had lower IQ scores compared to their normal-birthweight peers – possibly as a result of the neurological problems connected to prematurity.

Slim-fast for fat little Jimmy?

With the number of overweight children on the rise, US doctors are asking whether adult weight-loss medications such as Xenical (Orlistat) and Reductil (sibutramine), as well as the diabetes drug Glucophage (metformin), might work for kids. One study put 6 to 10-year-olds on the meal replacement product Slim-Fast and found liquid meals safe and effective. Children who replaced one meal a day with the drinks slowed their rate of weight gain slightly more than those who received 12 weeks of instruction on diet and exercise, with education and support for parents. Some 35 universities and other centres around the USA are studying sibutramine in children, with early results suggesting that more than a third of the children are losing substantial amounts of weight. In Britain, medication is not yet recommended for obese children as there are some concerns about possible negative effects on puberty and later eating behaviour.

Key discovery

Potty training?
No need to rush it

Tired of running after your little one with a portable potty and a mop? Relax. New research in the March 2002 issue of the US journal *Pediatrics* confirms what wise parents instinctively knew but doctors apparently didn't: Most children aren't ready to toilet train until after their second birthday, and boys are ready later than girls.

'The prevailing theory on toilet training was 18 to 24 months, but no one ever studied it,' says the study's lead author, Dr. Timothy R. Schum, associate professor of paediatrics at the Medical College of Wisconsin. His study of 126 girls and 141 boys between the ages of 15 and 42 months found that most children are ready to be toilet-trained between 24 and 30 months. 'This will be reassuring to parents that they can wait until their children are older' before beginning training, he says.

The survey also found that girls were about 32 months old before they stayed dry all night (boys were 37 months old) and about 33 months old when they could urinate completely by themselves (37 months again for boys).

'One thing we've come to realize is that there's a window of opportunity in potty training,' he says, 'between 24 and 30 months.' Miss that window, and you're likely to be buying Pampers for much longer than you'd hoped.

> **'One thing we've come to realize is that there's a window of opportunity in potty training – between 24 and 30 months.'**

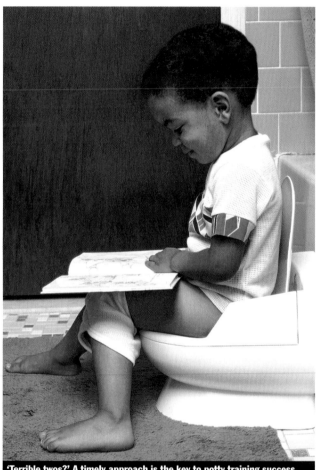
'Terrible twos?' A timely approach is the key to potty training success.

Take action

Three steps to a toilet-trained toddler

Dr. Schum is one of those rare researchers who not only studies an issue (in this case, potty training) but also develops a solution to the problem (in this case, a child you are convinced will leave school still wearing nappies). He calls his three-step programme the Parent-Coached Approach.

■ **READY:** Watch for signs of readiness in your child. They include staying dry for 2 hours, showing interest in the potty, being able to walk and pull pants up and down, following simple directions and indicating a need to use the bathroom.

■ **OUT:** Get your child out of nappies, sending the message that you're serious about toilet-training.

■ **COACH:** Remember, you and your child are a team. Your role is to be supportive and patient. Employ techniques such as praise, reminding your child to use the potty, offering rewards and being consistent.

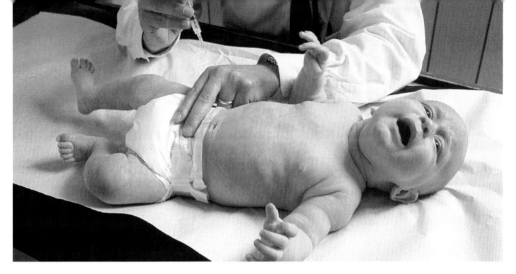

◀ The needles may cause tears, but multiple vaccines will not weaken, dilute, or overwhelm an infant's immune system.

Key discovery

Bring on the vaccines – baby can take them

Remember your fears and your baby's cry when those first shots were given? Now US researchers have made a finding that should put parents' minds at ease – babies' immune systems can easily handle all the vaccines and injections they receive in their first few months of life.

There has been growing parental concern in the USA about the increasing number of vaccines babies there receive – 11 to 20 in the first two months, compared to just the one combined diphtheria, tetanus, pertussis and hib (DTB-Hib) injection plus the polio immunization by mouth, that British babies get at the age of two, three and four months. So Dr. Paul A. Offit, director of the Vaccine Education Center at the Children's Hospital of Philadelphia, and his colleagues looked into the subject.

They reviewed current research on the effects of vaccines on the immune system and the ability of infants' immune systems to respond safely to multiple, simultaneous immunizations, they found that 'the infant immune system has an enormous capacity to respond safely and effectively to immune system challenges from vaccines,' Dr. Offit says. Their study was published in the January 2002 issue of the US journal *Pediatrics*.

Around the same time, a National Institute of Medicine panel came to the same conclusion, finding that multiple vaccines also do not increase a child's risk of developing Type 1 diabetes or other common childhood infections.

According to the US researchers, it's not the number of vaccines or even shots that's important, it's the number of antigens – foreign substances that trigger an immune response – in vaccines that matters. The smallpox vaccine, which was the first vaccine ever given to children, contained about 200 antigens, whereas all the childhood vaccines routinely recommended in the USA contain fewer than 130 antigens combined.

Babies are much tougher than we think, notes Dr. Offit. His research shows that infants have the theoretical capacity to respond to about 10,000 vaccines at once.

RESEARCH ROUND-UP

Measles vaccine sparing childhood misery

Combined with better hygiene and nutrition, the UK's public vaccination programmes have saved millions of children from suffering and death. Before the measles vaccine was introduced in 1968, some 250,000 cases were recorded annually in England and Wales, with as many as 85 fatalities. In 1999, 2,438 cases were recorded and two people died, both from the later effects of the disease caught in the 1980s or before. In 2002 there were fears of a resurgence in measles cases when intense adverse publicity linking the combined Measles, Mumps and Rubella (MMR) vaccination with autism prompted a sharp drop in uptake for children aged 16 months. It dropped from 76.2 per cent in December 2001 to 70.1 per cent in March 2002, though it rose to 72 per cent in April. For information on vaccines, look at the web site: www.immunisation.org.uk

WELLNESS

Here's a good reason to cultivate optimism – it could save your life. New evidence shows that a positive attitude can help protect you against heart disease and stroke.

Good news for grazers. A new study shows that more frequent eating lowers your cholesterol. Just make sure it's not all chips and crisps that you're putting away. The American Heart Association has issued a strong warning against high-protein diets. It says that they eliminate many healthy foods, depriving us of essential nutrients and possibly putting us at greater risk for all sorts of diseases of the heart, kidney, bone and liver.

Even hospitals come with a warning label these days – on both sides of the Atlantic. 'Speak Up' is the name of a US programme that educates patients about medical errors and how to avoid them. Speaking of warnings – cases of MRSA infection have almost trebled in Britain since 1992. But a promising new vaccine may soon protect against the deadly *Staphylococcus aureus* **bacterium.**

Key discovery
Coffee, tea or...Gatorade?

No one's surprised to hear that being strapped into a cramped airline seat for 8 to 10 hours is not healthy. Long flights have been linked to the formation of blood clots in the legs, a condition called deep vein thrombosis (DVT) – sometimes referred to as 'economy class syndrome'. Worse still, these blood clots can spread to the lungs, or, more frequently, a piece of a clot may break off and get lodged in a blood vessel there, preventing the lung from oxygenating your blood. This can result in a deadly condition known as pulmonary embolism.

But a study published in the *Journal of the American Medical Association* (JAMA) in February 2002 suggests that Gatorade, Powerade, and other brands of electrolyte beverages known as 'sports drinks' may reduce the risk of these blood clots.

The Japanese researchers who made the discovery compared the electrolyte drinks to plain water in 40 healthy young men on a nine-hour flight in economy class. Those who drank the sports drinks lost far less water – as a result of urinating less – than those who drank water. The amount of water held in the body, say the researchers, affects how thick or thin our blood is. Blood samples confirmed that the water drinkers had thicker blood in their feet, which could contribute to clot formation in the legs.

How it works The potassium, sodium and carbohydrates in electrolyte drinks stimulate rapid absorption of the fluid through the intestinal wall and into the bloodstream, according to the makers of Gatorade. This, and the added sodium, which helps with fluid retention, may be the reason such drinks keep us hydrated better. Plain water is more likely to be excreted in the urine. That does not, of course, mean that water is a poor source of hydration. But apparently sports drinks get absorbed a little more easily into the body.

'If one is to "dilute" the blood with electrolyte drinks, then it is possible to decrease the risk of blood clotting,' says Dr. Chi Van Dang, Ph.D., a blood disorders specialist at Johns Hopkins University in Baltimore.

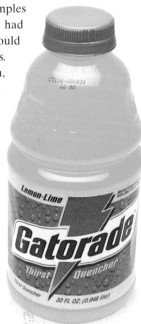

▲ ON LONG FLIGHTS, sports drinks can help the body retain fluid, preventing blood clots.

Take action

Clot-busting techniques

The risk of deep vein thrombosis is generally low for healthy people. But you can ensure better circulation on long flights or car journeys by taking a few simple steps.

■ DRINK UP Drinking lots of water (still a wonderful source of hydration), juices or sports drinks is especially important on planes because recycled cabin air is particularly dry, according to Dr. Chi Van Dang, Ph.D., of Johns Hopkins University in Baltimore. Drinking these beverages 'thins' the blood, helping to prevent clot formation.

■ WALK A MILE IN THE AISLE So you were hoping to put your feet up and let the plane do the work? Better to stand up and move around the cabin once in a while. That's probably the best way to protect yourself against clotting during prolonged travel, says Dr. Dang, as it increases the rate of blood circulation, pumping it from the legs back to the heart.

■ PLAY FOOTSIE If you can't get up, at least exercise your ankles by flexing and pointing your feet for about a minute every half hour or so. This action also mobilizes blood so that it doesn't collect in the lower legs.

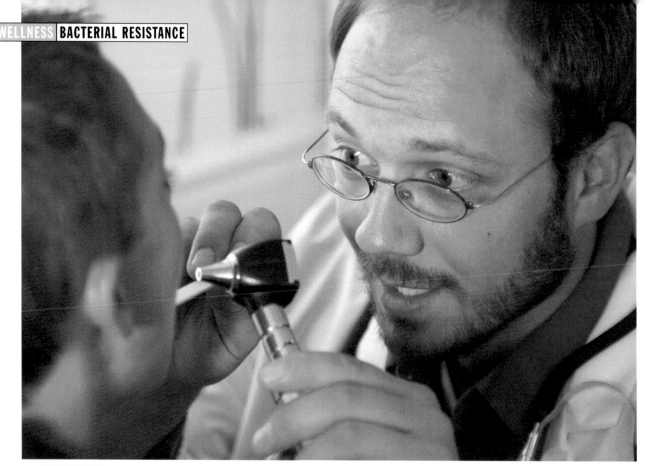

▲ A SORE THROAT can be very painful but if it's caused by a cold or the flu, antibiotics are utterly useless.

Key discovery
Antibiotics: resistance is on the increase

Is your throat red and swollen? Your doctor may give you a prescription for an antibiotic but it may not be necessary. Evidence from both the USA and Britain suggests that in many cases antibiotics don't help and may, in fact, do some harm.

A US study published in September 2001 found that 73 per cent of patients with sore throats from 1989 to 1999 were prescribed antibiotics by their doctors. Yet only 10 to 20 per cent of sore throats are actually caused by the bacterium *Streptococcus aureus*, which requires antibiotics. Most are the result of viruses which do not respond to the drugs.

The study also found that when antibiotics *were* prescribed, 68 per cent of the patients did not get the ones recommended for this disorder – traditional penicillin or erythromycin. Instead they received newer, more expensive 'broad spectrum' antibiotics, which are more likely to promote bacterial resistance, that is, the bacteria become immune to the drugs that are supposed to kill them.

Concerns about the overprescribing of antibiotics and increasing antibiotic resistance have also been aired in the UK. They were the subject of a report by the Select Committee on Science and Technology in 1998, which declared that the situation could pose 'a major threat to public health'.

The Association of Medical Microbiologists reported that in England alone between 1992 and 1994, GPs had been prescribing 'enough antibiotics to treat every man, woman and child in England for five days a year'.

Do without a prescription

If you have an extremely sore throat, your doctor can take a throat swab for micro-biological analysis. The test, which takes three days to run, will show whether you have a bacterial infection. If you don't, skip the antibiotics. Instead go home, rest, and do the following:

▩ **DRINK UP** Clear fluids will soothe the throat and help to thin the mucus at the back of the throat.

▩**GARGLE WITH SALT WATER** To soothe and heal, add half a teaspoon of salt to 1 cup of warm water and gargle with the solution. Repeat several times a day.

▩ **GET WET** Apply a warm, wet flannel to the neck to soothe swollen glands.

▩ **KILL THE PAIN** Take the recommended dose of paracetamol, ibuprofen or aspirin regularly. Their anti-inflammatory and analgesic properties help to relieve the fever and pain of a swollen throat. But do not give aspirin to a young child who has a fever because aspirin can increase the risk of Reye's syndrome, a rare but dangerous disorder.

▩ **LOOK TO LOZENGES** For temporary relief of sore throat pain, use a lozenge that contains phenol, lidocaine, benzo-caine, or amethocaine. Phenol has anti-septic properties, meaning the lozenge will kill off surface germs and keep the number of invaders in check. And both phenol and '-caine' ingredients numb nerve endings, easing the pain.

As a result, in January 2002, the British govern-ment was amongst the first in Europe to publish a strategy for tackling the problem. This includes persuading GPs to reduce antibiotic prescribing (which has already dropped by 23 per cent since 1998, according to the Department of Health).

But, as in America, a number of factors may influence doctors to over-prescribe antibiotics, according to the American study's co-author Dr. Randall Stafford, Ph.D. It can, for instance, be hard to resist patients who beg to be given *something* for relief. Also, drug manufacturers have been aggressively marketing new antibiotics, erroneously thought to be more effective.

'My great concern is that we're breeding a population of bacteria that no longer respond to traditional antibiotics,' says Dr. Stafford.

Progress in prevention

A crash course: belt up in the back

Drivers, when your backseat passengers are reluctant to fasten their seatbelts, ask them this: 'Are you trying to kill me?' Rear-seat car passengers put more than themselves at risk when they refuse to buckle up. The impact from a car crash – especially in a head-on collision – can catapult them forward, killing people in the front. Japanese researchers studied car crashes in their country that occurred between 1995 and 1999. They found that a huge 80 per cent of the front-seat passengers who were killed despite wearing seat-belts could have survived had their backseat passengers worn restraints.

'That's a fivefold increase in death rate,' says lead researcher Masao Ichikawa, community health lecturer at the University of Tokyo's Graduate School of Medicine. The findings, published in the British medical journal *The Lancet* in January 2002, provide a strong argument for a government to make rear seatbelt use mandatory, he says. It is now in Britain, but not in Japan and many US states.

If protecting your driver isn't incentive enough, how about the prospect of living with brain damage? Another recent study, presented in January 2002 at a meeting of the Society of Critical Care Medicine, found that unrestrained backseat passengers, though less likely than their drivers to die, are at greater risk of brain damage from an accident. The reason? Although there's more impact in the front of the car, air bags can help to protect those in the front against brain injuries, says the study's leader Dr. Lewis Kaplan of the MCP/Hahnemann University School of Medicine in Philadelphia. Backseat passengers, on the other hand, hit their heads on the seat in front of them, the side window, or the side post.

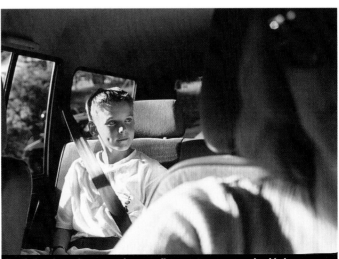

For their sake and yours, make sure all your passengers are buckled up.

Nutrition tip

Snack your way to lower cholesterol

I t sounds like wishful thinking, but it's turning out to be true. The more often you eat, the better off you are – at least cholesterol-wise.

A Cambridge University study, published in the *British Medical Journal* in December 2001, compared the eating habits and cholesterol levels of nearly 15,000 people aged 45 to 75. Researchers found that those who ate six mini-meals a day had cholesterol levels, on average, 5 per cent lower than those people who ate only once or twice a day. 'That's enough to drop heart disease risk by 10 per cent,' says study leader Dr. Kay-Tee Khaw.

The more frequently the subjects ate, the lower their cholesterol level, especially their LDL cholesterol, the harmful type. Previous short-term studies had yielded similar results. But this one spanned four years and is the first large study of its kind among the 'free living population' – people outside a controlled study – says Dr. Khaw.

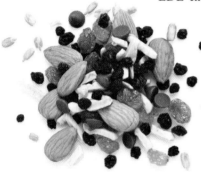

▲ NUTRITIOUS NIBBLES

Eating mini-meals and healthy snacks is better for your health than gorging at one sitting.

How it works It is believed that grazing is connected to the body's starvation mode. When we go too many hours without food, then eat voraciously, our body assumes the worst and treats each meal as if it's our last – storing more fat. This raises cholesterol levels. On the other hand, eating smaller meals throughout the day appears to prevent the body from hoarding energy in the form of fat. Eating more frequently also helps to keep our metabolism rate high, since the body must expend energy to digest food.

Take action The trick, says Dr. Khaw, is not to add meals to your daily routine, but to break up the meals you're already eating. 'Divide the same amount of food you would normally eat over more frequent, smaller meals,' she says. And, if you do find yourself eating more, just make sure it's fruit and vegetables.

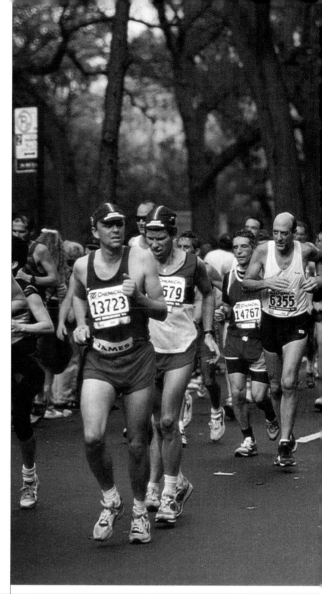

Key discovery

Going the extra mile? Consider your heart

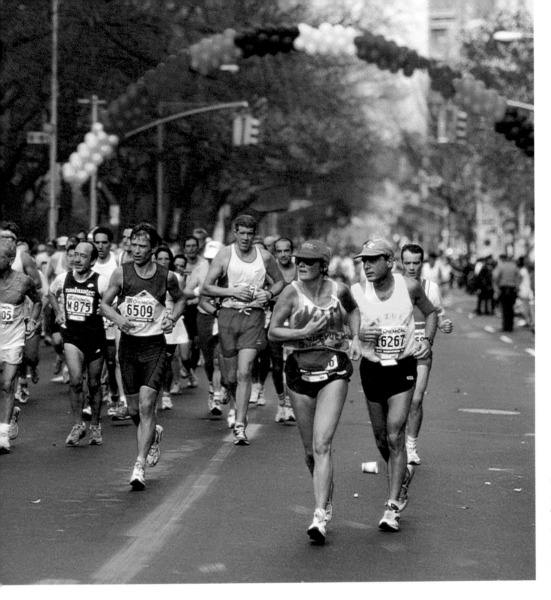

◀ In a recent study of 215,413 marathon runners, there were four exercise-related deaths from undiagnosed heart disease.

More of a good thing isn't always better, especially when it comes to running. The marathons (distance: 26 miles and 385 yards) run by millions of people each year may do the heart more harm than good, according to a study published in the *American Journal of Cardiology* in October 2001. The researchers tested the blood of healthy middle-age runners within 24 hours of completing the Boston Marathon and found a temporary increase in substances that trigger clotting and inflammation and thicken the blood – which increases the risk of a heart attack.

The clotting, say researchers, probably occurs as a result of excessive stress on both the blood vessels and the skeletal muscles – from pushing the body so hard. When runners over-exert themselves, the body will react by pumping out substances that create an inflammatory response. The inflammatory proteins can then increase the risk of blood clotting, says the leader of the study, Dr. Arthur Siegel, director of internal medicine at Boston's McLean Hospital.

Inflammation and clotting aren't enough by themselves to trigger a heart attack but may be dangerous for people who also have plaque build-up on their arteries or cardiac arrhythmia. About 1 in 50,000 marathon runners have heart attacks either during the race or within 24 hours – five times the normal incidence. But this doesn't mean you have to stop running marathons. Just train wisely.

Build up slowly Condition your muscles steadily but gradually by training for at least six months prior to a race.

See your doctor Know your medical history and current health status – whether you have high cholesterol, for instance. If you have any sort of heart condition, you should think twice before running a marathon.

Pop an anti-inflammatory Marathon runners who have concerns about their hearts should perhaps take an aspirin beforehand to help thin their blood during the race, says Dr. Siegel. But check with your doctor first to make sure that this is safe for you and won't interfere with any other medications you are taking.

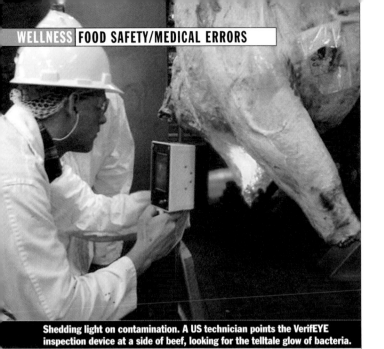

Shedding light on contamination. A US technician points the VerifEYE inspection device at a side of beef, looking for the telltale glow of bacteria.

High-tech help
Safer beef on its way to your dinner table

More than 42 million kilos of beef were recalled in the USA in 2002 because bacterial contamination was suspected. But a new device, called VerifEYE may be able to make meat safer to eat by detecting trace levels of manure on beef carcasses.

It works by shining a near-ultraviolet blue light on beef sides, to reveal the natural phosphorescence of chlorophyll, present in manure, which is a source of *E. coli,* the bacterium responsible for some 73,000 cases of food poisoning and about 60 deaths each year in the USA. Until now, the meatpacking industry has relied solely on the manual or visual detection of manure, which often goes unnoticed or is mistaken for specks of harmless dirt.

In Britain, new European regulations were introduced in 2002 that require all licensed 'fresh and poultry meat plant operators' such as slaughterhouses, cutting plants and cold stores, to carry out regular microbiological testing of carcases. The mandatory tests are designed to detect the bacteria on fresh meat that can cause food poisoning. In 1999, 82,943 confirmed cases of food poisoning in the UK were attributed to *Campylobacter* (61,713), *Salmonella* (19,801) and *E.coli* (1,429).

Progress in prevention
US Government advises patients to speak up

In a bid to help patients to protect themselves against the medical errors that in 1999 cost nearly 98,000 lives in the USA, the country's Joint Commission on Accreditation of Healthcare Organizations launched a new campaign called 'Speak Up' in March 2002. It encourages patients to make their voices heard with advice that includes the following:

■ Ask your surgeon to use a marker to identify the arm or leg to be operated on.

■ Be sure that your doctor or nurse has washed his or her hands.

■ Make sure you are being given the right medication. Enquire about the purpose of the drug and ask for written information including its brand and generic names.

■ Get a second opinion from a specialist if you are not confident that a recommended surgical procedure is best for your condition.

■ Tell your surgeon, anaesthetist, or nurse if you have allergies or have had a bad reaction to anaesthesia in the past.

■ Ask a relative or friend to go with you and serve as an advocate.

In the UK, the government set up the National Patient Safety Agency in 2001 to report on adverse incidents within the NHS. But such were the problems with its early pilot scheme that the preliminary figures were deemed to be 'unreliable' according to a report in the *British Medical Journal*. More than 27,000 adverse incidents were reported over a nine-month period in 2001 and 2002.

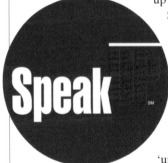

▲ To find out more about the 'Speak Up' programme, visit www.jcaho.org on the web.

ALSO IN THE NEWS

Cold comfort for needle phobics

Whether you are having blood taken or getting your annual flu jab, needles can be a pain. However, a new discovery supports the use of a simple trick that might bring comfort to the needle phobic. Sticking syringes in the freezer before use can decrease pain by 20 to 30

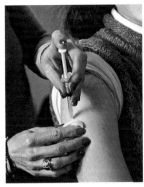

per cent. The reason is logical. 'Nerves that detect cold are the same ones that detect pain. They can only handle one stimulus at a time,' says Dr. Keith Denkler, the San Francisco plastic surgeon who tested the frozen-needle technique. It's the same concept as applying ice topically for pain relief, but Dr. Denkler says this works better because the chilled point affects the nerve cells deep below the surface, too. The results of his in-office research were published in the *Journal of the American Medical Association* in October 2001.

Calcium for your smile

If you're worried about osteoporosis, you're probably already taking calcium supplements to keep your bones strong. Now a study published in the *American Journal of Medicine* finds that the supplements may also help you to keep your teeth as you age. Compared with people who received a placebo (dummy pill), those who took daily supplements of calcium (500mg) and vitamin D (17.5mcg) for three years were only half as likely to have lost a tooth – even after being off the supplements for two additional years. Be careful not to exceed your recommended daily limit from food and supplements. For adults, that's 2,500mg of calcium and 50mcg of vitamin D.

Another reason to drink orange juice

Drinking two long 425ml glasses of orange juice a day for six weeks can reduce blood pressure, according to a study from the Cleveland Clinic in Ohio. The findings were presented in March 2002 at the American College of Cardiology's annual meeting. On average, the juice lowered systolic (the higher number) blood pressure by 7 per cent and diastolic (the lower number) by 4.6 per cent. Previous research has indicated that antioxidants and nutrients such as potassium and vitamin C – both found in orange juice – can lower blood pressure. But this is the first study specifically to show the merits of orange juice. But a word of warning. If you have diabetes, talk to your doctor before increasing your juice intake.

Two paths to a leaner future

In two recent unrelated studies scientists have made huge advances in understanding how to prevent and treat excessive weight gain. In the first study, published in the US *Journal of Clinical Investigation* in March 2002, researchers at the Johns Hopkins School of Medicine in Baltimore discovered how to genetically alter mice that, by middle age, have 70 per cent less body fat by weight than regular mice. The researchers 'knocked out' a gene that carries the blueprint for myostatin, a protein involved in the regulation of muscle growth. The mice without the myostatin gene gained much more muscle mass, turning them into 'mighty mice'. As a result – because more muscle leads to a faster metabolism – they gained much less fat as they aged.

Meanwhile, researchers at Baylor College of Medicine in Houston have engineered mice that have just half the body fat of regular mice and can eat nearly 40 per cent more – without gaining an ounce. The results of their study were reported in the journal *Science* in March 2002. The mice were altered to lack the gene that codes for an enzyme called ACC2. The enzyme controls the conversion of fat into energy. Researchers hope this new information will one day lead to the development of an ACC2 enzyme-blocking drug.

Sleepless in Seattle

Here's an eye-opener that may well have echoes here. Nearly a quarter of all Americans don't get enough sleep, and lack of it is making them cranky and sometimes even dangerous to themselves and others. A survey released in April 2002 by the US National Sleep Foundation linked lack of sleep, coupled with daytime fatigue, to anger, stress and pessimism. The 'walking tired' are more likely to seethe in traffic jams, fight with others and stuff their faces with food, the poll shows. Although US and UK experts recommend seven or eight hours sleep a night, only 30 per cent of adults polled met this requirement, 8 per cent

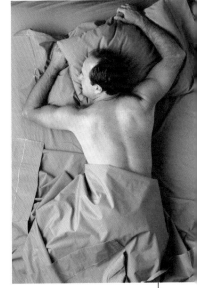

less than those polled a year earlier. American adults currently sleep an average 6.9 hours on weekdays and 7.5 hours at weekends.

Progress in prevention

Happiness is good for your health

Smile! A sunny disposition can work wonders, it seems. According to a Welsh study published in *Stroke* in January 2002, fatal strokes were three times more likely to occur in middle-aged men who were depressed or anxious than in men who reported no psychological distress.

A happy temperament may also have more influence on how well we recover from a stroke than the severity or the location of the stroke, says a study conducted at the University of Maryland and presented at the February 2002 meeting of the American Stroke Association. A stroke can leave patients with memory problems, slurred speech or weakness on one side of the body, leading to frustration, anxiety, anger, apathy or depression, say researchers. But the people who responded to humour and spent more time with family and friends became more outgoing, active and optimistic a year after a mild to moderate stroke. Their cheery outlook helped them to take steps to improve their condition, such as attending physiotherapy sessions and following dietary guidelines.

Another new study by the Harvard School of Public Health, published in the US publication *Psychosomatic Medicine* (Nov/Dec 2001) reinforces the happy and healthy link. Putting a positive spin on life could also almost halve your risk of developing heart disease, the study discovered by tracking 1,306 healthy US ex-servicemen for 10 years to see which ones would develop heart disease and other cardiovascular problems. The personality tests the servicemen completed revealed that those who were most optimistic were 44 per cent less likely to end up with heart disease than those at the most pessimistic end of the spectrum.

People who are happy in their marriage may also enjoy a health advantage. A recent University of Pennsylvania study found that patients hospitalized with congestive heart failure were more likely to be alive after four years if they had a good relationship with their spouse than if they had a contentious one.

How happiness helps It's hard to pinpoint the exact mechanism at work, but researchers speculate that optimistic people may be more likely to take better care of themselves. When you're happy, it's easier to stick to a diet, get regular exercise, take medicines faithfully and follow your doctor's advice. There is also a physical connection. Optimism seems to provide a buffer against chronic stress, which has been shown to wreak havoc throughout the body. And studies have demonstrated that depression and anxiety can cause changes in the autonomic nervous system, which controls breathing, heart rate, the contraction of blood vessels, and the production of adrenaline, a stress hormone. Also, in the Harvard study, pessimistic men were more inclined to overindulge in alcohol. While a little red wine a day is healthy for the heart, too much alcohol of any kind is obviously not.

▶ **A long life is a happy life – or is it the other way around? The new research gives us every reason to smile.**

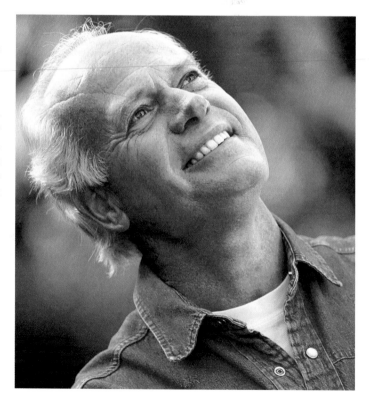

Fatal strokes were three times more likely to occur in middle-aged men who were depressed or anxious than in men who reported no psychological distress

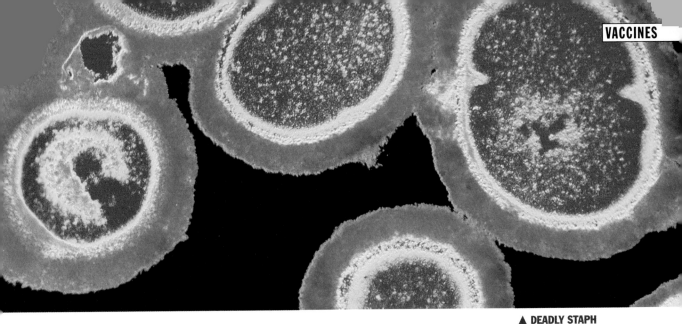

Drug development

MRSA menace: promising vaccine emerges

▲ DEADLY STAPH bacteria have outsmarted antibiotics. A new vaccine is the next defence.

In April 1999, a 63-year-old woman in Illinois in the USA was taken into hospital with a heart valve infection. A decade ago, she would probably have recovered after being treated with antibiotics. Instead she died.

The US government declared her the first patient to have unquestionably died from an MRSA (methicillin-resistant *Staphylococcus aureus*) infection that didn't respond to the antibiotic vancomycin. The worrying aspect was that this was one of the strongest drugs against the *S. aureus* bacteria. Increasingly, the germs are becoming resistant as a result of overuse of antibiotics throughout the Western world. In England and Wales, reported cases of MRSA infection leapt from just over 5,000 in 1992 to almost 14,000 in 2001.

But a new vaccine may provide a powerful antidote. In a study that appeared in the *New England Journal of Medicine* in February 2002, the vaccine StaphVax, reduced the number of MRSA infections by 60 per cent in patients whose immune systems were severely compromised as a result of advanced kidney disease.

The infections are particularly dangerous because the *Staphylococcus aureus* microbe tends to infect people who already have weakened immune systems. Staph infections can occur in any patient who receives frequent needle injections or who has to undergo surgery, such as a heart operation or a hip replacement.

Vaccinating patients who are at risk from MRSA infections before they become infected may eliminate the need for antibiotics altogether. As an added benefit, the vaccine appeared to temporarily strengthen the immune systems in 86 per cent of the patients, which may help to protect against other infections as well.

How it works The *S. aureus* germ – which has an outer coating made of a sugar-based polysaccharide molecule – can slyly work its way through the body without being recognized or attacked by the immune system. Meanwhile, the StaphVax vaccine is made up of a harmless, non-toxic carrier protein covered with the same polysaccharide molecule. Once injected, the patient's immune system forms antibodies against the vaccine. But because the vaccine has the same molecular shape as the *S. aureus* germ, the antibodies will bind to the germ if it ever enters the bloodstream. That action triggers the mobilization of white blood cells to attack the *S. aureus* bacterium, according to the study's co-author Dr. John Robbins, of the USA's National Institute of Child Health and Human Development in Bethesda, Maryland.

Availability It could be as long as three years before StaphVax becomes available in the USA as its maker, the Nabi Corporation has to repeat the clinical trial and produce similar results. The company also plans to begin clinical trials in Europe this year.

Diet debate

The protein diet controversy sizzles

The American Heart Association (AHA) has taken a stand on high-protein diets declaring that they are *not* part of a healthy lifestyle. The warning, in the US journal *Circulation* in October 2001, may surprise many people faithfully following plans such as the Atkins Diet, but the concern isn't new. These structured eating plans, says the AHA, provide little variety of foods, restrict healthy foods (mainly carbohydrates) that offer essential nutrients, and can generally lead to greater fat intake, especially of saturated fat, which raises cholesterol levels. High-protein diets consist largely of meat. In time, they compromise vitamin and mineral intake and increase risk for heart, kidney, bone and liver diseases. The British Heart Foundation agrees: 'People need a balanced diet that includes all food groups.'

But protein diets often produce the desired weight loss, which is why they have gained so much popularity in recent years. Here, to give both sides of the issue, are two of the most prominent figures in the great protein debate.

For

DR. ROBERT ATKINS

is a leader in natural medicine and nutritional pharmacology, and the founder and medical director of the Atkins Center for Complementary Medicine in New York City. He has cared for more than 65,000 patients in more than 40 years of practice. He has a national radio show in the USA, 'Your Healthy Choices', and his book *Dr. Atkins' New Diet Revolution* has sold more than 10 million copies, making it one of the top 50 best-sellers of all time.

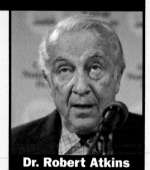
Dr. Robert Atkins

'Evidence shows that the more our society replaces dietary fat with carbohydrates, the more we see ... obesity and diabetes soar.'

Q: Who are the best candidates for high-protein diets?

Dr. Atkins: First of all, 'high-protein' is an inaccurate label. It's a 'controlled-carbohydrate' approach that incorporates more protein and fat and less carbohydrate than the standard diet. It's for anyone who is overweight, has diabetes, is insulin-resistant, or has high triglycerides and low HDL (the 'good' cholesterol). It's also safe and effective for people who have failed on portion-controlled, low-fat, low-calorie diets. Switching to a higher-protein diet creates a fat-burning energy system.

Q: Are carbohydrates unhealthy?

Dr. Atkins:: Not per se, but in a mixed diet with excess calories, carbohydrates can trigger large insulin output, which increases the risk of diabetes. In fact, evidence shows that the more our society replaces dietary fat with carbohydrates, the more we see the incidences of obesity and diabetes soar. Other research, including the Harvard Nurses study, even links high carbohydrate intake to increased risk of heart attack.

Q: Is it true that your diet plan's quick results are just from water loss?

Dr. Atkins: No matter the diet, all weight loss is initially due to water loss. However, the ensuing weight loss from a higher-protein diet is primarily from fat. Whereas a low-fat, low-calorie diet would break down muscle.

Q: Higher-protein diets can cause ketosis (an accumulation of chemical substances called ketones). Isn't that unhealthy?

Dr. Atkins: Ketosis is not an abnormal condition. The body has an exquisite capacity to regulate the level of ketones, just as it regulates body temperature and acid/base balance, never going out of a safe range. Only if a person has some abnormal metabolic condition, such as uncontrolled diabetes or alcoholism, will ketone accumulation become a problem. People confuse safe, benign ketosis with the abnormal metabolic ketoacidosis associated with diabetic coma. Studies show that people can be in a state of ketosis safely for long periods of time.

Q: Don't higher-protein diets lack sufficient nutrients?

Dr. Atkins: The Atkins Diet has four phases. When it is followed correctly, a person quickly moves past the introductory phase and enters the maintenance phase, which includes a liberal intake of a variety of nutrient-rich foods, such as vegetables, fruits, nuts and seeds, and whole grains.

Q: Won't the extra meat boost cholesterol levels?

Dr. Atkins: First of all, you can get protein and healthy fats from fish, poultry and nuts and seeds, which are all low in saturated fat. Even so, no research shows that saturated fat hurts cholesterol levels when carbohydrates are kept in check. In fact, triglycerides plummet and HDL increases.

Against

DR. JOHN MCDOUGALL

has been touting the benefits of low-fat, vegetarian cuisine for more than 20 years and has treated thousands of patients in his private practice. He's a best-selling author who's written *Dr. McDougall's Total Health Solution* and has a nationally syndicated TV show, 'McDougall, M.D'. He is also the founder and medical director of the McDougall Program, a 12-day, live-in plan at St. Helena Hospital and Health Center in California's Napa Valley.

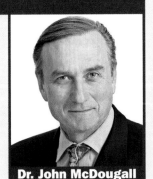
Dr. John McDougall

'Fat in the American diet is the biggest culprit for weight gain. It's already in the chemical form for storage and is almost effortlessly moved from the fork to our fat cells.'

Q: Is a high-protein diet a healthy option for anyone?

Dr. McDougall: No, these diets centre on unhealthy foods. The primary foods are meat, egg and dairy products, which are high in cholesterol, fat, animal protein and microbes. They also lack in fibre and carbohydrates and have serious vitamin and mineral imbalances. Meat, egg and dairy products are believed to cause many diseases, such as obesity, heart disease, adult-onset diabetes, certain cancers, kidney stones and kidney failure, constipation and arthritis.

Q: How does this diet harm the kidneys?

Dr. McDougall: Protein is metabolized by the liver and excreted by the kidneys into the urine. A high protein load causes damage to these organs. By their 80s, people in affluent societies often lose 30 per cent of their kidney function, which is believed to be the result of overworked kidneys from all the protein in our diet. In fact, one of the most fundamental treatments for patients with liver and kidney failure is to put them on a low-protein diet, like 4 to 8 per cent protein.

Q: How much protein should a healthy person eat?

Dr. McDougall: About 6 to 14 per cent of the average person's diet should be protein. We usually recommend about 10 per cent protein, 10 per cent fat, and 80 per cent carbohydrates. The popular Atkins Diet, on the other hand, can be more than 80 per cent protein or fat, and the high-protein diet plan called the Zone recommends 30 per cent protein.

Q: How do high-protein diets suppress the appetite?

Dr. McDougall: A diet too low in carbohydrates makes the body enter ketosis, the natural state that occurs when people are sick. It's the same metabolic changes that happen during illness. It does suppress appetite, but that's because your body thinks it should be resting and recuperating, instead of gathering and preparing food. In order to remain in sufficient ketosis to suppress appetite, carbohydrate intake has to be extremely low. For some, 60 calories – meaning one-third of a baked potato, one-third cup (50g) of rice, or one orange – could be their daily limit to remain in ketosis.

Q: Why do some people lose weight quickly on high-protein diets?

Dr. McDougall: The initial rapid results are misleading. Most of that weight loss is water loss, not fat loss. The ketones also exert a strong diuretic effect on the kidneys, resulting in large losses of fluid.

Q: Do carbohydrates cause weight gain?

Dr. McDougall: Not if you're eating complex carbohydrates and watching your overall calorie intake. Fat in the American diet is the biggest culprit for weight gain. It's already in the chemical form for storage and is almost effortlessly moved from the fork to our fat cells. Whereas, to convert carbohydrates into body fat, we burn 30 per cent of the calories in the conversion. Fat in the American diet also happens to be the biggest culprit in terms of its contribution to cardiovascular disease.

Q: Do carbohydrates raise insulin levels?

Dr. McDougall: Insulin is the hormone that pushes fat into fat cells. That's a problem only if you're eating lots of simple, refined carbohydrates, such as sugar, white flour, ice cream, cakes, etc. These are foods you shouldn't be eating in large amounts anyway. Complex carbohydrates, on the other hand, are healthy and fine to eat.

PART 3

YOUR BODY HEAD TO TOE

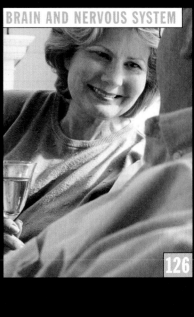

126

Is there a new cure that could change your life? The answer is
here. We've surveyed the medical literature – and questioned
top health experts – to find out what's new, what works and what
doesn't for more than 100 health conditions. Read about the latest
treatments, preventive techniques and screening tools for
everything from arthritis to vitiligo. Find out about an annual jab
that could put an end to osteoporosis, an astounding new cane
that is helping blind people to 'see' and a seemingly miraculous
experimental treatment for Parkinson's disease. And turn to the
special chapter on cancer for the latest life-saving information.

CANCER

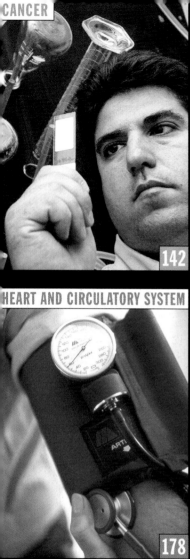

142

DIGESTION AND METABOLISM

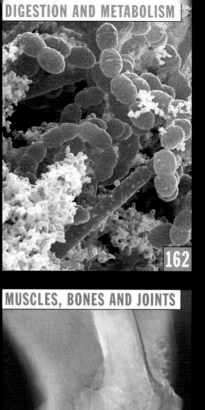

162

EYES AND EARS

170

HEART AND CIRCULATORY SYSTEM

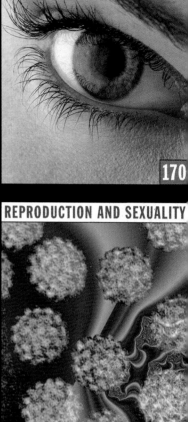

178

MUSCLES, BONES AND JOINTS

196

REPRODUCTION AND SEXUALITY

210

RESPIRATORY SYSTEM

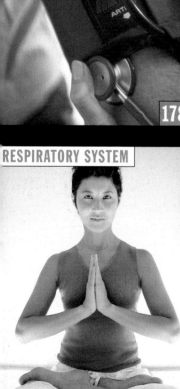

222

SKIN, HAIR AND NAILS

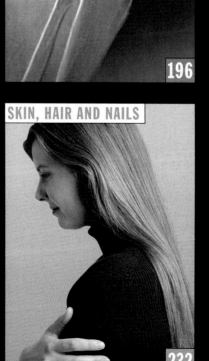

232

URINARY TRACT

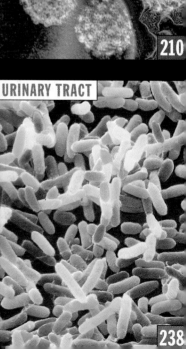

238

BRAIN AND NERVOUS SYSTEM

Is it fact, or science fiction? In 2002, monkeys with electrodes implanted in their brains were able to move a cursor on a computer screen using just their brain waves. The breakthrough might one day be great news for people with paralysis. And watch out: scientists have found a way to 'read' human memories. The technology is already used in the USA in criminal cases to separate truth from lies.

In other news, researchers have discovered that a simple compound can prevent long-term brain damage when administered to stroke victims by paramedics. And people with spinal cord injuries may have a better chance of retaining limb movement when they receive an experimental vaccine that halts tissue injury.

On the drug front, antibiotics show promise for easing symptoms of Parkinson's disease, and a common antidepressant can reduce hard-to-treat neuropathic pain. Finally, getting treatment for chronic depression could make you less vulnerable to illness.

Progress in prevention

Cheers! Moderate drinking protects the brain

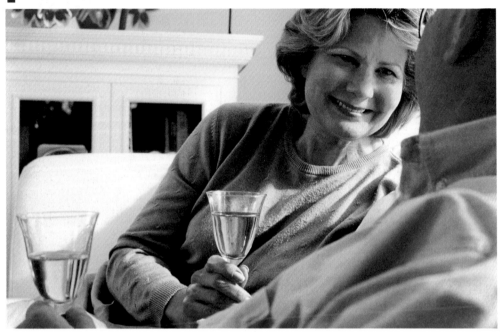

◄ A little wine or a couple of cocktails in the evening might help ward off cognitive problems such as Alzheimer's disease in later years.

In recent years, drinkers have found plenty of occasions to raise a glass to good health. Studies have shown that moderate alcohol intake lowers the risk for stroke, heart disease and even intestinal infections. Now there may be another reason to sip a little Chianti with meals.

A study in the British medical journal *The Lancet* in January 2002, reported that people who have one to three drinks daily are much less likely than non-drinkers to develop dementia, an age-related decline in mental ability.

Researchers at Erasmus University Medical Centre in Rotterdam, the Netherlands, kept track of nearly 8,000 men and women aged 55 and older. After six years, 197 of them had developed dementia, primarily in the form of Alzheimer's disease.

But those who quaffed one to three drinks a day – beer, wine or other alcoholic beverages – were about 70 per cent less likely to develop dementia and more than 30 per cent less likely to develop Alzheimer's. The benefits were even more pronounced among people who have the ApoE4 gene, a genetic mutation that dramatically increases the risk for Alzheimer's.

Alcohol offers a number of benefits. It thins the blood and helps prevent clots from jamming tiny blood vessels in the brain. It also improves circulation by raising levels of high-density lipoprotein (HDL), the beneficial form of cholesterol that removes artery-clogging low-density lipoprotein (LDL) from the blood. Alcohol also appears to stimulate the release of acetylcholine, a brain chemical involved in learning and memory.

Although red wine has received considerable attention for its health-promoting properties, the Dutch study suggests that all alcoholic beverages have similar health benefits. But the researchers warn that having more than three drinks daily may reduce rather than increase levels of mind-protecting acetylcholine. Heavy drinking also increases the risk of liver disease. The key – as with everything else in life – is moderation.

Key discovery

Everyday blues are sad news for health

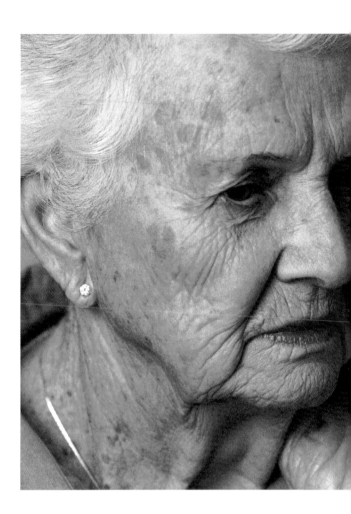

'**H**ow are you feeling?' is usually more of a casual greeting than a serious medical inquiry. But the answer can reveal a lot about your prospects for staying healthy – especially if you're older.

Previous studies have shown that serious depression weakens the body's immune system. But new research has found that even mild depression – the so-called 'blues' that millions of people experience at different times in their lives – suppresses immunity by reducing the ability of white blood cells to conquer infection.

Researchers at Johns Hopkins University in Baltimore and Ohio State University College of Medicine and Public Health in Columbus, USA, followed 78 older adults (average age about 72), 22 of whom suffered from mild to moderate depression at the start of the study. Eighteen months later, blood tests revealed that those who were depressed had a weaker immune response to laboratory-produced infections than those who weren't depressed.

Up to 57 per cent of older adults experience depression at some time in their lives – sometimes major, sometimes so mild that it's never brought to anyone's attention. This study suggests that the severity of the depression isn't as important as how long it lasts. A short bout won't increase the risk of infection. But even a mild depression that lasts months or maybe years may leave a person more vulnerable to illness.

Effective treatments for depression are readily available – but first, doctors have to learn to recognize the condition in its milder forms. They may find that the question 'Have you been getting sick lately?' is just as revealing as the traditional questions about mood.

This study suggests that the severity of the depression isn't as important as how long it lasts.

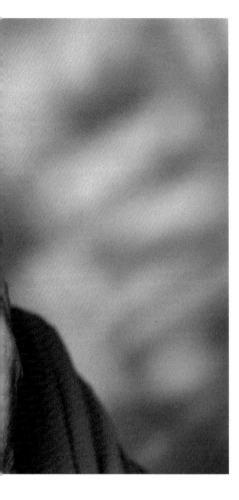

RESEARCH ROUND-UP

Can we turn off the depression switch?

People with mood disorders who feel as though symptoms such as fatigue or a general lack of enthusiasm come out of the blue may be exactly right. Scientists believe they have now discovered a chemical switch that 'turns on' depression.

Everything we do and feel is controlled by genes, which are constantly activating and deactivating the proteins that drive every one of the body's processes. US researchers have recently found that some genes, when they're switched on, activate protein segments that trigger symptoms of depression. When the same genes are turned off – by chemically deactivating a substance called cAMP response element binding protein (CREB) – symptoms of depression are reduced.

'We have identified CREB as a critical element in a chemical pathway that, when activated, can cause certain symptoms of depression,' says Dr. William Carlezon, director of the Behavioral Genetics Laboratory at Harvard University's McLean Hospital. CREB activates a peptide called dynorphin. The researchers found that blocking dynorphin in the brain appeared to have strong antidepressant effects; this may eventually lead to the development of new drugs for depression.

◄ Prolonged anxiety and depression, even when mild, can make older adults more susceptible to illness.

Take action

Six ways to beat the blues

Most people with minor depression don't need anti-depressants. These approaches can help.

■ **MAINTAIN AN ACTIVE SOCIAL LIFE,** whether it's with friends, neighbours or fellow church members. Research has shown that people who stay active socially suffer less depression than those who spend a lot of time alone.

■ **STAY IN TOUCH WITH YOUR FAITH** Whether or not you go to church, having a belief in powers greater than yourself can help depression resolve more quickly.

■ **EAT A HEALTHY DIET** and only drink alcohol in moderation. Excessive alcohol consumption – more than two drinks a day for men or one drink a day for women – increases the risk of depression.

■ **TRY TAKING 300MG ST. JOHN'S WORT DAILY** The herb can sometimes help minor depression, but check first with your GP for possible side effects.

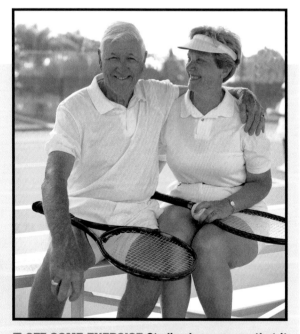

■ **GET SOME EXERCISE** Studies have proven that it really helps. Thirty minutes of aerobic exercise, for example, boosts levels of the mood-elevating brain chemical serotonin by 77 per cent.

High-tech help
Better lie detector 'fingerprints' the brain

Police and prosecutors have always tried to get into the minds of criminals in order to solve cases. And in the USA in recent years, to help separate truths from lies they've relied on polygraphs, which map blood pressure, pulse and other physiological measures of stress. But polygraphs are notoriously unreliable and the results rarely admissible in US courts. Now a new technique, called brain mapping or brain fingerprinting, makes it possible to actually scan the brains of suspects in search of incriminating memories.

How it works The human brain produces distinctive electrical patterns, called P300 waves, when it encounters familiar words or images – a picture of your spouse, for example. The waves are not produced if you look at a picture of a stranger. Specialists in brain fingerprinting can use the cutting-edge technique of recording P300 waves to determine if a suspect recognizes details from a crime scene – details that only the criminal would know, such as the murder weapon or the room where the crime occurred.

In more than 150 scientific tests, brain fingerprinting has proved to be 100 per cent accurate, says Lawrence Farwell, Ph.D., the inventor of the technique and chairman of Brain Wave Science in Fairfield, Iowa. It doesn't determine guilt or innocence, Dr. Farwell adds. But it can tell investigators whether or not specific information is stored in the brain of the suspect. Unlike fingerprints or DNA evidence, which is only available in about 1 per cent of cases, the brain's memories are always there.

Availability Its use in Britain – if ever – may be years away, but a judge in Iowa has ruled that the technology is admissible in court there and some experts anticipate that it will eventually supplement, or even replace, traditional lie detector tests. But what happens, for example, if a suspect is guilty, but simply doesn't remember details of the crime scene? 'There's always a margin of uncertainty with technology, but the accuracy of brain fingerprinting is accepted in the scientific community,' says Dr. Farwell.

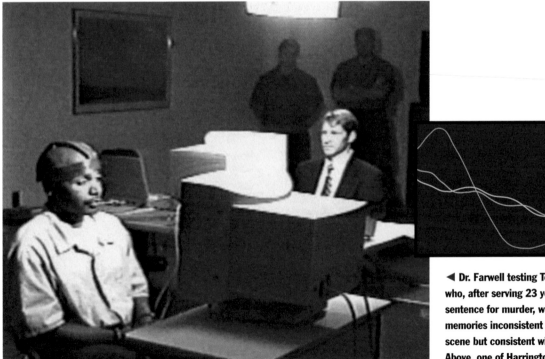

◀ Dr. Farwell testing Terry Harrington, who, after serving 23 years of a life sentence for murder, was found to have memories inconsistent with the crime scene but consistent with his alibi. Above, one of Harrington's brain scans.

BEHIND THE BREAKTHROUGH

A US inmate pins his hopes on brain waves

Terry Harrington has spent more than half his life in prison for the murder of a retired policeman in 1977. His conviction hinged on alleged eyewitness testimony – that was later recanted when the witness was confronted with compelling evidence of Harrington's innocence.

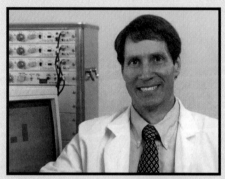

The technique's designer – Dr. Farwell.

Lawrence Farwell, Ph.D., made that evidence possible when he designed a way to 'read' a person's memory. Dr. Farwell's investigations in this area began when he was working on technology that would give speech to vocally paralysed people. He noticed in test subjects a kind of brain signal he was not familiar with. Intrigued, he set off to study the brain waves used in brain mapping, also known as brain fingerprinting. Along the way, Dr. Farwell received funding from the CIA.

In the Harrington case, alibi witnesses testified that Harrington was at a concert and later driving around town with friends at the time of the murder. The defence team approached Dr. Farwell to help with an appeal. By mapping Harrington's neurological response to words and phrases relevant to the murder, Dr. Farwell could determine that he had no memories of it. 'We can conclude with 99.99 per cent confidence that the critical details of the crime are not stored in his brain,' says Dr. Farwell. 'It's like finding that his fingerprints or DNA don't match those from the crime scene.' And Harrington did recognize information relating to his alibi. But he was refused a new trial and now the case is being appealed to the Iowa Supreme Court.

Drug development
Antidepressant banishes 'ghost' pain

When you whack your thumb with a hammer you know it's going to hurt. But neuropathic pain (sometimes called 'ghost' pain) isn't predictable. Stimuli that shouldn't hurt, like a puff of air on the skin, can trigger excruciating, burning pain.

'The body is telling us that something is wrong but we haven't understood what it is,' says Frank Porreca, Ph.D., professor of pharmacology and anaesthesiology at the University of Arizona Health Sciences Center in Tuscon.

British and American doctors have typically used a class of medications called tricyclic antidepressants to treat neuropathic pain – though in the UK, they're not formally licensed for this use. But these drugs don't always work well and may produce side effects such as weight gain and sexual dysfunction. Now there may be an alternative – bupropion, which seems to be more effective and much less likely to cause side effects. This antidepressant is also used to help people quit smoking – a beneficial effect that was noticed when the drug was first being developed. Bupropion, is, in fact, only licensed in the UK for that use under the trade name Zyban.

A study published in the US journal *Neurology* in November 2001 enrolled 41 people with neuropathic pain. After six weeks of treatment with bupropion, 73 per cent reported that their pain got better – and about a third said it was 'much improved'. Some of the subjects in the study experienced a dry mouth or other side effects, but these were generally considered to be more tolerable than those caused by tricyclics.

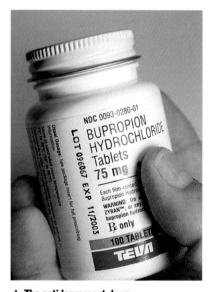

▲ The antidepressant drug, bupropion, can help to relieve neuropathic pain, too – and help people to give up smoking.

The US researchers had deliberately excluded people with depression from the study. As a result they felt they could justifiably attribute the benefits of the drug to its pain-killing effects rather than to its antidepressant quality.

High-tech help
From mind to computer, empowering paralysed people

Any monkey can be taught to play video games, but three bright primates at Brown University in Providence, Rhode Island, in the USA went one step further; with the help of wires that transmitted their brain waves to a computer, they were able to move a cursor just by thinking about where it should go. The experiment, reported in March 2002 in the journal *Nature*, suggests that people with spinal cord injuries or diseases that cause paralysis may one day be able to perform daily tasks such as answering emails or switching on lights by using brain power.

How it works Researchers implanted an Smartie-sized cluster of 100 electrodes into each monkey's cerebral cortex, an area of the brain that controls hand movements. They monitored the monkeys' brain signals while the creatures played a primitive video game with joysticks. Millions of neurons control the hand and arm, but the scientists found that they needed just a few signal samples, taken from about a dozen neurons, to design computer software that translated thought patterns into hand movements. They then wrote a computer program to turn those brain signals into data that could control cursor movements even when the joysticks were turned off.

'We substituted thought control for hand control,' explains John P. Donoghue, Ph.D., chair of the Department of Neuroscience at Brown, and the project's senior researcher. 'A monkey's brain – not its hand – moved the cursor.' The experiment worked so well, in fact, that the monkeys could play the game nearly as fast with their minds as they had with their hands.

The next step will be to use the same technology in people. With the proper software and signalling devices, people with paralysis may soon be able to work on computers or operate electronic appliances. A more challenging goal will be to use brain signals to control muscle movements, moving an arm or gripping a cup of coffee.

Availability Approval for human studies may be granted within the year in the USA, according to Dr. Donoghue. 'The electrodes are no more disturbing than having a pacemaker,' he notes. 'Once they're put in place, people won't even be aware of them.' Some experts predict that human neural implants could be ready in five to 10 years. One current limitation is that the electrodes may, over time, damage brain tissue or get jarred out of place. A solution may be wireless devices that are permanently implanted.

> ## 'A monkey's brain – not its hand – moved the cursor.'

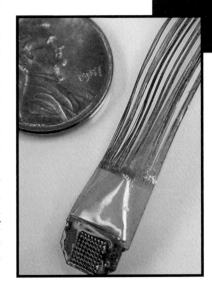

▶ Dr. John Donoghue in his lab. Below is one of the cables used to conduct brain signals to a computer; each one has 60 to 100 electrodes.

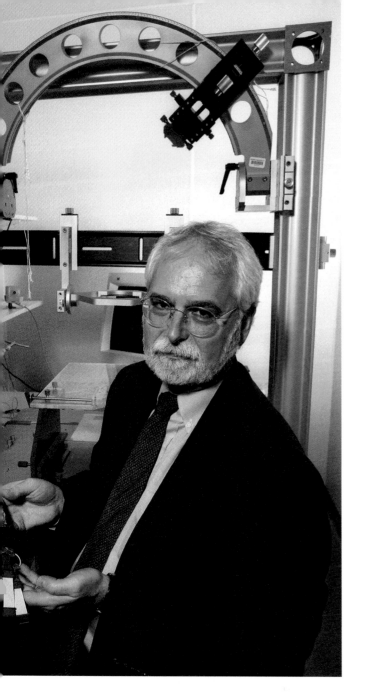

High-tech help
Plastics may repair spinal injuries

The future for spinal cord injuries may be plastics – more specifically, a newly invented film that appears to transmit nerve impulses with the same lightning speed as natural nerve membranes.

Researchers at St. George's Hospital Medical School in London have developed a hole-filled plastic film that allows ions of potassium and sodium to pass from one side to the other, just as ions pass through natural nerve membranes. It's the back-and-forth movement of ions, which changes the electrical charge on either side of the membrane, that allows impulses to travel from one end of a nerve to the other. With a thickness of 10 micrometres, the plastic film is 1,000 times thicker than natural nerve membranes – but the exchange of ions occurs just as rapidly. This means it's theoretically possible that the film could some-day replace injury-damaged nerves and permit people to regain normal function. The findings were published in *Biophysical Journal* in April 2002.

The film has to be perfected, however. For reasons that are not clear, potassium ions pass through the tiny pores more quickly than sodium ions. Future research will focus on making the film more 'nerve-like', in part by fine-tuning the pores to allow different ions to pass through at similar rates.

RESEARCH ROUND-UP

Vaccine helps to prevent paralysis

Spinal cord damage doesn't stop after the initial injury. Nerve cells and fibres surrounding the damaged area begin to break down as the degenerative process spreads outward. One way to stop this, according to researchers at the Weizmann Institute of Science in Rehovot, Israel, is to administer a vaccine containing protein fragments culled from the central nervous system. The vaccine appears to stimulate parts of the immune system that help curtail tissue-damaging inflammation. In a recent study reported in the US *Journal of Clinical Investigation*, laboratory animals with spinal cord injuries that would cause rear-limb paralysis were divided into two groups. Those that received the vaccine recovered limb movement dramatically, while untreated animals became paralysed. The vaccine won't work in cases involving a complete break in the spinal cord, but it does appear to prevent secondary degeneration in surrounding tissues – which can be worse than the original injury. The scientists hope to test the vaccine on people within a year.

Key discovery
Mind over muscle – just think yourself stronger?

It's the hammock-lover's dream come true. Just *thinking* about exercise can make you stronger.

Researchers at the Cleveland Clinic Foundation in Ohio in the USA divided 30 healthy young people into three groups. One group imagined flexing their little fingers. Another group focused on their elbow flexor muscles, while the third group did no imaginary exercises.

The results were fascinating. In the first group, strength in the little finger increased by 35 per cent. In the second group, elbow strength was up 13.4 per cent. And in the third group (the control group), no change was detected.

Brain recordings of the study participants showed highly visible electrical activity in certain brain regions during the mental exercises. After the training, further brain scans revealed greater and more focused activity in the prefrontal cortex in the front of the brain – an area associated with meditation.

The US researchers, who presented the study results in November 2001 at the Society for Neuroscience's annual meeting in San Diego, hope the findings will one day help people who have suffered strokes and spinal cord injuries.

Don't sell your gym membership just yet, though. Thinking about exercise is still no substitute for doing it. The authors say that the strength increase they recorded wasn't actually the result of muscle growth, but better signalling from the brain to the existing tissue.

If only you could do housework and gardening by just thinking about it …

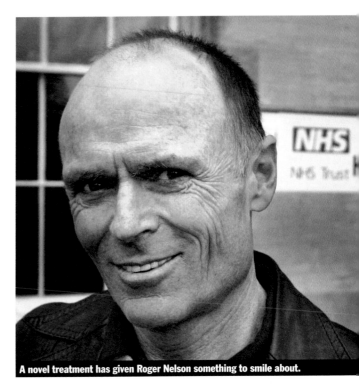

A novel treatment has given Roger Nelson something to smile about.

Drug development
New Parkinson's treatment is a laughing matter

Researchers have a variety of ways to measure the success of an experimental treatment, but laughter is surely one of the most unusual. Yet laughter – more specifically, the renewed ability of a man with Parkinson's disease to laugh at a joke for the first time in years and to smell the mouthwatering aroma of a Sunday roast – said more about the success of a preliminary new treatment for the disease than all of the blood tests or imaging scans in the world.

Parkinson's is linked to a loss of brain cells that produce the neurotransmitter dopamine, a chemical messenger responsible for transmitting signals within the brain. The lack of dopamine causes nerve cells to fire erratically, leaving patients unable to control their movements. Although a variety of medications provide relief from symptoms, none can stop the disease's progression.

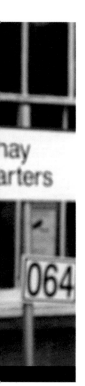

RESEARCH ROUND-UP

New clue in Parkinson's mystery

Doctors have long puzzled over why levodopa, the primary drug treatment for Parkinson's disease, is effective for only about five to ten years. Now they may have the answer. Researchers in Australia discovered that certain dopamine-producing cells in the base of the brain and in the brain's cortex, responsible for control of movement, the five senses, memory, language, thought and intellect, are missing in Parkinson's patients, not just inactivated or dead as earlier suspected. In fact, Glenda Halliday, Ph.D., an associate professor at the Prince of Wales Medical Research Institute, Sydney, discovered that 80 per cent of the nerve cells in the cortex disappear during the first ten years of the disease. Levodopa, intended to help these cells transmit messages better, therefore becomes ineffective. The finding is expected to lead to new treatments for the disease – for instance, ones that stimulate other areas of the cortex to take over before the cells die out. Dr. Halliday's results were expected to be published in late 2002.

Another stem cell success

For years, researchers have hoped that stem cell transplants could treat – or even cure – Parkinson's disease. Now, a study using embryonic mouse stem cells suggests the possibility may become a reality. Stem cells are unspecialized cells (usually harvested from foetal tissue) that can develop into any variety of specialized cell as they divide. In this study, mouse embryonic stem cells were transformed into neurons – brain cells that transmit chemical messages – and then transplanted into a mouse with Parkinson's disease, where they released dopamine, formed new nerve cell connections, and reduced symptoms of the disease. The study was published in the July 4, 2002, issue of the science journal *Nature*. It was one of the first studies to demonstrate that embryonic stem cells can generate dopamine-producing neurons to effectively treat the symptoms of Parkinson's disease.

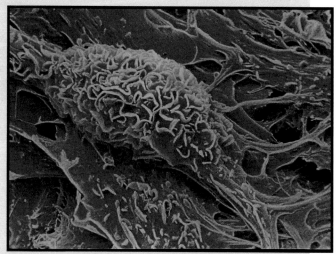

Embryonic stem cells can give rise to any type of cell – from blood to nerve to muscle cells.

In the experimental treatment, a chemical called a growth factor was pumped into the brains of five British patients to encourage the production of dopamine. The story appeared in many British newspapers in April 2002, and the results raised hopes for a new long-term treatment for a disease that affects an estimated 1.6 million people worldwide, including such well-known figures as boxer Muhammad Ali and actor Michael J. Fox.

How it works A team of surgeons at Frenchay Hospital in Bristol inserted tubes into the patients' brains and connected the tubes to pumps in their abdomens. The pumps were configured to send continuous levels of a naturally occurring chemical – glial derived neurotrophic factor (GDNF) – into the brain. GDNF is a growth factor required for the correct development and manufacture and maintenance of the dopamine production cells that die off in Parkinson's disease. After only a month or two on the drug, the patients' symptoms improved dramatically, exceeding all expectations.

Availability The results are very preliminary. Researchers don't know whether the improvements will last, or if symptoms will continue to improve. An earlier study of GDNF on 25 patients in the USA found no benefits – possibly because in that trial too little of the drug reached the dopamine-producing cells. Even if the treatment does prove successful, researchers said, it will not become available for at least four or five years.

Still, at least one of the five patients has rediscovered some of life's small pleasures. Roger Nelson, a former marketing director, is laughing at jokes again and can handle playing cards well enough to resume his bridge hobby. As he told the press, 'It has had a positive effect in very many little ways.'

Key discovery

Adult stem cells repair Parkinson's damage

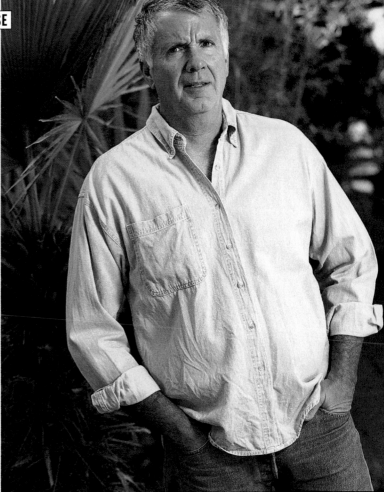

For years, one side of the debate over foetal and embryonic stem cells has centred on their potential to treat or even cure people with Parkinson's disease and other brain disorders. But opponents see ethical obstacles. 'A shameful day' was the pro-life campaigners' comment last autumn when Britain was awarded the contract to create Europe's first stem cell bank. And the issue has severely restricted research in the USA. Now there's exciting preliminary evidence that stem cells harvested from adults. – which skirts the controversy – have the potential to drastically reduce Parkinson's symptoms.

Embryonic stem cells are the remarkable master cells that can develop into specialized cells, such as brain, liver or kidney cells – virtually any cell that's needed – and divide indefinitely in the laboratory, producing generation after generation of similar cells. The cells are taken from fertilized eggs – often those created during IVF that would otherwise be discarded. Adult stem cells, on the other hand, are found in blood or bone marrow, and some brain tissue, in adults (and, despite the name, in children, too).

In April 2002, scientists from Celmed BioSciences reported that they had successfully used neural (nerve) stem cells from a Parkinson's patient's brain to reduce his symptoms by more than 80 per cent. This is the first indication that neural stem cells can be successfully used to treat Parkinson's disease.

How it works The patient, 59-year-old Dennis Turner, of San Clemente, California, is a nuclear reactor engineer and fighter jet pilot who was diagnosed with Parkinson's at 49. In 1998, Dr. Michel Levesque, a neurosurgeon with Cedars-Sinai Medical Center in Los Angeles and a CelMed vice-president, had removed 50 to 100 cells from Turner's brain during a routine brain biopsy, then cultured them in the laboratory for several months until they grew to

several million cells. About 20 per cent of those cells became the type that secretes dopamine. (The death of these cells causes Parkinson's.) In March 1999, Dr. Levesque injected the cells into six locations in Turner's brain. One year after the procedure, Turner's symptoms improved by 83 per cent.

Availability The researchers warn that their work is still extremely preliminary, particularly since their study involved only one patient. Additionally, Parkinson's symptoms normally ebb and flow, so improvement in one patient doesn't mean the procedure works. Also, Turner's improvement continued even after the transplanted cells stopped making dopamine, something that puzzles the researchers. Still, Turner is thrilled with the results. As he told the *Washington Post* in April 2002, 'Two years ago I couldn't put my contact lenses in without a big problem. Now it's no problem.' Another advantage: because the cells came from his own body, he doesn't have to take anti-rejection medication, which is required when cells or tissue from one human is transplanted into another.

The CelMed researchers have received US government permission to conduct further human trials of this treatment.

▲ Stem cells taken from his own brain improved Parkinson's symptoms significantly for Dennis Turner.

Drug development

Antibiotic protects brain, restores nerves

Parkinson's disease, which affects more than 120,000 people in Britain, occurs when damaged nerve cells in the brain produce less and less dopamine, one of the chemicals known as neurotransmitters that carry brain signals to muscles. Over time, muscles throughout the body lose the ability to contract and relax normally, causing tremors and muscle stiffness.

The current medications that are used to treat Parkinson's disease can slow, but cannot stop, the progression of symptoms. But a recent experiment with a common antibiotic suggests there may be another approach.

A US study reported in the December 2001 *Proceedings of the National Academy of Sciences* found that the antibiotic minocycline, a member of the tetracycline family, reduced inflammation and damage in dopamine-producing cells in the brains of laboratory mice. The mice were first given a chemical that induces changes similar to those caused by Parkinson's.

How it works In this case, the benefits aren't linked to the drug's antibiotic action. Minocycline has long been thought to have anti-inflammatory effects, so it makes sense that it would guard against inflammation that damages nerve cells in the brain. But the drug also had another, unexpected effect – it seemed to protect dopamine-producing cells from nitric oxide, a molecule linked to cell destruction. It also temporarily restored some nerve function in the mice in the hours after it was administered.

Availability Minocycline by itself will never be a treatment for Parkinson's disease. The researchers had to use enormous doses in the animal studies because very little of the drug passes into the brain. They also note that the benefits seen in animal studies don't always appear in humans. But the study showed that it may be possible to treat Parkinson's in a quite new way. The next step may be to develop tetracycline-like drugs that have been stripped of their antibiotic component but still reduce inflammation and can pass easily into the brain.

Nobel-winning work from the 1950s

Arvid Carlsson of Sweden, one of three researchers sharing the 2000 Nobel Prize in medicine, was honoured for work in the late 1950s. His findings greatly influenced current wisdom about how brain cells use an important chemical – dopamine – to communicate.

Foundational findings
Dopamine, Carlsson discovered, acts as a chemical messenger between brain cells, especially in the basal ganglia, a major centre for muscle movement. In Parkinson's disease patients, the nerves supplying dopamine to the basal ganglia die, causing muscle tremors and rigidity.

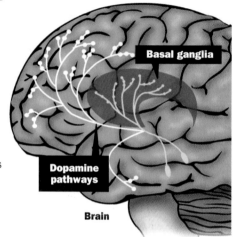

Essential communication
L-dopa is a naturally occurring precursor to dopamine.

Because of Carlsson's work, Parkinson's patients are still given L-dopa as a drug that brain cells convert to dopamine.

The dopamine is held in storage vesicles. Nerve impulses empty the vesicles, sending dopamine across the synapses between cells.

Receptors in the neighbouring cell take up the dopamine and pass the impulse into the cell.

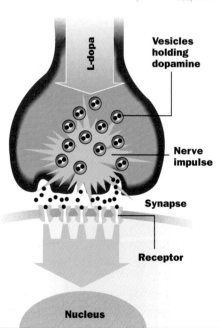

Key discovery

Orange pigment linked to the blues

Doctors have long been taught that bilirubin, the orange-yellow pigment that results from the breakdown of haemoglobin, the main pigment in red blood cells, is a useless waste product. But a study published in the US journal *Biological Psychiatry* in March 2002 suggests that it plays a key role in mood, especially for people with seasonal affective disorder (SAD), the 'winter blues' that affect two to three per cent of Britons but about 10 per cent of adults in low-light regions of the northern United States.

How it works In the first study of its kind, Yale University researchers took blood samples from volunteers with and without SAD. At the start of the study, the SAD patients had lower levels of bilirubin than the subjects who didn't have SAD. Over two weeks, some of the SAD subjects were exposed to bright lights for an hour a day, a standard treatment. The result? Their bilirubin levels rose and their symptoms declined, so researchers concluded that people with low levels of bilirubin may be more susceptible to SAD than those with normal levels.

Dr. Dan Oren, lead investigator of the study and an associate professor of psychiatry at Yale, can only speculate as to the role bilirubin might play in controlling mood. The pigment is known to be light sensitive. It's also capable of crossing the blood-brain barrier. And it's a potent anti-oxidant. It's possible that bilirubin may reduce a person's susceptibility to the symptoms of SAD by blocking the effects of cell-damaging free radicals, harmful oxygen molecules found throughout the body.

Availability The new research may one day provide clues to the causes of SAD, which in turn may lead to more effective treatments. In the meantime, researchers aren't sure yet whether low bilirubin actually causes SAD, or whether it's merely a biological 'marker' – a sign that something else in the body causes mood problems as bilirubin declines.

> **Researchers concluded that people with low levels of bilirubin may be more susceptible to SAD.**

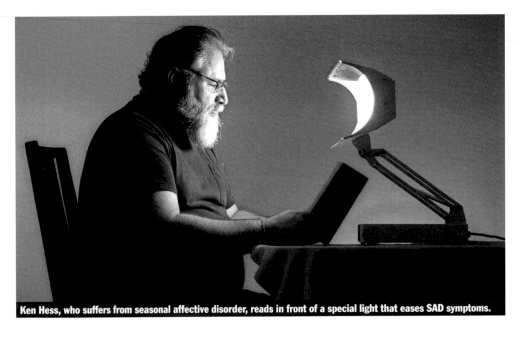

Ken Hess, who suffers from seasonal affective disorder, reads in front of a special light that eases SAD symptoms.

ALSO IN THE NEWS

Cool clothes may lead to new drugs for MS

About 80 per cent of people with multiple sclerosis have an increase in fatigue, muscle weakness and other symptoms during the warm months or when they engage in body-warming activities, because a rise in body temperature causes weak nerve impulses to get even weaker. Why? A new study suggests that heat triggers the release of nitric oxide, a chemical that hampers the transmission of nerve signals. Researchers at University Hospital in Groningen, Holland, found that people with MS who wore refrigerated waistcoats had a 41 per cent decrease in blood levels of nitric oxide, and a corresponding increase in energy, balance, and muscle strength. Patients who wore only slightly cooled waistcoats had no such improvements, nor changes in nitric oxide levels. The study, in the US journal *Neurology* in September 2001, suggests it may be possible to develop a drug that lowers nitric oxide levels and duplicates the beneficial effects of cooling.

MRI scans: coffee could skew result

Just a few cups of your favourite morning pick-me-up could upset one of the most sophisticated medical tests. Brain scans – functional magnetic resonance imaging (MRI) scans – can be used to measure the amount of blood that is circulating in different parts of the brain. Scientists at Wake Forest University School of Medicine in Winston-Salem, North Carolina, wanted to know if caffeine, which is known to affect blood flow, could interfere with the results of the test. They gave volunteers 250mg of caffeine – roughly the amount contained in two to three cups of coffee – and then scanned their brains. They did the same after giving the volunteers dummy pills (placebos). They found that caffeine reduced blood flow by as much as 25 per cent in some areas of the brain – more than enough to significantly skew test results. In the future, patients may be advised to abstain from coffee or other caffeinated beverages before the tests, or they will be asked how much coffee they drink regularly. This will allow doctors to calculate the extent to which changes in blood flow might be attributed to caffeine.

New uses for milk thistle

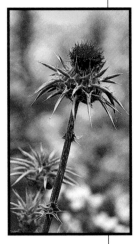

A recent animal study conducted at State University of New York (SUNY) Upstate Medical University in Syracuse suggests that the herb milk thistle has powerful effects – but not the same ones touted by herbalists. Scientists at SUNY's neuroscience and transplantation and immunology laboratories tested an extract of milk thistle, along with herbs such as echinacea and St. John's wort. They discovered that milk thistle stimulated the growth of neurites, branches of nerve cells that allow cells to communicate and that also play a role in cell regeneration. Milk thistle also seemed to stimulate immune response. If it proves to have the same effects in humans as it does in animals, it may lead to new treatments for spinal cord injuries, Alzheimer's or other neurological maladies. Herbalists have traditionally recommended milk thistle for hepatitis, other liver diseases, gallstones and psoriasis.

Brain works better when hands do the talking

University of Chicago psychologists have concluded that using hand gestures may help us to think better. Previous research has shown that listeners retain more information when the speaker uses hand gestures, but it now appears that the gestures may help the speaker as well. In a study published in the November 2001 issue of *Psychological Science*, 40 children and 36 adults were asked to solve maths problems. Then they were given a list of letters or words to memorize. Next they were asked to explain their maths answers – sometimes while using hand gestures, sometimes without. At the same time, they were asked to recall the list of items they had memorized. When people gestured while they spoke they could recall 20 per cent more words and letters than when they kept their hands still – possibly because gestures can help information processing, leaving more of our brain power available for memory recall.

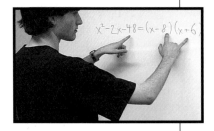

Key discovery
'Brain freeze' may prevent permanent stroke damage

Clot-busting drugs are, at present, the only effective treatment in the hours just after a stroke. But they have to be given quickly, preferably within 90 minutes, to give patients a decent chance of making a full recovery. The problem is that most people don't get the drugs for more than two hours after the onset of symptoms. The delay can be devastating because, as neurologists point out, 'time is brain' for stroke patients. What's desperately needed is a drug that can be given immediately by paramedics, even if they aren't completely sure whether someone has had a stroke.

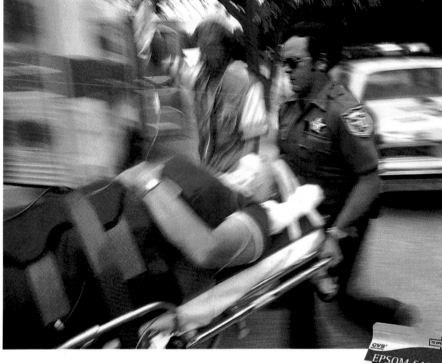

As it turns out, a remedy may be already available – and you may even have it at home. Britain's Medical Research Council (MRC) is funding a multi-centred study into the effectiveness of magnesium sulphate, better known as Epsom salts, to temporarily 'freeze' the brain, limiting stroke damage and buying time until doctors can take over. The Glasgow-based research team plan to report in October this year and initial results from one Los Angeles centre look encouraging.

How it works A stroke sets off a cascade of chemical activity in the brain, culminating in an overload of calcium, which triggers the death of nerve cells. Magnesium sulphate blocks the flow of calcium into the neurons. It also dilates blood vessels, which promotes blood flow to brain areas that would otherwise be cut off. In early 2002, researchers at the University of California, Los Angeles, completed a study in which para-medics, in consultation with physicians and nurses, gave injections of magnesium sulphate to stroke patients. It was given, on average, 23 minutes after paramedics arrived, compared to the two to three hours it usually takes for emergency doctors to begin treatment. The injections resulted in what researchers termed a 'dramatic' recovery in 25 per cent of the patients, all of whom had suffered ischaemic strokes, the kind that involve a blockage of blood flow to the brain. The drug may also have a smaller benefit in those who suffer haemorrhagic stroke, which involves a burst blood vessel in the brain.

Availability More studies must be completed before its effectiveness is widely accepted. But magnesium sulphate does show promise and, unlike other stroke drugs, is unlikely to cause side effects. And, if a stroke is misdiagnosed and the medicine is given, it won't do any harm.

▲ **Magnesium sulphate, better known as Epsom salts ('salt' in the USA) is more than just a laxative. It can help to prevent brain damage in stroke victims when given intravenously by paramedics.**

RESEARCH ROUND-UP

Speed counts for stroke

Tens of thousands of brain cells die each minute after a stroke. A clot-busting drug – tissue plasminogen activator (TPA) – stops extensive damage and preserves mental function, but only if it's given before brain cells are destroyed. A new study, reported in February 2002 at the annual meeting of the American Stroke Association, found that patients given TPA within 90 minutes of the first appearance of stroke symptoms were almost three times more likely to make a full recovery than those who didn't get the drug. The study, which looked at 2,776 patients in 18 countries, also found that people given the drug in the second 90 minutes after a stroke were about 1½ times more likely to recover than those who did not get the drug at all. Only about 2 per cent of stroke patients currently get TPA, mainly because they arrive at the hospital too late for effective treatment.

Robot works with stroke patients

Physiotherapists, take note – a robot may be taking over your job, at least for treating stroke patients with long-standing impairments. Lasting stroke symptoms such as muscle weakness and reduced mobility become harder to treat as time passes, but a tabletop robot called MIT-Manus might be the answer. Developed by researchers at Massachusetts Institute of Technology in Cambridge, the robot exercises the arm much as a physical therapist would. At the International Stroke Conference in February 2002, MIT scientists reported that long-term stroke patients

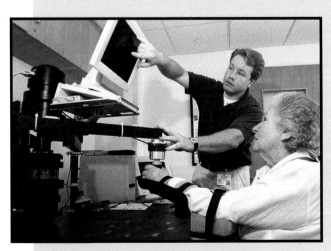

A stroke survivor undergoes therapy with the MIT-Manus, and watches her progress on the monitor.

who worked with the robot for six to eight weeks had a 5 per cent improvement in muscle strength and mobility. Robot therapy can produce improvements of 10 per cent when it's used with patients who have had more recent strokes – and the benefits have been shown to persist for up to three years.

Say 'ahh' to stop a stroke

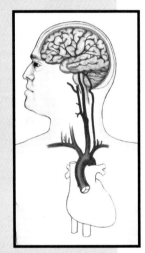

Dental X-rays do more than reveal cavities; they can also suggest how likely you are to have a stroke – if the dentist knows what to look for. Dental X-rays called panoramic radiographs include a view of the carotid arteries, large blood vessels on either side of the neck that carry blood to the brain. When researchers at State University of New York, Buffalo, examined the X-rays of 2,752 dental patients, they found that 5 per cent had noticeable calcium deposits in the arteries. Such deposits occur only in people with advanced atherosclerosis, or narrowing of the arteries, one of the principal risk factors for stroke. People who have plaque in the carotid arteries are twice as likely to die from heart attack or stroke as those without the deposits.

Implants keep blood flowing

The only way brain cells can survive a stroke is if doctors are able to restore normal blood flow before the damage is done. But even that doesn't always work when surgery to repair ruptured blood vessels is performed after a type of stroke known as a sub-arachnoid haemorrhage, in which blood from a damaged blood vessel accumulates at the surface of the brain. The repaired arteries often develop vasospasms – muscular contractions that cause them to clamp down and starve the brain of blood. Japanese researchers may have found a solution. In a study of 20 patients, reported in the US journal *Stroke* in April 2002, surgeons in Tokyo implanted rice-sized pellets next to arteries that they suspected might develop vasospasms. The pellets contained nicardipine, a calcium channel blocker used to treat high blood pressure. None of the arteries adjoining the pellets went into vasospasm, although six of the patients did develop problems in arteries farther away.

CANCER

Cancer research is proceeding so rapidly that doctors may soon be able to treat the disease as confidently as they now deal with high blood pressure or diabetes. Some highlights: the amazing promise of angiogenesis inhibitors, compounds that starve tumours of their blood supply, is beginning to be realized. And researchers have used the new science of proteomics to 'fingerprint' ovarian cancer so that it can be detected earlier, with just a drop of blood. There's a highly effective new radio wave treatment for kidney cancer, and targeted new radiation therapies for breast cancer and prostate cancer that cut down on side effects. More and more people will be undergoing chemotherapy at home instead of in a hospital or clinic. And early research indicates that meditation may help to boost cancer patients' immune systems.

Key discovery
Common virus linked to brain cancer

Researchers at Temple University in Philadelphia have linked a virus that infects nearly 70 per cent of children by the time they're 15 to the development of medulloblastoma, the most common type of malignant brain tumour in children, accounting for a fifth of all childhood brain tumours. Each year about 60 children in the UK are diagnosed with this aggressive, difficult-to-treat, and often fatal cancer.

The virus in question, called the JC virus, manufactures a protein that tells other cells to divide very rapidly. It's a turn-on switch for cancer, notes Kamel Khalili, Ph.D., lead author of research published in February 2002 in the *Journal of the National Cancer Institute*. When he and his colleagues took the gene with the code for this viral protein and inserted it in mice, the animals developed a brain tumour similar to a human brain tumour.

'We thought, "This is a human virus that has [cancer] potential in animals. Maybe it's associated with human tumours",' Dr. Khalili says. And he was right. In studying tissue samples from children who died of brain tumours, Dr. Khalili and his colleagues discovered that many medulloblastomas contain the JC viral protein.

The virus doesn't directly cause the tumour in humans, notes Dr. Khalili. If it did, nearly every child would have brain cancer. Several other factors, both genetic and environmental, must be present to trigger the development of the tumour. And some medulloblastoma cells didn't contain the viral protein at all, suggesting that the JC virus may not be involved in all medulloblastomas.

The next step, Dr. Khalili says, is to continue studying the biology of the virus to learn how it induces tumour growth. Then their efforts will follow two paths. One will be the development of a vaccine against the viral protein. The other will be an effort to identify or devise drugs that interfere with the way the virus works and halt its dangerous effects on brain cells.

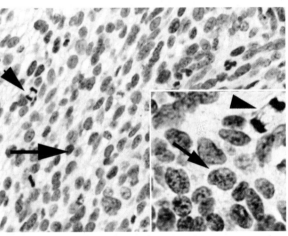

▲ A microscopic slide of human medulloblastoma. The arrows point out cells that contain JC virus proteins that cause cells to divide too rapidly – a hallmark of cancer.

The JC virus manufactures a protein that tells other cells to divide very rapidly. It's a turn-on switch for cancer...

High-tech help
Targeted radiation, minus the needles

U ntil very recently breast cancer patients who underwent a lumpectomy had two choices after surgery: to undergo seven weeks of daily radiation, or to have needles that delivered targeted radiation inserted in the breast for seven days. But now a new radiation delivery system called MammoSite has been approved for use in both Europe and the USA, and it delivers 10 minutes a day of targeted radiation for five days – without needles.

'The most important thing is that it's comfortable for the patient,' says Dr. Frank Vicini, clinical associate professor in the department of radiation oncology at William Beaumont Hospitals in Royal Oak and Troy, Michigan, who conducted clinical trials of MammoSite. The availability of a simple, relatively painless radiation therapy may spur more women to choose breast-sparing lumpectomy – and more doctors to recommend it – instead of mastectomy as a treatment for early-stage tumours.

> **Simple, relatively painless radiation ... may spur more women to choose breast-sparing lumpectomy ...**

How it works Either during the lumpectomy, or up to 10 weeks afterwards, surgeons implant a balloon-like device in the cavity created by the removal of the tumour. A tiny catheter extends from the balloon to the outside of the breast. A day or two after surgery, a radioactive seed about the size of a grain of rice is attached to a wire and inserted through the catheter into the balloon, where it delivers the prescribed levels of radiation for about 10 minutes. After five daily treatments, the balloon is deflated and removed.

Availability Five-year studies already show that targeted radiation delivered by up to 18 needles in the breast is as effective as whole-breast radiation, with less severe side effects. But few centres have offered the procedure because it was difficult to learn and could be painful for the patient.

Now, MammoSite radiation should be available at most US cancer centres in 2003, says Dr. Vicini. It has also been approved in Europe and phase two clinical trials will start at two UK cancer centres this year.

Treatment with MammoSite

At the time of the lumpectomy, or later on an out-patient basis, the MammoSite delivery system is placed into the surgical cavity and inflated; the catheter exit site is dressed and the patient is sent home. After a brief recovery period of several days, the radiation source is introduced via the catheter into the balloon, where it irradiates the tumour cavity for about 10 minutes a day. The procedure is repeated for 4 or 5 days, after which the balloon is deflated and the catheter is withdrawn.

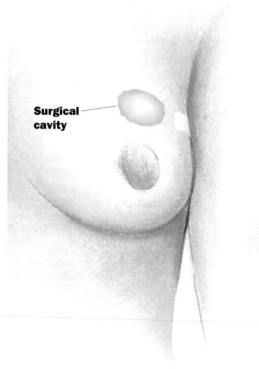

Surgical cavity

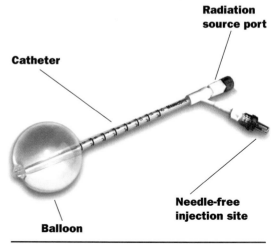

Radiation source port

Catheter

Needle-free injection site

Balloon

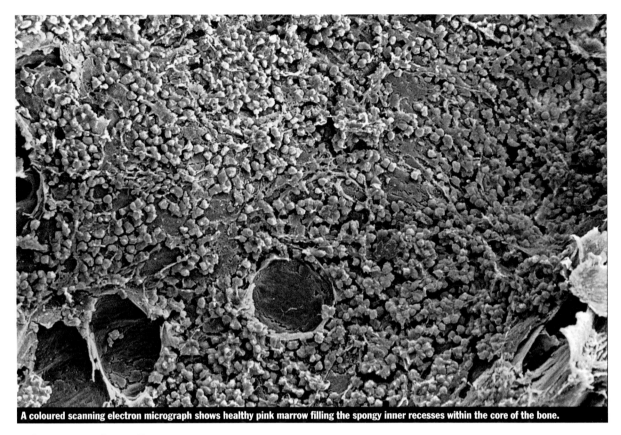

A coloured scanning electron micrograph shows healthy pink marrow filling the spongy inner recesses within the core of the bone.

Diagnostic advance

A better way to predict breast cancer's spread?

One of the most terrifying aspects of a breast cancer diagnosis is the fear that the cancer may have already spread from its original site. Even finding 'clean' lymph nodes, generally considered to be evidence that the cancer is confined to the breast, isn't a guarantee; 20 to 30 per cent of women with cancer-free lymph nodes have a recurrence of cancer elsewhere in their bodies.

But a large-scale study presented at the American Society of Clinical Oncology meeting in May 2002 suggests that doctors can predict the return of cancer by looking for cancerous cells in the patient's bone marrow, the spongy substance in the centre of the bone that manufactures blood cells. Most often, breast cancer spreads to this area.

In this study of more than 1,500 women, German researchers found that women whose cancers had spread to the bone marrow by the time of breast surgery were four times more likely to die or experience a relapse four years after surgery than those free of cancer cells at that site. Overall, women with breast cancer cells in their bone marrow have about a 50 per cent chance of dying from a recurrence of the disease.

It's also possible that the persistence or disappearance of cancerous cells in the bone marrow during the course of chemotherapy or radiation therapy (as evidenced by a second bone marrow test) might indicate how well the treatment is working. A small pilot study suggests that it does, says lead researcher Dr. Stephan Braun, and he and his colleagues are planning to conduct a larger study soon to find out more.

How it works To test for cancer in the bone marrow, doctors insert a needle into the woman's hip bone and withdraw a sample of the marrow. Some surgeons have begun taking the sample immediately after breast cancer surgery, while the patient is still anaesthetized.

RESEARCH ROUND-UP

Another reason to breastfeed

Researchers may have finally explained the dramatic increase in breast cancer rates over the past century. In a groundbreaking study published in July 2002 in the British medical journal *The Lancet,* epidemiologists at Oxford University in England analysed information collected by 200 researchers from more than 47 studies involving some 150,000 women worldwide. The conclusion: how long women breastfeed, and how many children they have, could be the two most important factors influencing their risk of breast cancer – even more important than their genes.

According to the epidemiologists, the risk of breast cancer dropped 4.3 per cent for every year the women breastfed. They also concluded that women in

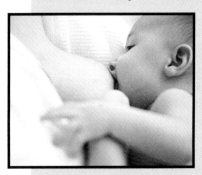

developed nations could cut their risk by 5 per cent if they nursed each child six months longer. Even women who had not breastfed previously would cut their risk by 7 per cent with every additional child they had. Currently, such women have two or three children and nurse for two to three months on average. In developing nations, on the other hand, women typically bear six or seven children and nurse each child for two years. That may explain the fact that Western women have a 6.3 per cent chance of developing breast cancer by the age of 70, compared to 2.7 per cent for women in poorer countries.

Hodgkin's survivors unaware of breast cancer risk

Many women treated with chest radiation for Hodgkin's disease (a type of cancer of the lymph glands) don't realize that they have an increased risk of developing breast cancer later in life, according to a study by researchers at the Dana Farber Cancer Institute in Boston, USA. Overall, women who have had Hodgkin's are three times more likely to develop breast cancer than women in the general population.

The Dana Farber study, published in April 2002 in the *Journal of Clinical Oncology,* questioned 90 women who had been treated at least eight years earlier with chest radiation for Hodgkin's. Of these, 40 per cent considered their risk for breast cancer to be equal to or lower than that of other women their age and less than half reported having had a mammogram in the

previous two years. During the four years of the study, ten of the women developed breast tumours, all of which were detected by mammograms.

New drug for breast cancer

In the USA, women for whom tamoxifen (Nolvadex) fails to stem the growth of breast cancer now have another option. In April 2002, fulvestrant (Faslodex) was approved to treat postmenopausal women with breast cancers that are sensitive to reproductive hormones. These hormones, oestrogen and progesterone 'feed' the tumours by latching onto certain receptors on tumour cells.

Fulvestrant, injected once a month, works by binding to, blocking and degrading the oestrogen receptors on cancer cells. The drug also helps to stop the growth spurt that natural oestrogen typically causes in cancer cells by preventing this hormone from attaching to the receptors. Fulvestrant is also less likely to cause the side effects known to occur with tamoxifen, such as hot flushes and an increased risk of endometrial cancer. A submission for a European licence for the drug will be made this year.

Better than tamoxifen?

The largest breast cancer treatment study to date finds that women taking anastrozole (Arimidex) were less than half as likely as those taking tamoxifen to develop a new cancer in the other breast. The study, presented in March 2002 to the European Breast Cancer Conference in Barcelona, was paid for by AstraZeneca, the manufacturer of Arimidex, and involved 9,366 postmenopausal women with early-stage breast cancer. After three years, 14 women in the Arimidex group developed a new tumour compared to 33 women in the tamoxifen group – a 58 per cent difference.

Arimidex belongs to a new class of cancer drugs called aromatase inhibitors. These drugs work by blocking the production of oestrogen in the body. (Tamoxifen works by preventing oestrogen from latching onto receptors on the surface of cancer cells.) Some doctors think that aromatase inhibitors could eventually replace tamoxifen as the drug most commonly used to prevent cancer recurrence.

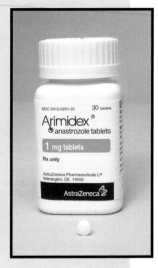

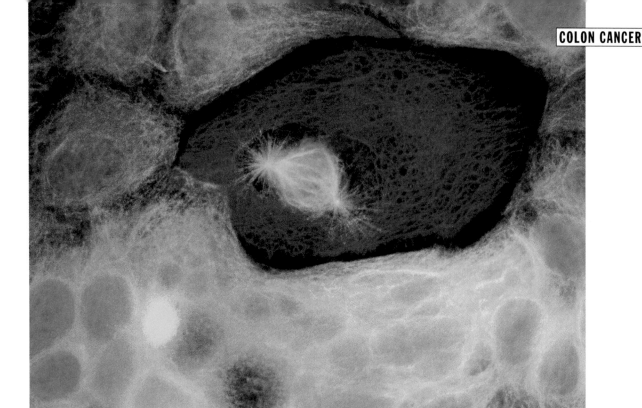

▲ In this immunofluorescent light micrograph of human colon cancer cells, the large nuclei (stained blue) are actively engaged in the rapid cell division characteristic of cancer cells.

Diagnostic advance

Painless test for colon cancer

While everyone agrees that detecting colon cancer early is the key to its cure, the means of detecting it – colonoscopy, sigmoidoscopy, and barium enemas can be uncomfortable and painful. Now, however, researchers at Howard Hughes Medical Institute in Chevy Chase, Maryland in the USA, have developed a technique that can test stool samples for a gene that triggers colon cancer.

How it works The APC gene, discovered in 1991, is a tumour suppressor gene, which inhibits the tendency of the genetic code in some cells to mutate and turn into cancer. When something goes wrong with the APC gene, cells have free rein to become cancerous. The new test spots cancer-causing mutations in this gene. 'These mutations initiate the cancer, so they're present in every cancer cell from the beginning,' says institute investigator Dr. Bert Vogelstein, senior author of a study on the test published in January 2002 in the *New England Journal of Medicine*.

Dr. Vogelstein and other scientists worked out a way to isolate human DNA from stool samples. They then developed a new analytical method, called 'digital protein truncation' which could identify the APC mutations. The process, says Dr. Vogelstein, was the equivalent of looking for the proverbial needle in a haystack. But separating the 'haystack' into smaller and smaller mounds made finding the 'needle' that much easier.

Using the test, scientists detected the APC mutations in 61 per cent of people with colorectal cancer, half of those with benign tumours (adenomas), and none in healthy people. With more testing, researchers think they can probably increase the test's sensitivity to at least 70 per cent. The best part is that there are no false-positives (detecting cancer when there is none), a mistake that leads to unnecessary testing and anxiety for the patient.

Availability Dr. Vogelstein and his colleagues are planning larger studies and hope that the test can be considered for potential clinical use in the near future. It could be used in conjunction with another test that will be available in the USA in 2003. Developed by Exact Sciences, that test searches stool samples for mutations in three genes that are commonly found in colon cancer.

147

High-tech help
Promising drugs rob tumours of blood supply

After years of anticipation, the promise of angiogenesis inhibitors – drugs that destroy a tumour's blood supply – is being realized at last. Interestingly these include thalidomide; it was precisely this ability to prevent the growth of blood vessels that resulted in the tragedy of thousands of deformed babies when the drug was used in the Sixties to treat morning sickness.

Thalidomide is already being used in the USA to treat multiple myeloma and, together with other angiogenesis inhibitors, is the subject of studies in the UK and across the world from Italy to Japan.

Among the most promising of these drugs is angiostatin. Results from one of its first clinical studies, presented at the May 2002 American Society of Clinical Oncology meeting, showed it is safe for patients with advanced cancers who are also undergoing radiation therapy. The small study, involving 20 patients, also found that most responded to the treatment; their tumours either stopped growing temporarily, while they received the drug, or regressed in size.

Another study reported at the meeting found that the drug was also safe for women with advanced breast cancer. They experienced less pain, were able to use less pain medication and required fewer blood transfusions while taking angiostatin, compared to women not taking it.

Much earlier, in May 1998, in a front-page *New York Times* article, Nobel laureate James Watson (famous, along with Francis Crick, for the discovery of the double-helix structure of DNA in 1953) had been quoted as saying that Boston researcher Judah Folkman would 'cure' cancer within two years. Watson was referring to Folkman's work with angiostatin and another such drug, endostatin. Stock in EntreMed, the company testing the drugs, skyrocketed, and a media frenzy ensued.

How to starve a tumour

For small cancerous tumours to grow and spread, they need their own blood supply. Towards that end, tumours release a signalling molecule that stimulates the growth of new blood vessels. As these new vessels proliferate, the tumour thrives. Angiogenesis inhibitors block the growth of these vessels, starving the tumour.

Small localized tumour

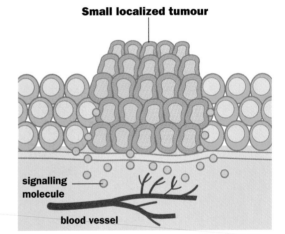

signalling molecule

blood vessel

Angiogenesis

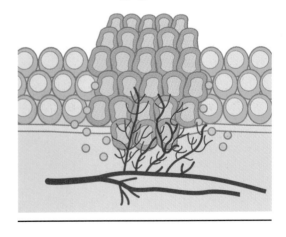

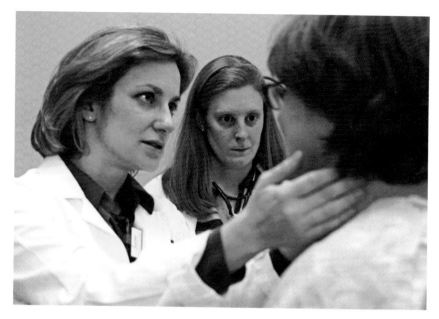

◀ Dr. Nevena Damjanov (left) examines a patient undergoing treatment. Dr. Damjanov is involved in the clinical testing of angiogenesis inhibitors.

While these medications don't directly kill a cancer, 'if we can stop tumour growth, we can stop a cancer from killing you' says Dr. Damjanov.

Watson protested that he'd been misquoted and stories began to appear about the preliminary nature of the research, which, up to that point, had involved only laboratory animals.

The story dropped off the front page, but the research continued and at least 15 angiogenesis inhibitors, including angiostatin and endostatin, are now in clinical trials in the USA and are being studied closely elsewhere.

How it works 'All tumours grow to a very small size by getting their blood supply from outside the tumour,' says Dr. Nevena Damjanov, an oncologist at the Fox Chase-Temple Cancer Center in Philadelphia. After that, they have to create their own blood supply by growing blood vessels, a process called angiogenesis. Drugs like angiostatin, and thalidomide, kill those blood vessels, effectively starving the tumours.

Angiostatin activates increased levels of a 'death receptor' on blood vessel cells, triggering cell suicide. Another drug called CAI prevents calcium ions from entering blood vessel cells, which suppresses vessel growth. While these medications don't directly kill the cancer, says Dr. Damjanov, 'if we can stop tumour growth, we can stop a cancer from killing you.'

Availability Angiogenesis inhibitors are being tested for use against a variety of cancers. but most are in early trials and will not be available for some years. Nor are they safe for everyone. Because they arrest all blood vessel growth in the body, they could be dangerous to people with coronary artery disease or other conditions that require blood vessel growth.

RESEARCH ROUND-UP

AIDS drugs may be effective for cancer

The class of AIDS drugs known as protease inhibitors may find a new role as a cancer treatment – one less toxic than chemotherapy – if early trials in mice prove relevant for humans. Protease inhibitors block protease enzymes, which play a role in tumour growth and angiogenesis (the process by which tumours create their blood supply system). Italian researchers thought that protease inhibitors might prove beneficial in cancer treatment because people with AIDS who took these drugs were much less likely to develop a form of AIDS-related cancer called Kaposi's sarcoma (KS). When researchers tested two protease inhibitors in mice with KS, the drugs kept the lesions at bay. The researchers reported their results in the March 2002 issue of the journal *Nature Medicine*.

Key discovery
Chemo at home – possibilities grow

A growing number of chemotherapy drugs – including tamoxifen and imatinib mesilate (Glivec) – are now available in pill form, opening the door to home chemotherapy. Changes in the molecular structure of the drugs and the development of drugs that metabolize slowly made these pill versions possible.

Although in the UK home chemotherapy is currently confined to a few private 'intravenous access' companies and a handful of nurse-led NHS projects, there is evidence that its safety and acceptability are growing. In the USA it is much more popular and there are government moves there to make it affordable for those who do not have adequate medical insurance coverage.

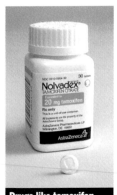

Drugs like tamoxifen, now available in pill form, permit chemotherapy at home.

Home chemotherapy can benefit patients and carers, according to a study published in the *British Medical Journal* (BMJ) in July 2001. It found that men and women with colorectal cancer who received the treatment at home stayed on the chemotherapy longer than those who received treatment at an outpatient clinic. Of those who went to the clinic, 14 per cent dropped out of the treatment, compared to only 2 per cent of the home care group. The latter group also reported higher levels of satisfaction with their care.

'Home care probably allowed the nurses to establish a better relationship with patients,' the researchers conclude. And, of course, it's only natural that patients would feel more secure and at ease in their own homes versus a clinical setting.

In the same issue of the *BMJ* an editorial highlighted the psychological benefits to both patients and carers that have emerged from other trials. The increasing availability of the drugs in pill form could, in some cases, make home treatment even more feasible, though the *BMJ* editorial suggests that further research on patient selection and the cost effectiveness of such a service is required.

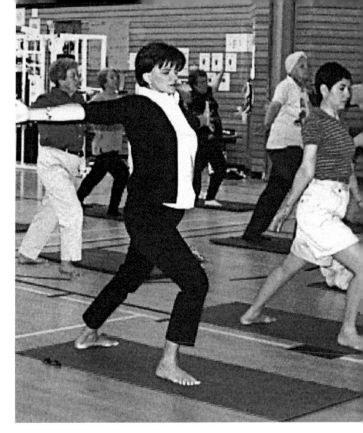

Key discovery
To boost immune system, give peace a chance

Sitting calmly and focusing on the moment at hand, a process called mindfulness meditation, can provide a host of psychological and physical benefits. They include lowering blood pressure, reducing anxiety, depression and stress, and even helping infertile couples conceive. Canadian researchers are now exploring its benefits for cancer patients.

Researchers at the University of Calgary enrolled 59 men and women with prostate or breast cancer in an eight-week mindfulness meditation training course and asked them to spend at least 45 minutes a day on a combination of meditation and yoga. Although final results aren't yet in, the researchers found interesting immune-system changes, says lead researcher Linda E. Carlson, Ph.D., assistant professor of psychosocial oncology. There was a noticeable change in the levels of cytokines (chemical messengers that immune cells secrete in small amounts to communicate with other

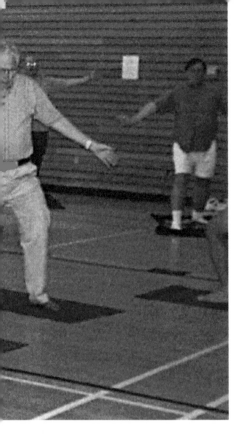

◄ A yoga class for cancer patients led by Dr. Linda Carlson, who also sits with her groups in mindfulness meditation sessions.

cells), suggesting that meditation can affect the immune system in some way. The researchers still don't know what this means to individuals with cancer.

'This is an interesting preliminary finding because no one has ever looked at the effect of meditation on the immune system in people with cancer,' says Dr. Carlson. She also notes that high levels of pro-inflammatory cytokines are typically associated with depression, so meditation may be helping with mood. Dr. Carlson is also measuring levels of stress hormones and blood pressure, and hopes to see changes there, too. Her findings are to be published in the journal *Psychosomatic Medicine* this year.

Mindfulness meditation uses the concept of moment-to-moment awareness to help you simply *be* where you are, rather than thinking about the past or future. People are taught to focus on their breathing to help them to achieve a calming sense of detachment from thoughts and emotions.

Earlier studies at the university found that people with cancer who participated in a mindfulness meditation-based stress reduction programme significantly improved in terms of overall mood and symptoms of stress; the greatest improvements involved the relief of depression, anxiety and anger. 'This is striking,' notes Dr. Carlson, 'since these are among the most frequently reported psychological symptoms that cancer patients identify as problems.' As one patient said, 'In times of pain, when the future is too terrifying to contemplate and the past too painful to remember, I have learned to pay attention to right now.'

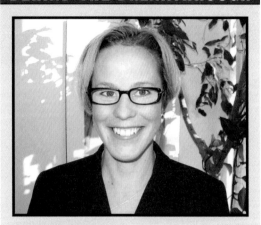

BEHIND THE BREAKTHROUGH

She practises what she preaches

Every morning, Dr. Linda E. Carlson meditates for 30 minutes – at work. It's part of her job, since she runs a daily meditation session for the staff at University of Calgary's division of psychosocial oncology.

Dr. Carlson began to meditate and practise yoga as a graduate student, when a classmate and former Buddhist monk introduced her to the disciplines. But she never expected it would become such a large part of her professional life. An internship at Calgary in 1997 changed all that. 'They were doing meditation with cancer patients a couple of days a week. I thought, "This is great!" I'd always wanted to find out how to incorporate meditation into the clinical side of things,' she says.

Today, she's a full-time faculty member, funded by the Canadian Institutes of Health Research New Investigator Award for the next five years. Her mission: to explore the clinical side of meditation with cancer patients. It's an area the doctors at the centre had little time to pursue, but because 70 per cent of Dr. Carlson's time is protected for research, she can design and run studies such as the one examining immune function and meditation.

Her involvement transcends science, however. She also instituted weekly drop-in meditation classes for cancer patients, increased the number of overall classes, and added a Saturday morning silent retreat.

'For a lot of people, it's a whole change in their perspective and priorities and the way they look at life,' says Dr. Carlson of the classes. 'They learn patience, acceptance, and how to let go. It's a very different approach from the conventional way people tend to go about things in the world.'

Key discovery

Cord blood best for stem-cell transplants

Often used as a cancer treatment, stem-cell transplantation involves a host of potential problems. First, chemotherapy drugs kill off the patient's bone marrow, leaving a barely viable immune system that can't protect against even the most trivial infection. Doctors then must find donors whose tissue type matches that of the recipient, and transplant donor stem cells to create new bone marrow. They can use stem cells that come from either bone marrow or from cord blood (the blood remaining in the umbilical cord after a baby's birth). According to a new study, that choice makes a difference.

A danger of stem-cell transplantation is the possibility of graft-versus-host disease (GVHD), in which the transplanted cells perceive the patient's body as foreign and begin attacking it. This is basically the opposite of organ transplant rejection, in which the body senses the new organ as the foreign invader.

One of the first large-scale studies to look at both bone marrow and cord blood stem cells found that cord blood transplants produce less GVHD. They also seem to 'take' more slowly, which in theory could lead to a higher failure rate. Yet in this study, presented in December 2001 at the annual meeting of the American Society of Hematology, researchers found no overall differences in the survival rates between cord blood and bone marrow transplants.

A major advantage to using cord blood is the potential for greater availability. If doctors would obtain cord blood for storage at more births, there would be a good supply of stem cells, says study author Dr. Mary Horowitz, professor of neoplastic diseases and scientific director of the International Bone Marrow Transplant Registry at the Medical College of Wisconsin. The sheer number of cord blood stem cells would then improve the odds of finding a match.

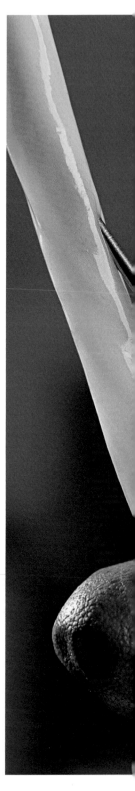

SHOULD YOU BANK YOUR BABY'S CORD BLOOD?

The full-colour brochures know just which heartstrings to tug. 'Think of the Future.' 'Protect Your Unborn Child.' Which parents-to-be could resist?

And so in the USA a growing number of couples are banking their babies' cord blood in case their children ever require stem-cell transplants. In the UK too, there is one private company, Cryo-care, that offers couples, for around £1,000, the opportunity to store their baby's cord stem cells for 20 years in case the baby or its siblings develop an illness that could be treated by cord blood transplantation.

The commercial move has provoked criticism from the Royal College of Obstetricians and Gynaecologists. And In

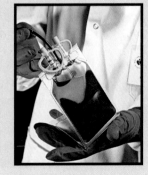

the USA, medical experts point out that unless there's a family history of genetic diseases, such as severe anaemia, immune disorders or some cancers, there's only a one in 10,000 chance of ever needing a stem-cell transplant. Parents there are urged instead to donate their babies' cord blood to a public bank, so that it will be available to any appropriately matched person.

Some NHS hospitals now collect cord blood with the informed consent of parents, says John Toy, medical director of Cancer Research UK, who was also wary of the new private initiative and 'nervous that parents might be exploited at a time when they are emotionally buoyed'.

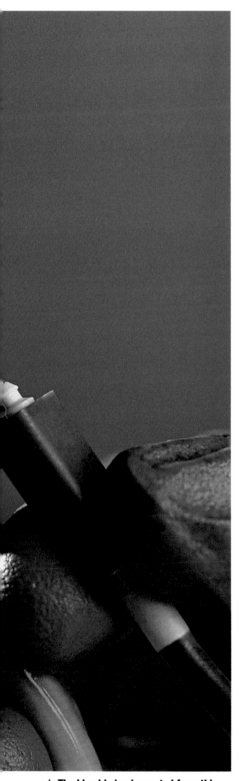

▲ The blood being harvested from this umbilical cord is rich in stem cells, which can be used to treat a variety of diseases, such as leukaemia. It will be stored in liquid nitrogen until it's needed.

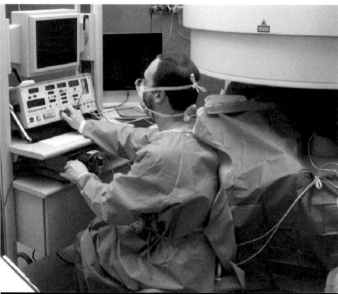

A physician uses radiofrequency ablation to 'cook' part of a tumour, killing cells.

High-tech help
Radio technology blasts away kidney cancer

D octors in the USA are experimenting with radio waves to blast away kidney tumours, which have traditionally been treated by surgery to remove part or all of the kidney. The procedure, called radiofrequency ablation – uses high frequency radio waves to essentially 'boil' tumours to death. Researchers and doctors from the Research Institute at University Hospitals of Cleveland and Case Western Reserve University in Cleveland reported promising results using this technique at the November 2001 annual meeting of the Radiological Society of North America. Their findings were so positive, they said, that radiofrequency ablation may become a first-choice treatment for all kidney cancers.

How it works Radiofrequency energy is fed to the tumour through a small needle with an electrode on its tip. The doctor inserts the needle directly into the tumour through the skin, using images from magnetic resonance imaging as a guide. After 10 to 30 minutes of contact with the tumour, the radiofrequency energy 'cooks' a part of the tumour, killing the cells. If necessary, the needle can then be moved to another section of the tumour. The dead cells eventually shrink and are absorbed by the body.

The patient needs only to be lightly sedated and no hospital stay is required. In the Cleveland study, the procedure completely destroyed the tumours in 10 of 11 people, and in only one did a tumour recur.

High-tech help
New oral cancer test comes to light

A new product is shedding light on oral cancer. In February 2002, the US company Zila Professional Pharmaceuticals acquired world marketing rights to ViziLite, a kit that costs $15 (£9.50) in the USA and can help dentists and oral surgeons diagnose oral cancer more definitively. After the patient rinses with a special solution, the dentist shines a small light in the person's mouth for about 10 minutes. Normal cells absorb the light's wavelengths and abnormal cells reflect them, causing them to appear bright white. ViziLite was approved in the USA in 2001 but is not yet available in the UK.

In Britain, another test made by Zila that can detect precancerous oral lesions, invisible not only to the naked eye but even under a microscope, has been approved since 2000 and is available under the dental insurance Denplan. OraTest, which is already distributed in more than a dozen countries, uses a dye called toluidine blue. When used as a mouth rinse, the dye stains the precancerous cells blue.

Cancer in the mouth and throat afflicts 3,500 people each year in the UK, eventually killing about half this number. There are about 45 new cases per million of the population each year in England, and twice that number in Scotland. Five-year survival rates in the UK are just under 50 per cent and dentists are commited to improving this figure. Tobacco users and heavy drinkers are at increased risk for oral cancer.

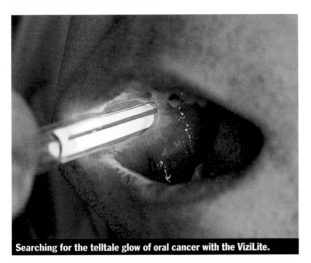

Searching for the telltale glow of oral cancer with the ViziLite.

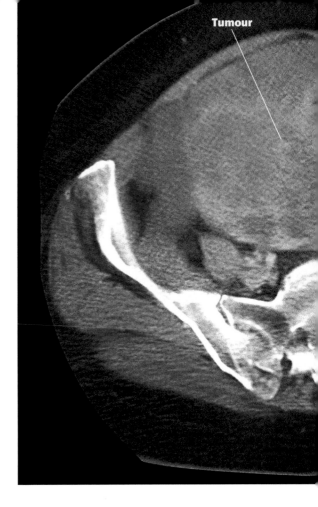

Tumour

Drug development
New weapon in war on ovarian cancer

There is rarely good news concerning ovarian cancer, which in the UK accounts for some 5 per cent of all female cancers with some 7,000 cases annually. Most occur in women over the age of 50, but the disease can affect younger women as well. Survival is typically just 30 months after diagnosis because disease is usually advanced before signs appear. But an experimental drug is cause for new hope. Called oregovomab (OvaRex), the drug, made from mouse antibodies, targets a protein produced by most ovarian cancers.

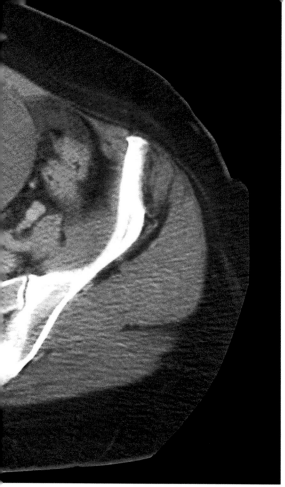

▲ A large ovarian tumour is revealed on a cross-sectional MRI scan of a woman's abdomen.

RESEARCH ROUND-UP

Chemo cocktail for ovarian cancer

Sometimes you just have to see old favourites in a new light to appreciate their worth. That's what researchers at the Rotterdam Cancer Institute in the Netherlands found when they combined two drugs already used to treat other types of cancers, and gave the mixture to women with ovarian cancer. Ninety-eight women received the chemotherapy drugs cisplatin and etoposide. Nearly 80 per cent improved and all signs of the cancer disappeared in more than half of the women. Researchers told the Reuters news agency in January 2002 that, although they were worried that the women would be too ill to cope with the treatment because of the advanced state of their disease, 'they suffered relatively few side effects'.

The quest for screening tests

Whatever the stage of the disease, women who have ovarian cancer have elevated levels of a protein called osteopontin, according to researchers from several Boston hospitals. The finding, published last April in the *Journal of the American Medical Association*, paves the way for a screening test to identify the disease in its earliest stages. Combined with tests for other protein markers for the disease, including prostasin, an osteopontin test could be nearly 100 per cent effective.

How it works OvaRex was initially developed to help diagnose rather than to treat ovarian cancer, explains Dr. Alan Gordon, director of gynaecologic oncology research for US Oncology at the Sammons Cancer Center of Baylor University Hospital in Dallas. The drug is an antibody to CA-125, a protein on the surface of many ovarian cancer cells. It was intended to 'tag' the protein and show up on a nuclear medicine scan.

'What happened then was that the patients who were given the antibody to CA-125 in an effort to visualize the tumours actually did better than you would have expected them to do,' Dr. Gordon says. In other words, these late-stage cancer patients were living longer than expected. Immediately, the experiments with oregovomab took on a whole new mission.

Researchers think the drug acts as a vaccine to stimulate the immune system to fight off the cancer. It does this by attaching itself to the cancer. Because OvaRex is a mouse antibody, the immune system readily recognizes it as foreign, so it mounts a strong attack against the drug – and the cancer. OvaRex also appears to work even when given in combination with chemotherapy drugs. Initially, says Dr. Gordon, researchers worried that if they made the immune system stronger, it would effectively fight off the chemotherapy drugs. But that doesn't seem to be happening. And, since the drug has no side effects (beyond an occasional allergic reaction), it's safe to give to every woman with ovarian cancer in order to identify those in whom it works best.

'I can give a woman something that may be effective and not have any problems and that has a chance for helping her,' says Dr. Gordon. 'That's wonderful.'

Availability OvaRex has undergone clinical trials in the USA and could be approved in 2005. In Europe, trials are also due to begin soon.

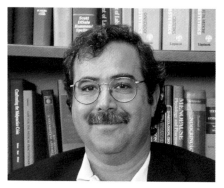

▲ Dr. Alan Gordon of the Sammons Cancer Center, whose research with oregovomab (OvaRex) may pave the way for new therapies for ovarian cancer.

Diagnostic advance

Scientists 'fingerprint' ovarian cancer for easy identification

When ovarian cancer is caught early, it's highly treatable. But usually the disease remains hidden; by the time it's diagnosed, chances of survival are quite slim. Enter the new science of proteomics, the study of the proteins that govern every biological process in the body. (See related article on page 16.) It's being used to 'fingerprint' cancers so that they may one day be diagnosed, at their earliest stages, from just a few drops of blood. Scientists have already fingerprinted ovarian cancer and shown that computers can use that fingerprint to correctly identify stage one ovarian cancer.

The results were reported in the February 2002 electronic version of the British medical journal *The Lancet*. The paper was written by Dr. Lance Liotta, Ph.D., of the National Cancer Institute (NCI), and Dr. Emanuel Petricoin, of the US Food and Drug Administration (FDA). Their work presents cancer researchers with an entirely new paradigm, says Dr. Petricoin. Instead of focusing on one biomarker

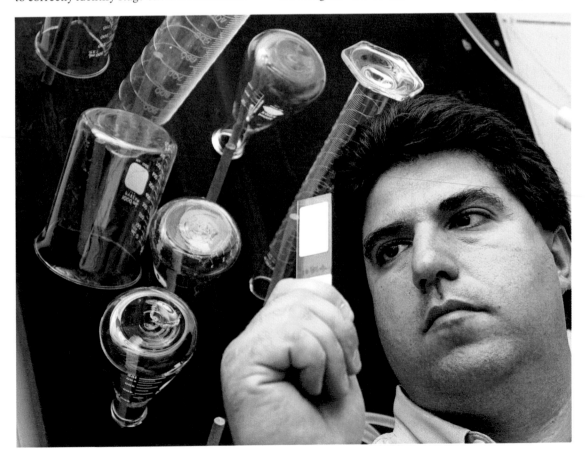

▼ Government scientist Dr. Emanuel Petricoin ponders the unique protein pattern of a specific type of cancer in a laboratory at the National Institutes of Health in Bethesda, Maryland.

The researchers and computer correctly identified 50 out of 50 ovarian cancers and 63 out of 66 non-cancers.

for cancer – for example, the blood protein marker CA-125 for ovarian cancer or the PSA (prostate specific antigen) marker for prostate cancer – researchers can now examine multiple patterns of proteins in the blood, looking for a match.

How it works The scientists examined blood samples taken from women with and without ovarian cancer to establish the protein patterns – specifically, the unique arrangement of amino acids that make up each type of protein – which indicate ovarian cancer. Once they had 'fingerprinted' the patterns of protein common to ovarian cancer, they then tested a computer's ability to detect these patterns (and thus the cancer) from blood samples taken from another set of people with and without cancer. The result: the researchers (and computer) correctly identified 50 out of 50 ovarian cancers and 63 out of 66 non-cancer samples. The researchers are exploring the use of this technology in prostate cancer too, and plan to focus eventually on the more common tumours such as breast, colon, and lung.

The technology can do more than simply diagnose early cancers. One clinical trial currently underway is testing whether it can reliably detect a recurrence of ovarian cancer before any symptoms appear. More than 80 per cent of ovarian cancers reappear after treatment. 'A simple test that identifies the presence of a recurrence of the tumour would be a valuable clinical tool,' says Dr. Elise Kohn, of the pathology laboratory at NCI, the lead researcher on the clinical trial.

Availability Although proteomics is still in its infancy, the science is expected to advance very quickly. Still, in terms of practical applications, it may be years before it can be used routinely for diagnostic testing and treatment. And, according to Drs. Petricoin and Liotta, it will most likely be used in conjunction with – but will not replace – existing technologies, such as diagnostic imaging, biopsies, and other conventional tests.

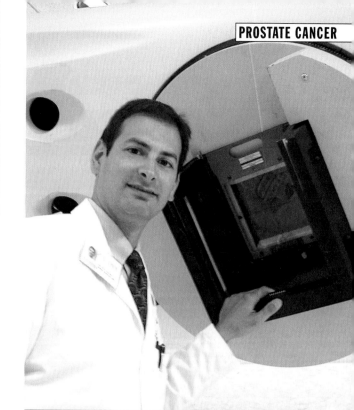

Dr. Horwitz, of Fox Chase Cancer Center, demonstrates the linear accelerator that can irradiate tumours with pinpoint accuracy.

High-tech help
Zapping prostate tumours with unprecedented precision

Part of the problem of radiation therapy used to treat prostate cancer is that a few stray beams may hit the bladder or penis, possibly causing incontinence or impotence. To discover a way to deliver radiation within a hair's breadth of the tumour would be a breakthrough indeed.

That's what doctors at a few cancer centres around the USA are now able to do by using a highly sophisticated technology called Intensity Modulated Radiation Therapy (IMRT), which is currently being evaluated in the UK as well.

How it works By using a complex computer programme in combination with a high-tech linear accelerator (a machine that delivers radiation), radiologists can now send 60 to 80 pencil-thin beams of radiation directly into a specific point of the prostate, avoiding the nearby bladder, rectum and sexual organs. The strength of the beams can be adjusted so that the dose is strongest where the tumour is thickest, and weakest near healthy tissue, minimizing the risk of damage to the healthy tissue.

'Tumours are not perfectly round,' says Dr. Eric Horwitz, associate professor in the department of radiation oncology at Fox Chase Cancer Center in Philadelphia. 'They come in all sizes, shapes and thicknesses and sometimes they intertwine with organs, making them a challenge to destroy with radiation. We precisely calibrate the computers and equipment so that we can reach the target with minimal interference to other organs.'

Studies presented at the American Society for Therapeutic Radiation and Oncology meeting in November 2001 found that patients experienced fewer side effects when treated with IMRT than they did when treated with an alternative type of radiation delivery method, called 3-Dimensional Conformal Radiation Therapy, or 3-DCRT.

One caveat: cancer experts note that treating a smaller area of tissue could make the cancer more likely to return. This could happen if undetected microscopic tendrils from the main tumour had reached out beyond the treated area.

Availability Because the complex equipment used to generate the radiation beams is so costly, only a few large US medical centres currently offer the therapy. And in Britain it has not yet undergone all the necessary clinical trials. But some US experts predict it could become standard treatment for prostate cancer within a few years.

Careful with that radiation beam

This cross-sectional CT scan shows the close proximity of the prostate to neighbouring organs like the bladder and rectum, and the nerves that govern urination and sexual function.

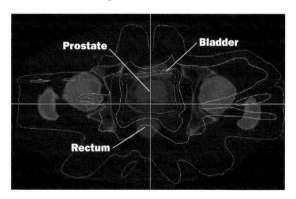

Prostate · Bladder · Rectum

High-tech help
Test may take guesswork out of spotting melanoma

It's scary to think that diagnosing one of the deadliest cancers around is often a guessing game. But that's true of melanoma, an often-fatal form of skin cancer that is responsible for 80 per cent of skin cancer deaths.

'It's subjective,' says Dr. Rhoda Alani, assistant professor of oncology, dermatology, molecular biology and genetics at Johns Hopkins Medical School in Baltimore, USA. No test is available to tell if the growth is in fact cancer. So pathologists generally err on the side of caution and say the sample is cancerous, resulting in surgery, the only treatment for melanoma. 'That's good in that you're saving people's lives,' says Dr. Alani. 'However, you're also subjecting them to something that's not a trivial surgery.'

Dr. Alani and her colleagues now think they may have found a genetic marker that can provide a definitive diagnosis.

Irregular borders and colouring are typical of melanoma.

How it works The researchers discovered that a protein that is produced by the Id1 gene acts like a switch, turning off a tumour suppressor gene and thus allowing cancer cells to grow unchecked. The researchers published their findings in two journals in 2001, including the August issue of *Cancer Research*. Even better, notes Dr. Alani, the Id1 protein is expressed at very early stages in the cancer, before it becomes invasive and while the odds of treating it successfully are at their best.

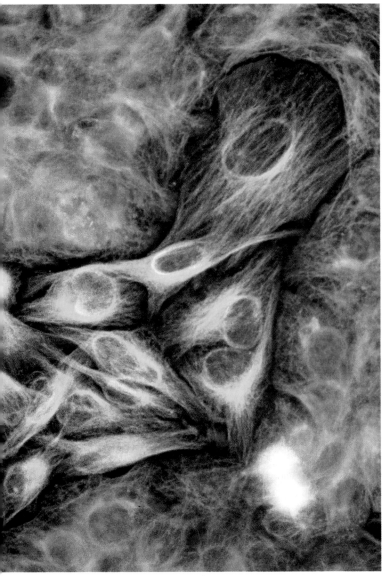

'The hope is that if this turns out to be true, each time someone takes out tissue they think is cancerous, they'll send it off to be tested for the expression of this gene. If it's positive, we'll treat it as cancer and take out more tissue,' she says. 'If it's negative, we'll just say it's an irregular mole so we don't need to do more surgery.'

▲ An immunofluorescent light micrograph showing melanoma cells (orange) invading normal skin cells (green). Melanoma cells divide and grow much faster than healthy tissue.

Availability Dr. Alani and her associates have been working to find a simple and reliable way to test for the gene – one that could be used by small labs in doctors' surgeries as well as in academic centres. Once they develop such a test, they plan to examine thousands of melanoma samples to see if the gene expression is consistent. Ideally, she says, the test could be in US pathology labs within two years.

Take action

Life-saving strategies for skin cancer

Cases of melanoma have doubled in the UK in the past 30 years; around 5,700 cases are now diagnosed each year. Though most common in people aged 40-60, it is the third most common cancer in women under 35 and the fifth in men under 35. Yet it can be easily prevented with a few simple steps that most people ignore.

1 Stay out of the sun in the heat of the day. If you can't, wear a broad-brimmed hat and sunglasses with ultraviolet (UV) light protection.

2 Don't assume sunscreen will protect you. While it does guard against sunburn and premature wrinkling, it may not stave off melanoma and shouldn't be your sole line of defence. When you use it, use it correctly. Apply it liberally, reapply it often, and put it on at least 15 minutes before you go outside.

3 If you're prone to freckles, sunburn easily or have light-coloured hair or eyes, keep sun exposure to a minimum and examine your skin regularly for signs of any mole that's changed size or shape. If you find one, ask your doctor for advice.

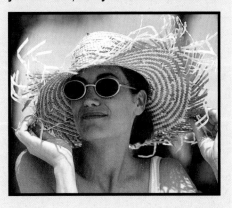

ALSO IN THE NEWS

Drug may prevent lung cancer

Everyone knows that quitting smoking is the best thing you can do to prevent lung cancer. But if you smoked for any length of time, your lungs still took a beating – and you're still more likely to get lung cancer than someone who never smoked. That's why it's so exciting that a drug called anetholtrithione (Sialor, Sulfarlem), commonly used to treat dry mouth, appears to prevent pre-cancerous lung tissue from developing into full-blown cancer. For six months, researchers at the University of British Columbia in Vancouver kept track of 101 current and former smokers who were diagnosed with a pre-cancerous condition called bronchial dysplasia. Anetholtrithione slowed the rate at which the pre-cancerous condition turned into cancer by 22 per cent compared to a placebo (dummy pill). The drug, not currently available in the United States or the UK, is widely used in Canada and continental Europe.

Instant test for bladder cancer

Most visits to the doctor include providing a urine sample. Soon, that simple act may be all that's required to identify bladder cancer – even before you leave the surgery. Currently, tests for bladder cancer take several days to yield results. But the NMP22 BladderChek test, approved in Britain and the USA in August 2002, provides immediate answers. It works much like a home pregnancy test. A technician puts four drops of urine on a small disc, and the resulting lines indicate whether you have bladder cancer. The test detects certain proteins that are elevated in bladder cancer cells and released into the urine. Approximately 125,000 new cases

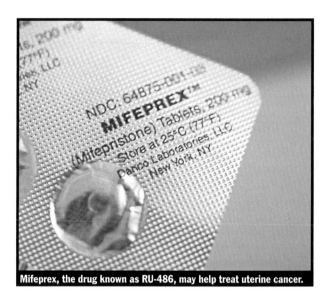

Mifeprex, the drug known as RU-486, may help treat uterine cancer.

of bladder cancer are diagnosed worldwide each year. If the disease is caught in its early stages, the five-year survival rate is 90 per cent.

Treatment for endometrial cancer

The controversial drug mifepristone, commonly referred to as RU-486 or 'the morning-after pill,' has been used to help abort a foetus in the very early stages of pregnancy. But the drug may also have a use as a treatment for endometrial cancer, which involves the lining of the uterus. It is the fifth most common cancer in women in the UK with more than 4,800 cases diagnosed each year. In 2002, M.D. Anderson Cancer Center in Houston, Texas launched the first clinical trial in the United States to study mifepristone in women with endometrial cancer. Because the drug blocks the action of the hormone progesterone (which causes the uterine lining to grow), researchers hope that it will slow tumour growth. Mifepristone has already shown promise in shrinking uterine fibroids and treating endometriosis. In some small trials, it also has shown promise against ovarian and metastatic breast cancer.

New approach to gastrinoma

Gastrinoma is a rare tumour, usually in the pancreas, that secretes excess amounts of the hormone gastrin. This causes Zollinger-Ellison syndrome, a disorder involving severe peptic ulcers. Current treatments are not very effective. But a recent study found that the drug octreotide (Sandostatin), used to treat the severe diarrhoea and other symptoms that occur in conjunction with certain intestinal

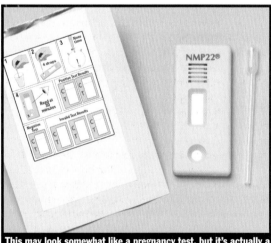

This may look somewhat like a pregnancy test, but it's actually a simple urine test for bladder cancer.

In one study of Glivec, tumours shrank in more than three-quarters of all cases, and more than half the tumours shrank at least 50 per cent.

tumours, may shrink the tumour or slow its growth. The study followed 15 men and women with malignant gastrinoma who received octreotide every 12 hours before they were placed on a long-acting form of the drug. Tumours in 8 of the 15 responded; seven tumours stabilized and one decreased in size. The authors suggest that octreotide treatment should replace chemotherapy as the standard treatment.

New hope for liver cancer patients

A new US treatment for inoperable liver cancer shows exceptional promise. The non-surgical outpatient procedure called TheraSphere delivers millions of microscopic radiation-imbedded glass beads into the main artery leading into the liver through a catheter placed in the femoral artery in the thigh. Patients can return home the same day. The beads, one-third the diameter of a human hair, remain in the body and lose their radiation in two weeks. Generally, people diagnosed with primary liver cancer live an average of four months after diagnosis without surgery. But the 16 patients treated with TheraSphere during a

Glivec (Gleevec in the USA) is exciting cancer researchers both sides of the Atlantic as studies have produced dramatic results.

study at the University of Maryland's Greenebaum Cancer Center, in Baltimore, survived an average of eight months. 'We expect that more than 40 per cent will still be alive a year after treatment,' says Dr. Ravi Murthy, an interventional radiologist and member of the pioneer research team. The treatment is also being used for colon cancer.

More uses for Glivec

Licensed in the UK for the treatment of chronic myeloid leukaemia in November 2001, shortly after its approval in Europe, imatinib mesilate (Glivec) has been hailed as a breakthrough cancer drug. Now, reports about its possible use in numerous other cancers are emerging. In July 2002, Glivec was also licensed here for the treatment of inoperable and malignant gastrointestinal stromal tumours, or GISTs, rare intestinal cancers that are virtually untreatable when advanced. In one large-scale US study of Glivec in people with GISTs, tumours shrank significantly in more than three-quarters of all cases, and more than half the tumours shrank by at least 50 per cent. Clinical trials are now under way in the USA to test Glivec against cancers of the brain, lungs, breast, prostate and abdomen. But there have also been reports that some leukemia patients have become resistant to the drug after taking it daily for about a year, suggesting that it may need to be combined with other medications to do most good.

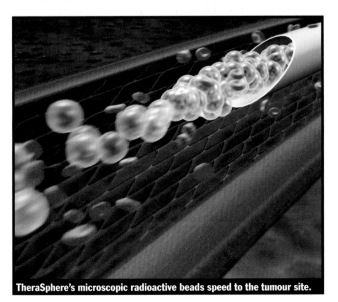

TheraSphere's microscopic radioactive beads speed to the tumour site.

DIGESTION AND METABOLISM

Do you eat live yoghurt? Maybe you should. New evidence shows that probiotics – the 'living drugs' in fermented foods and supplements – can boost the immune system, reduce diarrhoea in infants, and stem some of the complications of inflammatory bowel disease. For people with Crohn's disease, a new drug offers the relief of traditional steroids without the steroid side effects. And scientists have pinpointed one of the genetic mutations that causes Crohn's, paving the way to better treatments.

Do you take insulin for diabetes? You've probably heard about insulin pumps that give people a break from injections. Now there's a new and improved pump you can even wear in the water. Further good news for diabetics – scientists have developed an experimental protein that boosts natural insulin levels in people with Type 1 diabetes. Finally, there's welcome relief for haemorrhoid sufferers – a new surgical technique eliminates the problem with a lot less pain than traditional procedures.

Key discovery

Crohn's mystery solved — flawed gene blamed

Crohn's disease is an intestinal inflammation that rages and recedes with maddening unpredictability. The cause has always been a mystery – but the recent discovery of a genetic mutation will eventually permit doctors to test for the disease. The discovery may also pave the way for better treatments.

How it works Two teams of researchers, working independently, found that 16 per cent of Crohn's patients have a 'mistake' on a gene called Nod-2. People who have one flawed copy of Nod-2 are 50 per cent more likely to develop Crohn's than those with the normal gene. Those with two flawed copies are 17 times more likely to get it.

The Nod-2 gene controls a protein that helps specialized immune cells called monocytes recognize bacteria in the body. In some people with Crohn's, proteins produced by the flawed gene are about 3 per cent smaller than they should be. This tiny difference causes monocytes to miss their bacterial targets when they go into battle. Another part of the immune system steps in as back-up, but it strikes with too much force. The result is intense inflammation and devastating tissue damage.

Since the flawed gene occurs in only about 15 per cent of Crohn's patients, other genetic mutations are probably also involved in the disease. This may explain why the symptoms of Crohn's, such as diarrhoea, fever, and intestinal scarring, vary widely from person to person.

'Eventually, we will be able to predict how the disease will behave based on different genetic mutations,' says Dr. Samuel Meyers, clinical professor of medicine at Mount Sinai School of Medicine in New York City. 'This will allow us to customize therapy for different patients.'

Availability It will be years before the discovery of the Nod-2 gene leads to improved treatments, says Dr. Meyers. The immediate focus of research will be on identifying other Crohn's mutations and on developing practical screening tests to identify the mutation.

Typical area of Crohn's inflammation

Crohn's disease is marked by chronic inflammation that ravages the walls of the lower segment of the small intestine (ileum) or large intestine (colon), but it can affect any part of the digestive tract, from the mouth to the anus.

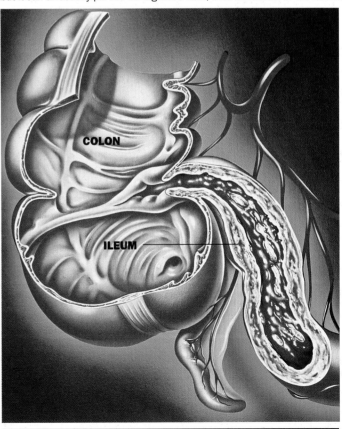

COLON

ILEUM

Drug development
A safer way to treat Crohn's

Prednisone and related drugs called corticosteroids have long been the gold standard for treating inflammatory bowel disease. Stopping inflammation is critical because it literally destroys intestinal tissues. But using prednisone could be likened to putting out a fire but tearing down the house to get to it. For although prednisone quells inflammation very quickly, the side effects, which include high blood pressure, osteoporosis and an increased risk of infections, can sometimes outweigh the benefits.

One drug, licensed in Britain in 1996 and 2001 in the USA, appears to offer the best of both worlds. Budesonide (Entocort CR) is a nonsystemic steroid, that works locally on the intestines with little impact on the rest of the body; it has the inflammation-fighting powers of prednisone but few of the side effects.

How it works Taken once daily, budesonide releases its active ingredient in the intestines. There, it quickly eliminates the inflammation that flares up during active phases of Crohn's disease, colitis and other inflammatory bowel diseases. From the small intestine, the drug is absorbed into the bloodstream and transported to the liver, which acts as the body's chemical processing plant. Unlike prednisone, however, budesonide is broken down almost immediately by the liver into inactive substances. This means that very little of the drug stays around long enough to cause systemic side effects. Five scientific studies of approximately 1,000 patients showed that budesonide provides steroid-like relief with only a fraction of the typical steroid side effects.

Budesonide also appears to block inflammation as effectively as nonsteroid drugs. In a study reported in the *New England Journal of Medicine,* 69 per cent of patients given budesonide were in remission after eight weeks, compared to 45 per cent of those taking mesalazine, a standard treatment for Crohn's.

Availability Budesonide, available on prescription, is approved for the treatment of mild to moderate Crohn's disease. Doctors have found, however, that it is sometimes effective in more severe cases – such as prior to surgery, when it may be combined with conventional steroids to reduce inflammation to the lowest possible levels.

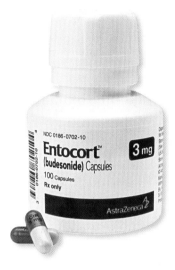

▲ A special coating protects budesonide capsules from stomach acid, so they dissolve entirely in the intestine.

RESEARCH ROUND-UP

New drugs offer some hope

A new class of medications, anti-TNF antibodies (TNF stands for 'tissue necrosis factor'), appears to reduce inflammation as well as or better than traditional treatments and may, in some cases, cause the disease to go into remission. One anti-TNF antibody, infliximab (Remicade), is already on the market but in Britain is advised only for severe active Crohn's disease as it has been associated with the development of TB and worsening of heart failure.

Another may be on the way. The British firm Celltech has announced that in 2003 the drug, called CDP 870 for now, will enter the final trials needed before it can be approved in Europe and the USA. CDP 870 carries more human antibodies than infliximab and may have fewer side effects. In earlier studies, Crohn's patients who took CDP 870 showed improvement in as little as one week.

Take action

Simple ways to reduce Crohn's symptoms

These five low-tech, non-medical, do-it-yourself techniques will help alleviate the symptoms of Crohn's disease:

■ **EAT A LOW-FAT DIET** Fatty foods may trigger diarrhoea or cramps.

■ **ADJUST DIETARY FIBRE** For some people, too much fibre makes symptoms worse. For others, too little fibre has the same effect. Make adjustments based on your individual reaction.

■ **EAT MINI-MEALS** 'Grazing' with multiple small meals is less likely to cause intestinal discomfort than fewer large meals.

■ **TAKE A MULTIVITAMIN** It helps replace nutrients that are lost because of intestinal damage.

■ **REDUCE STRESS** Stress can make Crohn's symptoms worse. Try exercise, deep breathing, or other stress-relieving techniques.

High-tech help
Go-anywhere insulin pump makes a splash

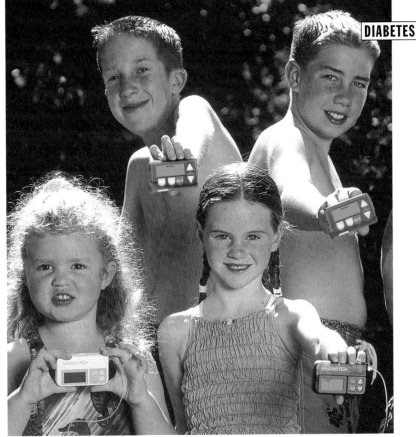

Insulin injections are a lifesaver for people with diabetes, but it's hard to love being a human pincushion two or more times a day. It can be more convenient to use an insulin pump, an electronic device that automatically delivers insulin for several days through a narrow tube. A new pager-size model that's more compact and easier to use, was introduced in the USA in February 2002 and should be available in Britain within a year or two. It's even waterproof – so users can shower or bathe without taking it off.

▲ The compact Paradigm pump is easy enough for a child to use and sturdy enough to withstand the rigours of normal activities – even swimming.

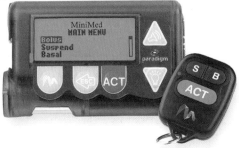

How it works Unlike injections, which deliver a full dose of insulin all at once, pumps constantly release small amounts, as the pancreas would do. By mimicking the natural flow of insulin, the pumps can help to prevent extreme blood sugar variations in between doses. They also provide very precise control, delivering insulin in amounts as small as 0.05 units. Good control is critical because glucose swings are the main cause of diabetes-related complications.

But it remains to be seen if the new device will encourage the use of pumps in Britain. In its 2001 submission to the National Institute for Clinical Excellence (NICE) requesting an appraisal of insulin pumps, Diabetes UK noted that in Britain only 0.1 per cent of patients with Type 1 diabetes use them, compared to 5 per cent in Sweden, Norway, Germany and the Netherlands. The UK reticence was initially born of safety fears in the 1980s, but the wide usage elsewhere suggests that these have now been addressed. Patients should discuss their use with their GP, says Diabetes UK, but it is aware that lack of experience of the pumps is 'a major concern for health care professionals'.

Insulin pumps are also expensive (the Paradigm costs more than £3000) but because of their ability to improve the quality of life for some patients, Diabetes UK believes they should be available here 'according to need and not ability to pay'.

RESEARCH ROUND-UP

Promising protein boosts insulin

The British medical journal *The Lancet* reports that injections of an experimental protein appear to increase natural insulin production in people with Type 1 diabetes. This could decrease their need for insulin injections. The protein also might be able to prevent the disease altogether if given early to people who are at increased risk of developing diabetes. Called DiaPep277, it causes cells to release cytokines, chemicals that make the immune system less likely to damage insulin-producing cells in the pancreas. One small study found that natural insulin levels in patients given DiaPep277 rose slightly over six months, while insulin levels fell in patients given placebos (dummy pills). If long-term studies show the protein is safe as well as effective, it could be on the market within five years.

Progress in prevention

New screening standards are set to help combat diabetes

Imagine having a bomb in your pocket and not knowing it. It's a terrifying image, and dangerously close to the truth for a million Britons and 8 to 10 million Americans with undiagnosed diabetes. About half will suffer permanent damage to nerve endings, blood vessels, or organs in the 7 to 10 years before the first symptoms appear. Now diabetes specialists in the USA are using tougher screening standards to detect the disease at the earliest possible stage. And Britain looks set to follow their lead. Caught early, diabetes can often be controlled or even reversed, with diet, exercise, and other lifestyle changes, without the lifelong need for insulin or other drugs.

How it works In the USA, people at high risk of diabetes, such as those with a family history of the disease, people who are obese or who have high blood pressure or heart disease, are now being advised to have a fasting blood glucose test at 30 instead of 45, as previously recommended. Taken after a six-hour fast, the test measures the amount of glucose per decilitre of blood. A normal reading is below 110. Anything higher suggests that diabetes may be developing. (In Britain, glucose per litre is measured, so a comparable 'normal' reading would be below 11.)

'We've found that people at the highest risk can reduce the incidence of diabetes by 58 per cent with modest lifestyle changes,' says Dr. Claresa Levetan, director of diabetes education at MedStar Health–Washington Hospital Center in Washington, D.C. 'But the only way this can happen is with early detection.'

In Britain, the UK National Screening Committee has advised the Department of Health that there is emerging evidence to suggest that it may be both clinically and cost effective to offer screening to people who have multiple risk factors for diabetes. However, definitive guidelines are unlikely to be issued until 2005. There is also currently no recommendation for an age at which those with multiple risk factors for diabetes should be screened, though it seems likely that this will be decided in 2003.

Complications of diabetes

Over time, untreated or poorly controlled diabetes can cause debilitating, even life-threatening complications. The inability of glucose to enter the body's cells literally starves and destroys the various organ systems at the cellular level, causing a host of widespread symptoms.

	PROBLEM	RESULT
Eyes	The small blood vessels of the retina (the light-sensitive membrane inside the eye) become damaged.	Decreased vision and ultimately blindness.
Blood Vessels	Atherosclerotic plaque builds up and blocks arteries that supply blood to major organs such as the heart and brain. The walls of the blood vessels become so damaged that they cannot transfer oxygen normally.	Poor circulation causes wounds to heal poorly and can lead to heart disease, stroke, gangrene of the feet and hands, impotence, and infections.
Kidneys	Blood vessels thicken and nephrons (kidney cells) are damaged. Protein leaks into urine. Blood isn't filtered normally.	Poor kidney function, which may ultimately lead to kidney failure.
Nerves	Nerves are damaged and destroyed because glucose isn't metabolized normally and blood supply is inadequate.	Leg weakness, reduced sensation, tingling pain in the hands and feet, chronic damage to nerves.

Surgical solution

New haemorrhoid surgery cuts pain and recovery time

A new surgical technique – hailed by surgeons in Britain and the USA – is proving to be a less painful way to remove haemorrhoids without the long recovery time of traditional surgery.

The spongy tissue that lines the anal canal is laced with blood vessels. When clusters of these veins become swollen – for example from straining during bowel movements – they may bleed or push downward into the anal opening. Haemorrhoids that occur an inch or more inside the anal opening are usually 'silent' because there aren't many nerves in the area. Haemorrhoids that form around the nerve-rich rim of the anus, however, can be intensely painful.

The traditional surgical treatment, a haemorrhoidectomy, involves cutting away the swollen veins. Patients often spend a night in the hospital, are out of work for two to four weeks, and require large amounts of sedatives. With the new technique – 'circumferential mucosectomy (stapled haemorrhoidectomy) – 99 per cent of patients are able to return to work within six days, and most don't require pain relief after the second day, says Dr. Eric G. Weiss, a colon and rectal surgeon at the Cleveland Clinic Florida in Weston, Florida. The technique, the subject of a randomized controlled trial reported in *The Lancet* in 2000, was introduced in the United States in 2001.

How it works Unlike in traditional surgery, the haemorrhoids are essentially left alone. The surgeon removes a strip of tissue 2-3cm inside the anal canal above the haemorrhoids, then pulls the loose ends together and fastens them with titanium staples. Stretching the tissue drags the haemorrhoids back into the rectal canal. 'There are very few nerve endings where the operation is performed, so there's little pain,' says Dr. Weiss.

Availability The technique is currently being evaluated at 11 medical centres across the United States, and will probably replace most traditional methods of haemorrhoidectomy in the next few years. It is also available at some British hospitals, although *The Lancet* report suggested that more data on long-term effects is required.

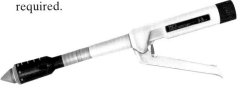

◀ In this technique, prolapsed anal tissue is pulled into this circular stapler device and excised, while the remaining tissue is stapled back in place.

ALSO IN THE NEWS

Researchers say: Go easy on ulcer cocktail

Antibiotics readily knock out *Helicobacter pylori*, the bacterium that causes most peptic ulcers. Standard treatment is to give a cocktail of drugs – amoxicillin, clarithromycin and metronidazole – for a full week. But a study in the February 2002 issue of the *Archives of Internal Medicine* suggests that giving the drugs for three days is just as effective <u>and</u> it's cheaper and less likely to cause side effects.

Can broccoli cure ulcers?

Dietary approaches to ulcer management were largely abandoned about 20 years ago, when doctors discovered that most ulcers are caused by a bacterial infection. But new laboratory studies suggest that food therapy may still play a powerful role.

In May 2002, French and American researchers reported in the *Proceedings of the National Academy of Sciences* that sulforaphane, a chemical compound in broccoli, Brussels sprouts and other so-called cruciferous vegetables, readily kills the ulcer-causing *H. pylori* bacterium. The sulforaphane extract killed antibiotic-resistant organisms as well, and it worked inside cells lining the stomach, reservoirs for the bacterium that conventional drug treatments have trouble reaching.

Even though sulforaphane extract was a clear winner in test-tube studies, it remains unknown if the compound will have the same effects in people. Nor is it certain that ulcer patients can get 'medicinal' doses of sulforaphane just by eating more vegetables.

'If future clinical studies show that a food can relieve or prevent diseases associated with this bacterium, it could have significant public health implications,' says Jed Fahey, M.S., a plant physiologist in the Department of Pharmacology and Molecular Studies at Johns Hopkins School of Medicine in Maryland, USA. Vegetables that contain sulforaphane could be especially helpful in poorer countries, where antibiotics are scarce and the ulcer-causing bacterium abounds.

Progress in prevention

Mainstream doctors are joining the culture club

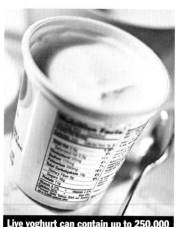

Live yoghurt can contain up to 250,000 million probiotic bacteria per serving.

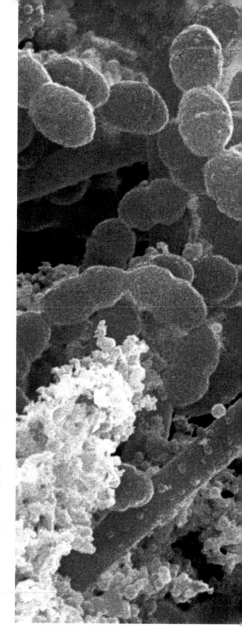

Pills, powders, or liquids that contain live, cultured bacteria – supplements called probiotics – have long been popular in the alternative-health community. But, it's only in the past few years that compelling scientific evidence has persuaded doctors to give these 'living drugs' a second look.

A study published in the *US Journal of Pediatrics* reported that a third of hospitalized infants given plain formula developed diarrhoea, compared with just 7 per cent of those given *Lactobacillus GG* probiotics. Another investigation, published in the December 2001 issue of the *American Journal of Clinical Nutrition,* found that the probiotic *Bifido-bacterium lactis* HN019 boosted certain immune cell functions in elderly patients. Researchers in Finland have also discovered that giving *Lactobacillus GG* to pregnant women, and then to their babies after birth, lowered the incidence of eczema in the children. And other studies have found that probiotics reduce the complications of inflammatory bowel disease and help prevent diarrhoea as well as vaginal and urinary tract infections.

Their benefits have long been suspected but now US doctors who would not have supported their use in the past are recommending them to patients, according to Dr. Samuel Meyers, clinical professor of medicine at Mount Sinai School of Medicine in New York City.

In Britain probiotics are used to treat gastrointestinal and vaginal infections but are not yet accepted as viable alternatives to conventional treatments for diarrhoea.

Take action

Ways to put more bio-yoghurt into your meals

Eating bio-yoghurt which contains live bacteria, is an excellent way to include some healthy probiotics in your daily diet. Here are four tasty ways to serve it:

1 Top your breakfast muesli with natural bio-yoghurt, instead of milk, for a healthy start to the day.

2 Blend bio-yoghurt with fresh or frozen fruit and milk to make a healthy smoothie.

3 Add fresh garlic, dill, parsley, or other herbs to make a dip. Then use pitta or vegetables instead of crisps.

4 Use natural bio-yoghurt in place of creamy, high-fat salad dressings by adding herbs and a little vinegar.

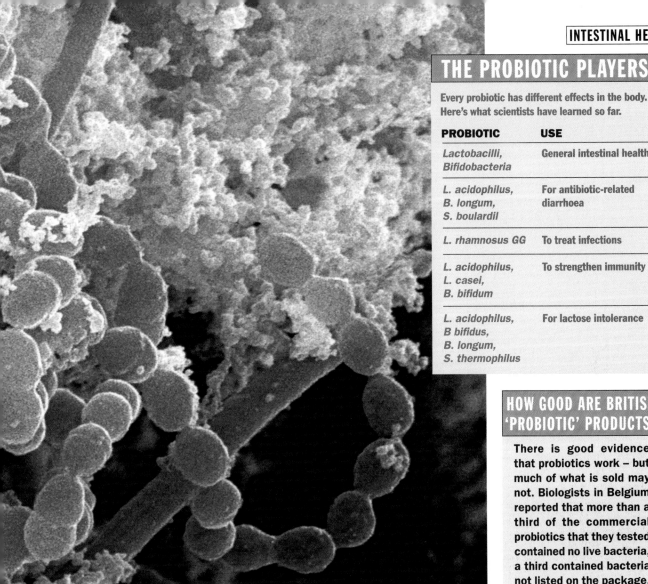

Every probiotic has different effects in the body. Here's what scientists have learned so far.

PROBIOTIC	USE
Lactobacilli, Bifidobacteria	General intestinal health
L. acidophilus, B. longum, S. boulardil	For antibiotic-related diarrhoea
L. rhamnosus GG	To treat infections
L. acidophilus, L. casei, B. bifidum	To strengthen immunity
L. acidophilus, B bifidus, B. longum, S. thermophilus	For lactose intolerance

HOW GOOD ARE BRITISH 'PROBIOTIC' PRODUCTS?

There is good evidence that probiotics work – but much of what is sold may not. Biologists in Belgium reported that more than a third of the commercial probiotics that they tested contained no live bacteria, a third contained bacteria not listed on the package, and only 13 per cent contained all those listed.

Jeremy Hamilton-Miller, professor of medical microbiology at the Royal Free Hospital in London, says he has 'no doubt whatsoever that probiotics are clinically effective' but also found that less than 40 per cent of the 50 British products he has tested over the past six years contained all the bacteria claimed. And he regrets that the probiotic with the best clinical track record – *Lactobacillus* GG – is not available in the UK. 'But that is a marketing matter,' he says. 'It's just too expensive.'

How it works The human body can usually maintain a balance between the beneficial and harmful bacteria in the intestines – there are some 1.3kg (3lb) of bacteria in our gut – but factors such as illness, ageing, high alcohol consumption, or the use of antibiotics can give 'bad' bugs the edge. Probiotics, taken either in supplement form or in foods such as live yoghurt, can restore the balance by replenishing beneficial bacteria. These 'good' bugs use up some of the food and other resources that symptom-causing bacteria need in order to thrive. At the same time, probiotics create healthful pH levels in the gut and produce germ-fighting compounds.

Availability Probiotics in supplement form are not yet as popular here as in the USA but are available in healthfood shops, from chemists, by mail order or on the internet. One example is the Multibionta Probiotic Multivitamin which contains probiotic cultures *Lactobacillus acidophilus*, *Bifidobacterium bifidum* and *Bifidobacterium longum* as well as vitamins and minerals.

▲ **A SUPER CLOSE-UP** view of the probiotic bacteria found in yoghurt. *Streptococcus thermophilis* is the spherical one; *Lactobacillus bulgaris* is rod-shaped – and yes, this stuff really is good for you.

EYES AND EARS

I n one of the most impressive breakthroughs of 2002, scientists have invented a whole new way for the blind to see. It's a 'bat cane' that, like the natural sonar that bats use to navigate, interprets echoes from ultrasound waves to give a three-dimensional map of your surroundings and warn you of obstacles in your path.

There's also welcome news about two dreaded thieves of good vision. Researchers have discovered that vitamin C and other antioxidants known as carotenoids protect against cataracts. And prescription drops for reducing pressure from fluid in the eye have now been shown to delay or even prevent the onset of glaucoma.

Finally, for people plagued by tinnitus, a new therapy in the works could help banish that persistent ringing in your ears for good.

Progress in prevention

Preventing cataracts: it's a food fight

A cataract is a vision-impairing cloudiness in the eye's lens. Cataracts are common in older adults – nearly half of those over 75 have them – and millions of operations are performed each year to replace the clouded lens with an artificial one. But the condition can be prevented before it reaches that point. The latest research on cataracts suggests three ways in which women in their fifties (and, presumably, men too) may reduce their risk:

1. Take a supplement of at least 362mg of vitamin C every day.
2. Eat plenty of brightly coloured fruits and vegetables rich in the plant chemicals known as carotenoids.
3. Don't smoke.

These findings were published by a New England research team in the March 2002 issue of the *American Journal of Clinical Research*. The most important discovery is that carotenoids prevent the less common but especially troublesome 'posterior subscapular' type of cataract.

▲ A healthy intake of antioxidant nutrients, along with not smoking, can help to keep your eyes clear of cataracts.

These cataracts affect vision more than other types because the opacity (cloudiness) is located farther back in the lens. The women in the study who ate a diet rich in carotenoids were much less likely to suffer from this type of cataract – as long as they were non-smokers. Smoking and diabetes are the two biggest risk factors for cataracts.

How it works Vitamin C, carotenoids and folate (a B vitamin also shown to reduce cataract risk) have something in common. They're all antioxidants, meaning that they reduce the damage that occurs as a result of normal chemical reactions in the body's cells. Such oxidative damage may contribute to cataracts. The researchers also noticed that vitamin C seems to retard the clumping of protein in the lens that creates the opacity.

The study examined the eye health and nutritional habits of 492 women between ages 53 and 73. The youngest women – those under 60 – reaped the greatest benefits from vitamin C. The under-60 subjects who took daily

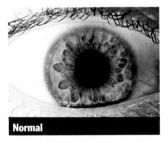
Normal

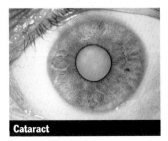
Cataract

171

supplements of 362mg of vitamin C had a 57 per cent less chance of developing the more common cortical (central external lens) cataracts over a 10 year period than those who took 140mg or less. A high intake of carotenoids reduced the risk of posterior subscapular cataracts for all ages.

In a separate study carried out in Baltimore, USA, researchers found that hormone replacement therapy (HRT) offered women some protection against developing nuclear and posterior subscapular cataracts.

Take action

Protective vegetables and fruits

Carotenoids are plant compounds that help to safeguard your precious vision. You can get your fill of these protective nutrients by eating plenty of these colourful fruits and vegetables.

- **RED VEGETABLES:**
  tomatoes and red peppers
- **ORANGE VEGETABLES:**
  carrots, pumpkin, butternut squash and sweet potatoes
- **ORANGE FRUITS:**
  mango, papaya and cantaloupe
- **DARK GREEN VEGETABLES:**
  spinach, watercress, kale, spring greens and broccoli

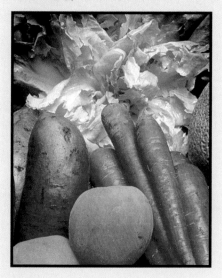

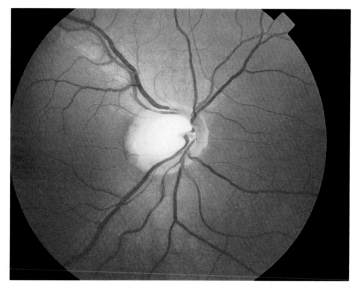

▲ GLAUCOMA can damage the delicate, light-sensitive, nerve-rich optic disc in the centre of the retina at the back of the eye.

Key discovery
Glaucoma gene identified

O pen-angle glaucoma – the most common variety of the sight-robbing eye condition – affects around 250,000 people in the UK and 33 million worldwide. It is a leading cause of blindness, and there is no cure. That's a gloomy picture indeed, but it got a lot brighter in February 2002 when University of Connecticut researchers announced they had identified the gene that causes the disorder.

The gene is responsible for producing a protein that the researchers believe has a role – as yet undefined – in preventing damage to the optic nerve, which connects the light-sensing retina to the brain. When the gene is defective, so is the protein, and the optic nerve loses its protection. The optic nerve is precisely what is damaged in glaucoma patients. That damage is the result of pressure from fluid build-up, which can happen even if the drainage channels in the eye are open – hence the name 'open-angle' glaucoma.

The researchers pinpointed the gene and four mutant variations by studying DNA samples of 54 families with the hereditary form of open-angle glaucoma. Although not all open-angle glaucoma cases are hereditary, the gene discovery is a major breakthrough for two reasons. One is that millions of people potentially at risk for glaucoma can be diagnosed much earlier. That's important because drugs or surgery can only halt the disease's progression – not reverse it – so early treatment means less permanent damage to the eye. Also, knowledge of the gene and the protein whose maintenance it directs will lead to a deeper understanding of how glaucoma develops. That should eventually mean better treatment and perhaps a cure.

Progress in prevention

Eyedrops prevent glaucoma

Increased pressure inside the eyeball caused by poor drainage of fluid into and out of the eye – known as, ocular hypertension, or elevated intraocular pressure (IOP) – has long been associated with glaucoma, the sight-robbing progressive eye disorder. Pressure-reducing eyedrops can reduce IOP, but until recently doctors did not know whether the eyedrops could stave off glaucoma.

That changed in June 2002 when results from a US study published in the *Archives of Ophthalmology* offered the first solid evidence that drops to reduce eye pressure actually prevent the onset of glaucoma.

Investigators from Washington University in St. Louis studied 1,636 people between the ages of 40 and 80, all of whom suffered from ocular hypertension but had no signs of glaucoma. Half were randomly chosen to receive daily pressure-reducing eyedrops similar to the beta blockers used to reduce high blood pressure (cardiovascular hypertension). The other half were not treated but closely monitored. After five years, only 4.4 per cent of those receiving the drops had developed glaucoma, compared with 9.5 per cent of the untreated group. In other words, the daily drops, which reduced eye pressure by only about 20 per cent, lowered the risk of glaucoma by more than 50 per cent.

'There are millions of people in the United States and other countries at risk of developing glaucoma because they have high pressure in their eyes,' says Dr. Michael A. Kass, the ophthalmologist who piloted the research. 'This study provides the first good evidence that treating those people may delay, or possibly even prevent, the blinding eye disease glaucoma.'

It is important to remember that a raised IOP does not always lead to glaucoma and glaucoma can be present in patients with a normal IOP. The number of people with elevated IOP is difficult to estimate, as the condition is often symptomless. Diagnosis is usually made during a routine eye test. The decision to prescribe eye-drops at this stage will depend on the individual's risk factors for developing glaucoma. Such prescriptions will probably become more commonplace as a result of this research, especially for people of African descent, whose risk of developing glaucoma is three to four times higher than the rest of the population. Since glaucoma develops slowly without symptoms, regular eye tests are recommended. In the UK anyone over 40 with an immediate relative who has glaucoma is eligible for free eye tests.

Eye pressure on the rise

The fluid that fills the front of the eye is produced by the ciliary body surrounding the lens. Normally this fluid flows (red arrows) through the pupil and into the anterior chamber, where it then drains through tiny canals into the sclera. If these drainage portals are blocked, pressure inside the eye increases.

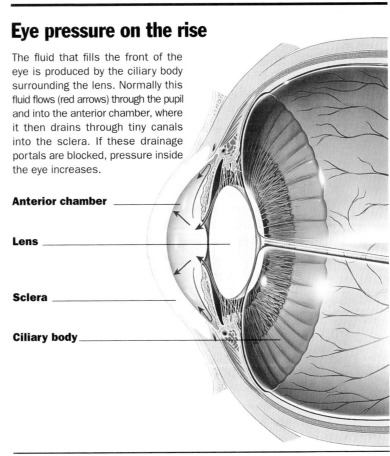

Anterior chamber

Lens

Sclera

Ciliary body

Progress in prevention

Oestrogen may impede hearing loss in women

It's no cure-all for ageing, but oestrogen – at least as it occurs naturally in a woman's body – does seem to have health-protective effects. Prior to menopause it appears to guard against heart disease. And now new research from South Korea makes a case that, even in postmenopausal women, it may protect against hearing loss.

'Our findings strongly suggest that oestrogen may have a favourable effect on the hearing sensitivity of post-menopausal women,' says study author Dr. Sung Hoon Kim. The results of the study were published in the journal *Obstetrics & Gynecology* in May 2002.

The Korean researchers measured levels of a form of oestrogen called estradiol in the bloodstream of 1,830 women over 50. About 10 per cent of the women had some degree of hearing loss. On average, those with hearing problems had lower levels of estradiol in their blood-streams than the others did. They were also older, on average, than the women without hearing problems. 'These findings suggest that hearing sensitivity in post-menopausal women is determined mainly by age and... estradiol level,' concluded the researchers. Around half of all people in the UK over the age of 60 and 93 per cent of those over 80 report some degree of hearing loss.

Although the Korean study established a connection between oestrogen levels and hearing health in women, it stopped short of concluding that undergoing hormone replacement therapy (HRT) after menopause will reduce the risk of hearing loss. HRT was not associated in the study with better hearing, possibly because only 3 per cent of study participants were actively taking the therapy. Meanwhile, HRT has come under intense scrutiny in the past two years. In fact, a recent study was halted because women taking hormones showed an increased risk of breast cancer, heart disease, stroke and blood clots.

RESEARCH ROUND-UP

Better hearing help on the horizon

Future hearing aids and cochlear implants may deliver even more help to the hard of hearing thanks to two recent discoveries about the way sound works in the human ear. Scientists from the Johns Hopkins Medical Institutions, in Baltimore, announced in May 2002 that they have finally pinned down exactly what kind of chemical reaction converts sound waves into electrical signals to the brain. The results raised some eyebrows, because it turns out that the tiny cells in the cochlea, deep inside the ear, send electrical signals to the brain by continually pumping out the chemical messengers, rather than emitting a bulk load at a time, as most messages to the brain are sent. The investigators hope this understanding will stimulate new research that could lead to more sophisticated hearing devices with improved range and accuracy.

Two months earlier, a research team from Harvard and MIT unveiled another of the ear's secrets: how it splits sound into 'tone' and 'pitch'. The investigators found that the ear separates sounds into two 'layers' and processes them separately – the tone layer being more important for basic speech patterns and the pitch layer determining how high or low a sound is. That could make a big difference for cochlear implant users, because current devices for the profoundly deaf aren't usually capable of discerning pitch.

The researchers hope their discovery will bring pitch perception to cochlear implant users and, along with it, a better ability to appreciate music and understand the speech nuances determined by pitch, such as indicating a question by a rising pitch at the end of a sentence.

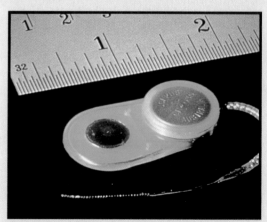

A new generation of cochlear implants that discern pitch as well as tone are on the horizon.

Drug development
Sight for sore eyes: vision-restoring drug on the horizon

A new drug promises to save the sight of many people suffering from a leading cause of blindness: the 'wet' form of age-related macular degeneration (AMD). The drug, manufactured by Genentech, goes by the name of rhuFab, and although it's still in the experimental stages, study subjects and their doctors have reported stunning early successes. So far, rhuFab has been able to prevent vision loss in volunteers when taken soon after AMD has been diagnosed. It's even returned nearly perfect sight to those on the brink of blindness.

If these results remain valid under more rigorous testing, it could mark a new era in the treatment of wet AMD. To date, prevention has been the principal strategy against the disorder, since the onset of symptoms is usually followed by blindness within months and there has been little that doctors can do about it – until now.

The wet form, which accounts for about 10 per cent of

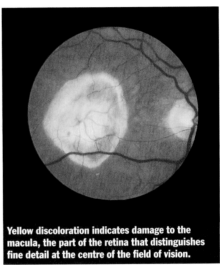

Yellow discoloration indicates damage to the macula, the part of the retina that distinguishes fine detail at the centre of the field of vision.

the 500,000 cases of AMD in the UK, results from the growth in the eye of faulty blood vessels that leak blood and other fluid (hence the term 'wet'). The leakage damages the retina, which is the eye layer that houses the vision receptors. The unfortunate process is known as choroidal neovascularization, or CNV, after the choroid, the name of the layer where the abnormal blood vessels form. This is the process that rhuFab is thought to reverse. The drug is not effective against the 'dry' form of macular degeneration, which is more common yet much less aggressive in damaging sight.

How it works It all started with the recent discovery of a protein called VEGF (for vascular endothelial growth factor), which encourages the formation of new blood vessels. RhuFab is an antibody fragment that binds to VEGF, preventing the protein from activating vessel-forming cells. RhuFab is injected directly into the

RhuFab has returned nearly perfect sight [even] to those on the brink of blindness.

jelly-like body that fills most of the eye. From there it passes through the retina to the area where the faulty vessels are growing. A shot in the eye may not be a pleasant prospect, but most would agree that staving off blindness is well worth it.

Availability The final results of the current US study (a combined Phase I and II multi-centre clinical trial) aren't expected until the second half of 2003 or 2004. That means that the treatment is only available to the current study volunteers. Some of the issues to be resolved include what dosages are needed, whether a series of eye injections is safe and whether the effect is temporary or long term. The drug will need to undergo clincial trials in the UK before it can be licensed for use here, so its practical application is some way off. A similar drug called EYE001 is also being tested in the US. Both drugs are thought to work against diabetic retinopathy, another blindness-causing condition that affects some 100,000 people in the UK.

Key discovery
A new therapy for toning down that ringing in the ears

If your taste in live music runs more to rock than Rachmaninoff, you've probably had the experience of a post-concert ringing in the ears that continues for hours after the last amplified note was inflicted. But for millions of people worldwide, hearing a noise that's not coming from any external source is an ongoing – and distressing – condition. It's called tinnitus, and although loud noises can trigger the problem, neither cause nor cure is known.

But a significant discovery announced by German scientists in March 2002 may lead to a new kind of therapy that could finally put tinnitus sufferers out of their misery. In a small pilot study, a research team from Heidelburg University found that 'tone training' appears to ease the incessant ringing. The patients were required to listen to closely matched tones with a pitch frequency similar to that of the phantom noises they hear in their heads. Subjects who learned to distinguish between the two tones – in four weeks of 2-hours-a-day training – experienced a 35 per cent reduction in tinnitus symptoms. Those who were asked to distinguish between unrelated tones showed no improvement.

Why would such an exercise work? The German researchers suggest that it might have to do with an abnormality in the brain of people with tinnitus. The areas of the brain's auditory cortex that respond to different sound frequencies should be more or less the same size, but the areas activated by the phantom sounds seem to be larger in tinnitus sufferers. Further research will attempt to confirm that tone therapy actually shrinks those areas and also try to find out whether extending the treatment for more than four weeks will result in further improvement.

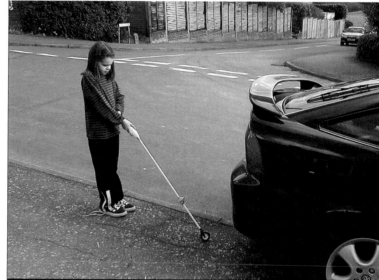

Ultrasound waves bounce off of objects near and far to create a virtual sonic landscape that can be 'seen' by the sense of touch via the 'bat cane'.

High-tech help
Brits pioneer bat canes — seeing with sound!

When it comes to getting around in the dark, bats are the undisputed experts. Borrowing a page from the winged mammals' noted navigational strategy, British scientists have devised a new kind of high-tech cane for people with impaired vision. Employing the same echolocation that bats use to detect and avoid objects in their flight path, the 'bat cane' provides the visually impaired with a map of their surroundings, making it much easier for them to negotiate their way through the physical world.

How it works The bat cane emits inaudible high-frequency ultrasound pulses at four angles in front of its user: left, right, straight ahead and upward. Sophisticated software reads the returning echoes of these pulses as they bounce off objects and converts them to vibrations that the user can feel in the hand while gripping a sensor device on the cane's handle. The vibrations are felt in a different finger depending on which direction the echo comes from. And the vibrations speed up as the object gets nearer. That's enough information for the brain to create a spatial map, virtually enabling the user to 'see' with sound.

According to its manufacturer, the bat cane can detect objects that are well beyond the reach of a conventional cane, thus enabling the users to increase their stride and, in general, enjoy greater independence and mobility. The bat cane needs no programming and runs on only a set of AA batteries.

Availability After several years of testing and development, the ultrasound cane is expected to hit the market by early 2003, with an estimated price tag between £350 and £750. It will most likely be available for purchase through such organizations as Guide Dogs for the Blind in the UK, and the American Council for the Blind in the United States. Those groups have been involved from the beginning in developing the ultrasound cane and will also provide the necessary training assistance to its potential users.

RESEARCH ROUND-UP

Squeezing out perfect vision

A tiny artificial eye muscle may soon do the work of conventional glasses, helping both the near and the far-sighted achieve perfect vision. Researchers from the University of New Mexico, in Albuquerque, announced in March 2002 that they were developing a 'smart eye band' that can be sewn onto the tough white outer part of the eyeball. From there, the device can temporarily squeeze the eyeball into the shape best suited for overcoming specific vision problems. For example, slightly elongating the eyeball brings close-up objects into focus, helping the farsighted to read.

The artificial muscle consists of a synthetic compound covered by a gold coil that is activated by a magnetic field. The user controls the action with a switch hooked like a hearing aid over the ear. With nothing more than a press of a button, you can change your focus from the newspaper in front of you to the action outside the window with no loss of clarity – and there's no looking around for where you left your glasses. The researchers hope the device will be available in three to five years.

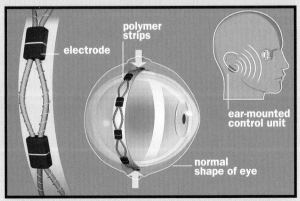

A negative charge in the electrodes causes the polymer strips to contract and reshape the eyeball so it can focus.

BEHIND THE BREAKTHROUGH

Batty idea leads to breakthrough

Ever wonder what a gaggle of professors talks about over morning coffee? In some cases, the conversation just might be a medical breakthrough in the making. That was certainly the case at Leeds University a few years ago when a biologist, an electronics engineer, a food scientist and a neurophysiologist sat down for an informal chat.

When the food scientist mentioned casually that ultrasound scanning can create a visual display to identify bruised apples, the neurophysiologist wondered aloud, 'If sound can be perceived visually, can it also be felt?'

'It sure can,' replied the electronics engineer. That inspired the neurophysiologist to begin thinking about a navigational aide for the blind, an idea that sat well with the biologist, who happened to be a bat specialist. And so the bat cane concept was born. But would it fly?

The professors formed a company called Sound Foresight, Ltd., to put their theoretical concept into action. 'We didn't want to just keep it confined to the realm of academia,' says Deborah J. Withington, Ph.D., the neurophysiologist of the group. 'We needed to get out into the real world and do something.'

That meant getting lots of input from the intended beneficiaries of the project: blind and partially sighted people. Three key decisions came out of that collaboration. 'First of all, we went with the basic concept of a cane, even though the ultrasound device could have been a wand, or anything, really,' Dr. Withington says. 'The new technology is a massive enough leap, and we decided it was better to introduce it in as familiar a form as possible.'

The second decision was to include ultrasound sensing of overhanging objects, something that traditional canes can't detect as they're swept in front of the user. 'Talking with visually impaired people made us realize that that's their biggest unaddressed problem – overhanging branches, for sale signs, that sort of thing,' Dr. Withington says.

The third discovery was a bit surprising. A common complaint among the volunteers – blind as well as partially sighted – was how ugly traditional canes are. 'People assume that aesthetic considerations as such don't matter to the blind, but they do,' Dr. Withington says. 'The group we talked to wanted a product that looks good. We saw the need to develop something a little sexier than the usual canes.'

HEART AND CIRCULATORY SYSTEM

Taming heart disease – the nation's number one killer – takes a team effort. Medical researchers have certainly done their bit in the past few years. They've uncovered evidence that cholesterol-lowering drugs can save a lot more people from heart attack and stroke than previously thought. They've aided older people by discovering how to relax stiff arteries. And surgeons have helped the younger-than-young by pioneering a successful surgical procedure to correct a heart defect in an unborn baby.

But science is also showing us what we can do on our own to protect ourselves. We now know, for example, that managing stress helps us to recover from heart disease as well as avoid it. And new research tells us that taming blood pressure that's even just a little above normal is important for staving off cardio-vascular disease. We even have new information about alcohol's heart benefits. Two drinks, it turns out, can be better than one – but zero's much better than three. Here's to your health!

Key discovery

When the heart stops, researchers cool it

If your heart stops for even a few seconds, the impaired blood flow that results can permanently damage your brain. But the very act of restoring that blood flow can cause even more brain damage. Catch-22.

Now German and Australian cardiologists have found a way around the dilemma. Their research shows that when mild hypothermia is induced in cardiac arrest victims – that is, when their body temperature is deliberately cooled to 33°C (91.4°F) for 12 to 24 hours – the victims are more likely to survive, and brain damage can be prevented.

The researchers didn't make this potentially life-saving discovery out of the blue. Animal studies had indicated that cooling could reduce neurological damage. And there are plenty of cases on record of near-drowning victims who were protected by the

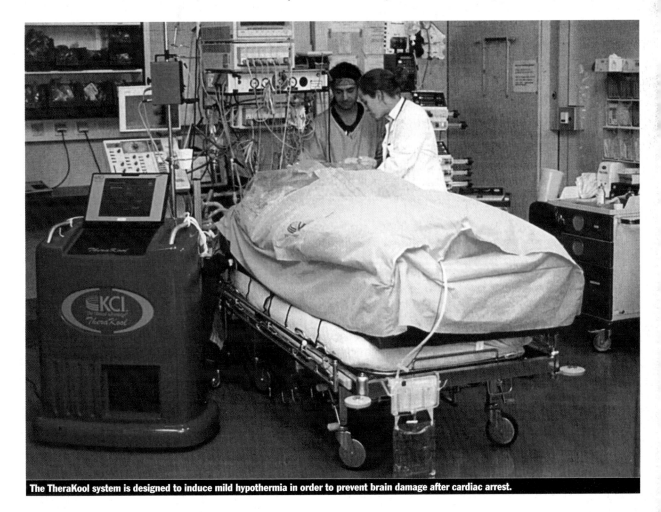

The TheraKool system is designed to induce mild hypothermia in order to prevent brain damage after cardiac arrest.

In the German study ... a much greater percentage of the cooled patients were able to live independently and hold a job.

cold when their hearts stopped after they fell through ice. So the investigators decided to compare the recoveries of cooled patients to those of patients who were not cooled, and they published their results in February 2002.

In the German study, 41 per cent of the patients who were iced down as their hearts were restarted died within six months, compared to 55 per cent of those who weren't. And a much greater percentage of the cooled patients (55 per cent vs. 39 per cent) were able to live independently and hold a job – indicators of more successful neurological recovery. In Australia, patients who had been iced down were more likely to be discharged from the hospital – a good indicator of recovery, since it means not only that you're alive but that doctors have determined you're able to function safely on your own again.

How it works Sudden cardiac arrest is the most severe potential consequence of heart disease: the heart stops pumping because the electrical impulses that control the heartbeat become irregular. A stopped heart starves the brain of oxygen-rich blood, which can kill off brain cells and result in permanent neurological damage within minutes. But restoring the heartbeat suddenly causes even more damage by triggering the over-release of an amino acid called glutamate, which kills nerve cells in the brain. Researchers believe that cooling the blood slows the release of glutamate, sparing the nerve cells.

Availability Casualty departments are equipped to induce hypothermia. But until general physician guidelines are formally revised, doctors are unlikely to do it routinely. The American Heart Foundation and similar bodies in Australia and some EU countries began preparing advisory statements in 2002. Meanwhile, Dr. Stephen Bernard, the Australian study leader, is testing a new hypothermia delivery system: an injectable, ice-cold saline solution. If that's successful – and early indications are good, he says – cooling of cardiac arrest victims could take place anywhere, in the vital minutes before they reach the hospital.

Home is where the heart is ... and the defibrillator?

Sudden cardiac arrest is a medical emergency brought on when the electrical impulses that control the heart go haywire, causing it to quiver rapidly instead of beat regularly. Blood stops flowing, and death is imminent unless CPR (cardiopulmonary resuscitation) is administered quickly, followed by shocking the heart back to its normal rhythm with a machine called a defibrillator. CPR is an important emergency measure that can buy a little time, but it cannot restore normal heart rhythm, which is why the defibrillator is crucial to survival.

You've probably seen TV doctors pressing the iron mitts of a defibrillator to the chest of a patient in a hospital. But recently, smaller 'mobile' versions known as automated external defibrillators (AEDs) have been developed, which some say can be used by untrained people. Those in favour of the devices reckon that if they were available in public places they could achieve faster defibrillation and so improve the survival rate of cardiac arrests.

However, other medical professionals argue that the usefulness of these machines is limited since most cardiac arrests outside of hospital occur beyond the reach of publicly accessible defibrillators anyway. In addition, the question of whether untrained bystanders would be able to use the devices effectively has yet to be answered.

A recent Scottish study looked closely at the locations of cardiac arrests that occurred outside of hospital over a seven-year period, and the overall effect of publicly accessible defibrillation on survival rates. Locations and outcomes were collected for over 15,000 patients with cardiac arrest. The

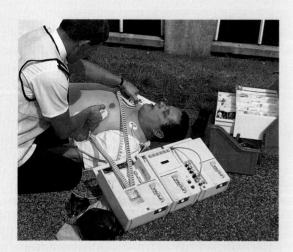

researchers found that the most likely location for a cardiac arrest to occur outside of hospital was in the patients' homes (and so out of reach of publicly accessible AEDs). Public access defibrillation was found to increase overall survival by just 1.5 per cent.

In America the machines are already on call for emergency use in sports stadiums and shopping malls, and in 2002 the American Heart Association urged fitness and health clubs to have them on hand. Now in the USA the debate has moved on to considering whether AEDs should be available in the home, with manufacturers of home versions seeking permission to sell them over the counter.

Dr. Gust H. Bardy, cardiologist and professor of medicine at the University of Washington in Seattle, is all for having AEDs at home. He thinks that ordinary people should be able to use the machines with minimal risk: 'One would have to alter the machine's electronics for the device to be dangerous. And that would be very hard to do.'

Dr. Arthur L. Kellerman, professor of emergency medicine at Emory University's School of Medicine in Atlanta, thinks otherwise. He says that there is no research available to tell us one way or the other if AEDs would be useful in the home, but until there's proof that they'll do some good, 'home use shouldn't be recommended'.

The machines are likely to cost more than £1500 and, says Dr. Kellerman, 'You're better off spending some of that money on what is known to save your heart: a health club membership, an exercise bike, a programme to quit smoking, hypertension and high cholesterol treatment.' Sound advice, indeed.

Key discovery
Blood transfusions prevent heart attack deaths

A surprising 40 per cent of people who suffer a heart attack after the age of 65 have anaemia. The condition – marked by an insufficient number of oxygen-carrying red blood cells – makes anaemia sufferers twice as likely to die from the heart attack. But the same US researchers who published those grim statistics in October 2001 also found a way to reduce the risk: blood transfusions.

The solution may sound obvious, because supplying blood (complete with red blood cells) via transfusion

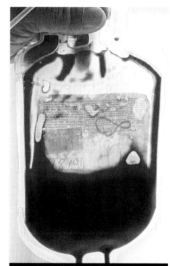

Iron-rich red blood cells can improve the odds of surviving a heart attack.

to anaemic patients is common. But the study – at Yale – was the first to link anaemia with heart attack death rates and to link blood transfusions with heart attack survival. Until now, less than a quarter of anaemic heart attack victims have received blood transfusions.

That may change as a result of the study, which reviewed nearly 80,000 heart attack cases in a 13-month period. The findings were striking: more than 38 per cent of the patients with severe anaemia died within 30 days of their heart attacks, compared with only 17.2 per cent of those with healthy red blood cell counts. But that 38 per cent figure dropped significantly for anaemic patients who received a blood transfusion in the hospital. Additionally, the analysis revealed that blood transfusions saved lives even among patients who were only borderline anaemic. Based on their findings, the study authors encourage changes in the clinical guidelines for treating heart attack victims.

Key discovery
Long live the fit

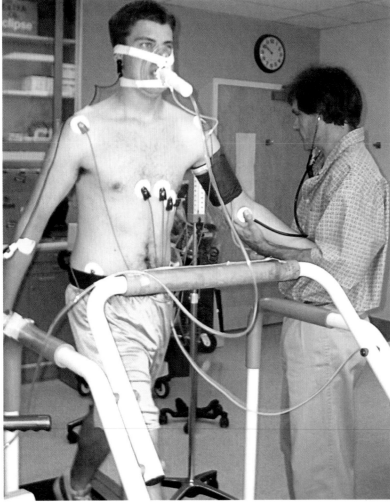

◄ The Stanford treadmill study showed that volunteers with the greatest capacity for vigorous exercise live the longest.

Darwin had it right: it's the fittest who survive. Study results published in March 2002 show that your stamina for exercise says more about how much longer you'll live than anything else but your age. Blood pressure? Smoking history? Diabetes? They're not as decisive as your peak exercise capacity as measured by your score on a treadmill test, investigators say.

How they did it Stanford University researchers looked at the records of 6,213 men who had undergone treadmill testing, then correlated their scores with their rates of death over the next 10 years. When the numbers were adjusted for age, the results were clear: the higher the score on the treadmill test, the lower the risk of dying, no matter what other factors (like smoking or diabetes) were involved.

The treadmill test isn't about how long you can exercise, but how hard. It measures your ability to perform under increasing degrees of difficulty such as a steeper incline or a faster speed. By calculating oxygen use, the technicians grade the subject's peak exercise capacity in units called METs (for metabolic equivalents). One MET is the amount of oxygen you use while sitting still. Eight METs are equivalent to a jog. The researchers found that with each additional MET in your maximum exercise capacity, your risk of early death drops 12 per cent.

What it means Researchers already knew that exercise lowers the risk for heart disease. They also knew that exercise capacity is a good indicator of the risk of early death in people who already have heart disease. But this study, which looked at subjects with and without heart disease, is the first to show that fitness predicts longevity for everybody. The message is clear: for a longer life, nothing is more important than exercise.

TAKING THE TREADMILL TEST

Stanford University's Jonathan Myers, Ph.D., headed the study that came up with an intriguing finding: the harder you're able to exercise during a treadmill test, the longer you're likely to live. He hopes the study will help convince doctors and patients alike of the importance of physical fitness in protecting against cardiovascular disease.

Q. What does your study tell us?

Dr. Myers: That we need to exercise. A recent large survey showed that only 23 per cent of physicians mention exercise to their patients on a typical visit. But exercise warrants as much attention as the more established risk factors for heart disease: smoking, high blood pressure, high cholesterol.

Q. How much exercise will improve treadmill results?

Dr. Myers: Get some moderate exercise for a half hour every day, or almost every day.

Q. That doesn't sound like much exercise.

Dr. Myers: We don't all have to be triathletes. In the study, the biggest improvement in mortality risk was between the lowest score and the second lowest score. That means if totally sedentary people – the least fit group – would just get up and do something for a half hour most days, they'd cut their risk of dying from cardiovascular disease almost in half.

Q. What kind of exercise should they do?

Dr. Myers: Anything that will increase your heart rate and metabolic rate will improve your treadmill test score if you do it regularly. Walking or jogging are good, but it can be things like washing the car or household chores.

Q. Does that hold true for both women and men?

Dr. Myers: I think it does. The data we analysed were from a VA [Veterans Affairs] hospital, so it was all men. But there is data out there that suggests that findings such as ours would apply to women, too.

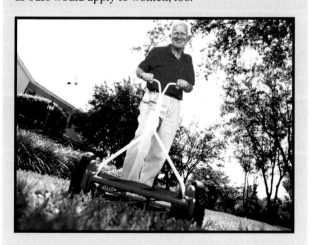

Surgical solution

In bypass surgery, the beat goes on

When a surgical procedure has been successful for several decades, the tendency is not to change it. But in the case of coronary bypass surgery, more and more surgeons are using a new technique that lets them reroute blood flow around blocked arteries without stopping the heart. Now, a UK study has confirmed what proponents of the 'beating heart' technique have been saying all along: it reduces complications, shortens hospital stays, speeds recovery and is every bit as safe and effective as the traditional method.

How it works Bypass surgery grafts a blood vessel from another part of the body onto the aorta (the major artery carrying blood out of the heart) to serve as a detour for blood flow around a clogged coronary artery.

In the past, surgeons found it necessary to stop the heart from beating during the delicate grafting procedure so they wouldn't be working on a moving target. To do that they place the patient temporarily on a heart-lung machine, which takes over the heart's blood-pumping role.

But now surgeons are able to graft while the heart is beating, with the help of a small device called a tissue stabilizer. It uses suction pods to steady the heart, immobilizing only the tiny section where the work is being done. No heart-lung machine is needed – which is why the method is also called 'off-pump' bypass surgery.

To study the technique, researchers at the Bristol Heart Institute randomly assigned half of some 400 bypass patients to traditional surgery and the other half to off-pump surgery. Follow-up showed that the off-pump patients were much less likely to experience irregular heart rhythms or chest infections – common complications of traditional

'The new method is better for the patient because it reduces the shortcomings of traditional open-heart surgery.'

bypass surgery. They were also more likely to be out of intensive care within a day and home from the hospital within a week. The results, published in April 2002, cheered 'beating heart' proponents on the US side of the Atlantic. 'The new method is better for the patient because it reduces the shortcomings of traditional open-heart surgery, and it's less invasive,' says Dr. Curtis Marder, a surgeon at Marquette General Hospital in northern Michigan, who has performed beating heart bypass surgery for six years. 'There's no difference in mortality, so there's no added risk involved.'

Availability The off-pump procedure is already performed at many sites across the US, where open-heart surgeons have been trained in the technique. The study authors hope their results will lead to greater use of the procedure worldwide.

PATIENT PROFILE

Without missing a beat

When James McMaster felt a heavy pressure in his chest while shovelling snow outside his rural Michigan home early one morning, he knew just what to do: he took antacid indigestion tablets.

'I'd had gas before, where you get pressure in the chest and it goes away with a couple of Tums,' he says. 'But this time it didn't go away.' So James tried a more advanced medication: aspirin. That didn't do the trick either.

As it turns out, what the 63-year-old retired plumber needed wasn't in his medicine cabinet but in an operating room at Marquette General 20 miles away. There, surgeons performed a quadruple coronary artery bypass operation, detouring blood flow around four arteries – one totally obstructed and three partially blocked. James didn't know it, but the surgical team chose to use the off-pump technique for his surgery, so his heart could beat naturally throughout the procedure instead of being stopped and its job temporarily given over to a heart-lung machine.

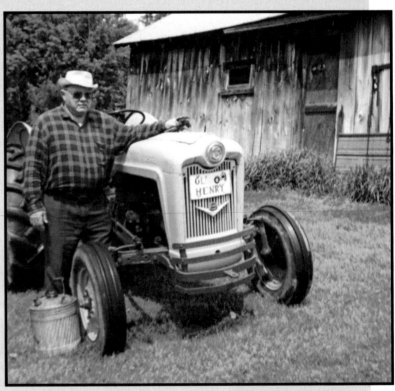

After quadruple bypass surgery with the 'off-pump' technique, James McMaster is as tough and ready for action as his trusty old tractor.

James is glad he wasn't put on the machine. 'Everything went well,' he says. 'I feel great and I'm feeling better every day.' Other than some shortness of breath for a month or so after the operation, James says he's had none of the problems that sometimes follow traditional bypass surgery – no chest infections, heart flutters, or disorientation. Best of all, he was discharged within four days of the operation. 'I was anxious to get out of there,' he says. 'Just lying in a hospital bed gave me more problems than my heart did.'

Key discovery
Treat the mind, help the heart

New research on heart attack victims indicates that the mind can help determine who survives and who doesn't. One team of investigators found that in depressed heart patients, a pessimistic outlook about recovery becomes a self-fulfilling prophecy. Another found that people with a positive personality are less likely to develop heart problems in the first place

The studies, presented to the American Heart Association's annual Scientific Sessions in November 2001, make a compelling case for the power of mood to lengthen lives.

Heart attack victims who become clinically depressed – and about one in five do – are known to be four to five times more likely to die from the heart attack than those who don't. What wasn't clear until now is whether this was a result of the depression itself or whether the depressed patients were simply sicker. By following patients for four months after their heart attacks, researchers at Johns Hopkins University in Baltimore found that the depressed ones were

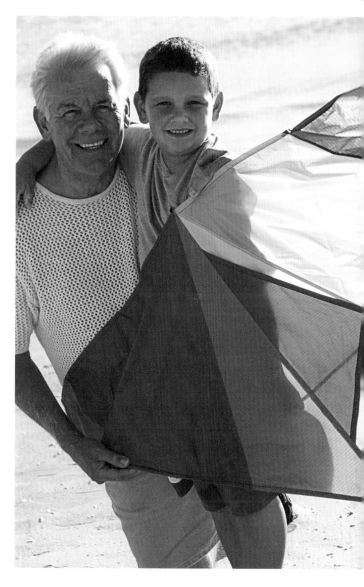

▶ Having a positive mental outlook and a zest for life turn out to be good for the heart.

less likely to adopt the sorts of healthy behaviour – such as diet adjustments, quitting smoking and taking prescribed medications – that would aid their recovery. It would follow, then, that treating the head could help save the heart.

The other research team, also from Johns Hopkins, came to a similar conclusion after following 586 people for seven years. These patients all had a family history of heart problems, but they themselves were healthy at the start of the study. Medical records and personality evaluations showed that those with positive mental outlooks were half as likely as the others to suffer cardiac events, such as a heart attack or serious chest pain.

British research roughly supports these findings. But exactly why a positive attitude is important remains a mystery – athough it undoubtedly adds to the quality of life. One possibility is that happy people release fewer stress hormones. Next, the researchers plan to find out whether engaging in pleasurable activities reduces heart disease risk – a study for which volunteers should be plentiful.

RESEARCH ROUND-UP

Prozac for the heart?
If depression is a risk factor for heart attacks, wouldn't antidepressants help prevent them? That's precisely what researchers at Pennsylvania University's School of Medicine found after tracking smokers over 28 months. Those who used drugs called selective serotonin reuptake inhibitors (antidepressants that include Prozac) were much less likely to experience a heart attack. The protective effect could come from the alleviation of depression, but it's also possible that the drug has anticlotting properties.

Alternative answers

Stress management saves lives – and money

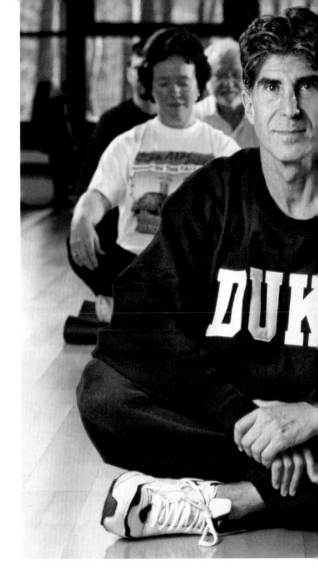

Plenty of research indicates that a stressed-out lifestyle invites heart disease – and doctors are not immune. The link between stress levels and high blood pressure was firmly established in a recent study of British GPs. To improve their long-term prospects, they and other potential heart patients should practise stress management techniques suggests a study by US psychologists at Duke University in Durham, North Carolina.

First, the researchers uncovered compelling evidence that patients with coronary artery disease who participated in stress management programmes were much less likely to need bypass surgery or angioplasty, to suffer a heart attack, or to die within five years, than those who didn't. This is the first study to confirm the benefits of stress management with respect to long-term heart protection, though earlier Dutch research has indicated its positive effect. Researchers involved also proved the financial benefit of stress management programmes: the average yearly medical costs of US heart patients who participate in such regimes are only about a quarter the costs of patients who don't. The results appeared in January 2002 in the *American Journal of Cardiology*.

How it works The stress management programme used in the Duke study consisted of four weekly classes in which patients were taught to recognize stress symptoms and then to react positively and realistically to the situations that cause them. What they learned in those four weeks seemed to protect them for the duration of the five-year study.

Exactly how emotional stress damages the heart isn't known for sure, but it could have something to do with the heart's increased need for oxygen in stressful situations. Also, over time, stress hormones prompt blood clotting (which can lead to a heart attack) and may eventually harden arteries, leading to high blood pressure and the build-up of arterial plaque, especially in the coronary arteries. Finally, stressed-out people are more likely to give in to bad habits such as overeating or smoking.

Take action

Ten ways to stop stress in its tracks

Stressed? Try these lifestyle strategies from Duke University psychologist James Blumenthal, Ph.D., a leading stress management researcher.

1 **TAKE CARE OF YOURSELF** Get adequate sleep and good nutrition.
2 **TAKE TIME FOR LEISURE ACTIVITIES** All work and no play is not healthy – physically or mentally.
3 **EXERCISE** Daily or almost daily exercise is recommended.
4 **LEARN TO SAY 'NO'** You can't please every one, so don't try.
5 **DELEGATE** Let other people share the load.
6 **PRIORITIZE** Concentrate on what's important and let trivial things go.

BEHIND THE BREAKTHROUGH

He showed them the money

Emotional stress is accepted as a risk factor for heart disease, but when it comes to treating medical conditions, psychology is still an outsider. Nobody knows that better than Geoffrey Reed, Ph.D., who is assistant executive director at the American Psychological Association and a member of the team that linked stress management therapy with better long-term recovery from heart disease.

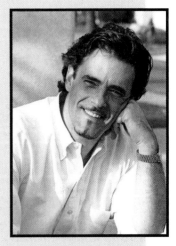

'In general,' he says, 'the medical community looks at psychological treatments the way they look at vitamins. They're not going to hurt you, but they won't contribute much either.'

Dr. Reed has dedicated much of his professional career to changing that thinking. So when he heard that Duke University Medical Center psychologist James Blumenthal, Ph.D., was researching the effects of stress management on recovering heart disease patients, he offered to add another dimension to the study that he knew would get attention from many concerned parties: medical costs. 'There's still some difficulty getting services like stress management programmes paid for on most health plans,' he says. 'They look at the numbers first.'

Dr. Blumenthal brought Dr. Reed and his colleagues on board, along with investigators from the accounting firm PricewaterhouseCoopers. In the end, the results from this unusual three-way collaboration clearly showed that putting heart patients on a stress management programme will not only protect them from heart attacks later on, but can also significantly reduce their medical bills.

Getting those results published in the *American Journal of Cardiology* was important to Dr. Reed's quest. 'If we publish this in a journal for psychologists, we're just telling them what they already know,' he says. 'To change the system, reaching other audiences is important. And cardiologists are more apt to accept psychological interventions because the link between behaviour and cardiovascular events like heart attacks is established.'

Dr. Reed's hope is that the results of this study will lead to more routinely prescribed stress management for heart patients. 'Some comprehensive cardiac rehabilitation programmes offer it, but not all of them,' he says. 'It's not as common as it should be.'

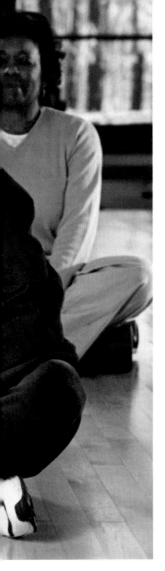

◄ Psychologist James Blumenthal, Ph.D., of Duke University, is one of the clinicians involved in studying the cardiac benefits of stress management techniques. Here he leads one of his study groups in meditation and relaxation exercises.

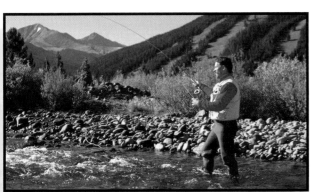

7 **PRACTISE RELAXATION** Try yoga, meditation or muscle relaxation techniques.

8 **CULTIVATE RELATIONSHIPS** A social support network is a buffer against stress.

9 **SHUN THE IRRATIONAL** Negative, unrealistic thinking increases stress.

10 **PURSUE YOUR PASSION** Find out what really inspires you in life, and then do it.

Key discovery

Statins' star rises even higher

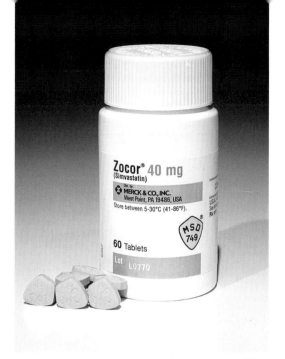

When the drugs known as statins do their job, they reduce the risk of heart attack and other cardiovascular problems by bringing down dangerously high levels of LDL (low-density lipoprotein), the blood cholesterol that can build up on the walls of the coronary arteries. But that turns out to be only part of their power. British researchers have discovered that at least one of the drugs – simvastatin, sold as Zocor – guards against heart attack and stroke even in people with normal cholesterol levels. They also found that statins protect people previously thought not likely to benefit from cholesterol-lowering treatment.

Those findings prompted the study leader to hail statins as 'the new aspirin', suggesting that a daily statin pill should be prescribed as a preventative treatment for those at risk of cardiovascular disease, just as aspirin often is now.

The research came out of the Heart Protection Study, which is a joint project between the Medical Research Council and the British Heart Foundation. It involved more than 20,000 people and as such is the largest trial of statin therapy ever conducted. Participants had varying cholesterol levels but all had a high risk of heart problems, stemming from previous 'vascular events' (such as heart attack or stroke), diabetes or other predisposing factors. After 5½ years, the patients who were taking a daily statin dose of 40mg suffered one-third fewer heart attacks or strokes than the non-statin group.

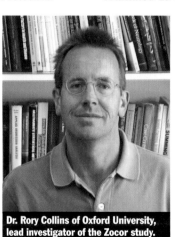

Dr. Rory Collins of Oxford University, lead investigator of the Zocor study.

How it works Simvastatin impairs the body's ability to manufacture cholesterol by inhibiting an enzyme in the liver. That makes it an effective medication for high cholesterol, a known risk factor for heart disease. But statins are not as a rule prescribed to people with marginal cholesterol levels, or to women, diabetics or people over 70. The reason? The evidence wasn't clear that these groups would benefit from a cholesterol-lowering drug. This study showed that they do.

'We've found that statins can protect a far wider range of people than was once thought,' says lead investigator Dr. Rory Collins, professor of medicine and epidemiology at Oxford University.

Availability Statins already are used by an estimated 25 million people worldwide. But the study leaders would like to see that number increase, claiming that if 10 million more people took statins, 50,000 lives would be saved annually. Says Richard Peto, Ph.D., an epidemiologist on the study team, 'Irrespective of the blood cholesterol levels, a statin should now be considered for anybody with a history of heart disease, stroke, other occlusive [involving blockage] vascular disease, or diabetes'. Such recommendations are supported by the low incidence of side effects with statins.

▲ Zocor is one of the increasingly popular statin drugs that have a great track record against heart disease.

Key discovery

For lower cholesterol, make it a double

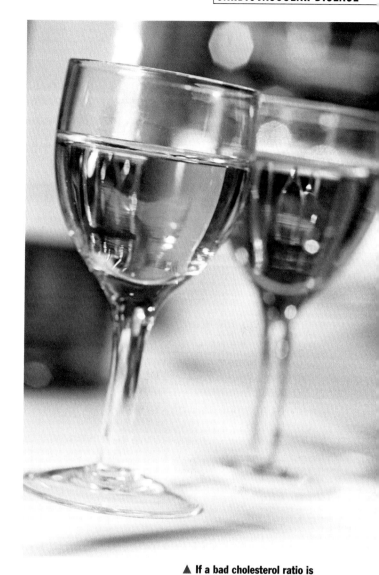

▲ If a bad cholesterol ratio is your problem, two drinks may be better than one – but three are worse than none.

Alcohol's heart-friendly reputation has just had a big boost, especially for postmenopausal women. Research published in the *Journal of Clinical Nutrition* in February 2002 revealed that having two alcoholic drinks in one day offers more than double the protection from cardiovascular disease than one drink provides. In the long term, having one drink a day lowers your risk by 5 per cent; having two cuts it by 10 to 13 per cent, according to the researchers.

In the study, one drink (15g of alcohol – what you will typically consume in a 330ml bottle of beer or a 125ml glass of wine) was shown to reduce levels of 'bad' cholesterol (low-density lipoprotein, or LDL) and triglycerides in the blood. That's good, because LDL can build up on artery walls, restricting blood flow and increasing your risk for heart disease. High levels of triglycerides are also a risk factor for heart disease. But a second drink protects in a different way: by raising levels of 'good' cholesterol (high-density lipoprotein, or HDL), which ushers harmful LDL out of the body.

How they found out The researchers followed 51 women at or near age 60 for three eight-week periods. The women all ate the same diet, but a third had two drinks a day, a third had one drink, and a third had none. Blood sample measurements showed that the alcohol brought down LDL cholesterol and triglycerides in both groups who drank. But only the women who had two drinks a day increased their levels of HDL cholesterol. The results are particularly significant for women over 50, since a woman's risk of heart disease rises sharply after menopause.

Keep in mind that alcohol can have other, negative effects. For instance, drinking too much can harm the liver. And the heart benefits stop with that second drink. A third does more harm than good, actually raising triglyceride levels.

In the long term, having one drink a day lowers your risk by 5 per cent; having two cuts it by 10 to 13 per cent.

Surgical solution
One small heart, one giant leap forward

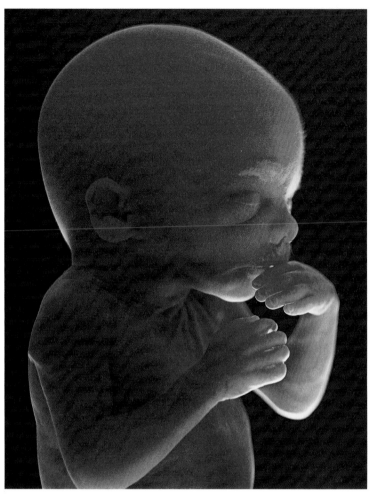

▲ In perhaps the most delicate of all operations with the most delicate of all patients, surgeons are now able to perform heart surgery on foetuses before birth.

Kirsty was just five months pregnant when a routine ultrasound scan revealed that her unborn baby was suffering from pulmonary atresia – a condition in which the pulmonary valve closes up – which generally requires immediate heart surgery at birth.

'It's the shock at first, because no one ever thinks their baby is going to be the one with the problem,' Kirsty told the *Sunday Express*. More scans and tests followed, then, six weeks later, doctors explained that the valve was closing fast; his heart circulation was failing. There were two choices – a Caesarean at 30 weeks, when he weighed only 1.3kg and might be too weak to survive the post-natal operation, or foetal surgery, giving him another two months to grow in the womb.

The parents had a week to decide. It was the first time this type of foetal surgery had been performed in the UK; it had been successful only once before – in Austria. It was an agonising decision, but they took the chance.

A pioneering team at Queen Charlotte's Hospital in London performed the operation. It was a success and five weeks later Jamie was delivered in June 2001.

How it works The pulmonary valve allows blood to pass from the right heart pump to the lungs. When the valve is too narrow, that side of the foetus's heart never fully develops. The team's task was to dilate the valve within the tiny heart of the 30-week foetus. With the help of ultrasound images on a monitor, the surgeons guided a hollow needle through the wall of the womb and into the foetal chest. It was removed through the surrounding plastic sheath and a balloon catheter fed through this across the pulmonary valve of the foetus. The balloon-like device was inflated to widen the passage through the valve before withdrawing the sheath. Blood flow improved immediately. Jamie was delivered weighing 2.5kg and much stronger at 35 weeks, but has had to undergo subsequent corrective surgery.

Availability Foetal heart surgery has been attempted since the 1990s to correct life-threatening abnormalities but had been considered a very risky undertaking. In *The Lancet* (November 2002) Dr. Helena Gardiner and colleagues describe the operations conducted in Austria and London. Similar surgery on a 23-week foetus was performed in Boston, USA in November 2001. The team in London performed a further three successful operations from 23 weeks in 2002 and all babies are doing well.

Drug development

Clogged arteries? This could help to unblock them

Because artery walls tend to stiffen with age, most people over 60 suffer from hardening of the arteries – or arteriosclerosis. But treatment aimed at relaxing the vessels is rare because the biochemical processes involved in the arterial stiffening were thought to be irreversible. That could soon change if a new drug called ALT-711 lives up to expectations. It is hoped that ALT-711 will be able to relax the walls of the arteries and increase their elasticity, so that the heart can pump blood more easily. That will reduce blood pressure and lower the risk for heart attack, heart failure and stroke. The drug is still being tested in the UK, but earlier trials in the US have sparked great interest.

> **It is hoped that [the new drug] ALT-711 will be able to relax the walls of the arteries and increase their elasticity**

When news of ALT-711's successful test was published in September 2001, the drug was immediately hailed as a break-through, and for good reason. As arteriosclerosis ranks as the top predictor of eventual death from heart disease, reversing it could be a lifesaver. Currently, people with the kind of high blood pressure associated with stiff blood vessels – known as isolated systolic hypertension – are typically treated with drugs such as ACE inhibitors (ACE stands for 'angiotensin converting enzyme') and beta blockers. Those drugs can fix the results of blood vessel stiffness but not the vessels themselves.

How it works ALT-711 may sound like a licence-plate number, but, according to American researchers, it's a novel compound that prevents blood sugar molecules from staying attached to the proteins that form artery walls. It does this by dismantling the chemical links between proteins and sugars known as advanced glycosylated crosslink endproducts (AGE or, simply, crosslinks) that cause arteries to stiffen. These crosslinks are most likely to form in diabetics and elderly people, so the drug is especially good news for them.

Availability Before any drug can be licensed in the UK, it must undergo rigorous testing which could take several years. Although its practical benefits might be some way off, ALT-711 offers real hope for the future.

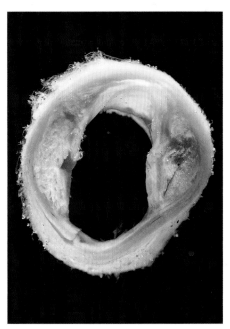

▲ A section through the aorta reveals fatty plaques, left and right, thickening and stiffening the walls.

Key discovery

Risky blood pressure: 'too high' just got lower

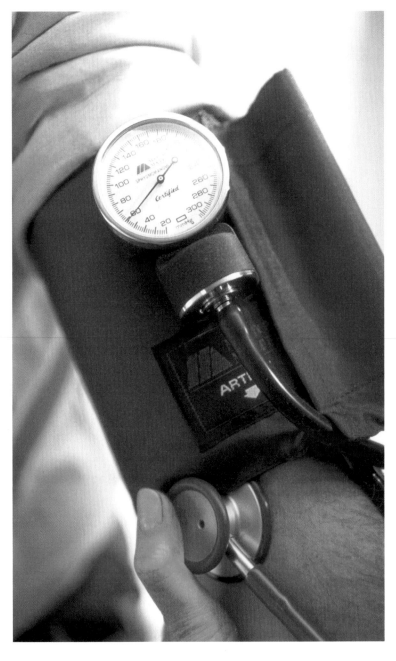

◀ **New research shows that the blood pressure grey zone between 130/85 and 140/90 is a risky place to be.**

There's a new message for the millions of people whose blood pressure is just a little high: the chances of having heart attack, heart failure or a stroke are greater than you may think. Recent results from the ongoing Framingham Heart Study in Boston, USA – which has had a huge impact wordwide – show that women and men over age 35 with 'high-normal' blood pressure run a 1½ to 2½ times greater risk of such cardiac problems than people with normal blood pressure.

Here's how it works. A 'normal' blood pressure reading is 129/84 or below, with the first number measuring the force of the blood on the arteries when the heart is contracted, and the second number measuring the pressure with the heart at rest. But a 'high' reading – indicating hypertension – is 140/90 or more. While hypertension is a warning signal for heart disease, the study found that people whose blood pressure readings fall between high and normal are also at increased risk.

How they did it Researchers have been gathering data on residents in the Boston suburb of Framingham since 1948. They found the high-normal blood pressure risks by following 6,859 heart-healthy people whose readings ranged from high-normal to 'optimal' (less than 120/80). After 12 years, 397 of them either died from heart disease or had a heart attack, heart failure, or a stroke.

By analysing the blood pressure data of the victims and of those who stayed healthy, the researchers determined that the chances of a woman suffering a heart attack, heart failure, or stroke in a 10-year period rises from 2.8 per cent with normal blood pressure to 4.4 per cent with high-normal blood pressure. In men, it goes from 7.6 to 10.1 per cent. And the risk increases sharply with age. The overall risk for women age 35 to 64 with high-normal blood pressure was

4 per cent; for the 65-and-over group it shot up to 18 per cent. For men, the overall risk went from 8 per cent in the younger group up to 25 per cent in the 65-plus group.

What it means Doctors were already urging patients with high-normal blood pressure to take action to bring it down to normal. The Framingham findings, published in the *New England Journal of Medicine* in November 2001, should prompt more people to heed that advice. Recommended changes include weight control, exercise, limiting alcohol intake, and cutting back on dietary fat, cholesterol and sodium.

Take action

Ten ways to limit sodium

Removing excess sodium from your diet can lower your blood pressure. But there's more to it than easing up on the saltcellar. Here are some lesser-known sodium sources to avoid.

1 Processed vegetables (pickles, sauerkraut, canned vegetable soup).
2 Treated meats (bacon, corned beef, canned fish, sausage).
3 Commercial sauces (salad dressings, condiments, gravies).
4 Additives (MSG, sodium bicarbonate, sodium saccharin, sodium nitrate, sodium benzoate).
5 Raising agents (baking powder, baking soda).
6 Over-the-counter medications (antacids, laxatives, sleeping aids).
7 Bread products (breadsticks, crackers).
8 Packaged desserts (pies, turnovers, cupcakes).
9 Fast food (virtually all of it).
10 Water (sports drinks, some bottled waters, tap water in some areas – contact your local water company or county council to find out).

Drug development
The fight against septicaemia

Septicaemia is a deadly cascade of bodily reactions to an infection. It might begin with an apparently minor injury and then progress to inflammation of the blood vessels' inner lining, then to abnormal blood clotting, and eventually to organ failure and death. In 1990 it claimed the life of Jim Henson, creator of the Muppets.

Efforts such as blood transfusions and kidney dialysis haven't put a dent in the 30 per cent death rate from septicaemia. Even administering antibiotics to get at the underlying infection has risks. The infection-causing bacteria themselves often contain toxins that can be released into the victim's bloodstream by the effect of the antibiotic. That causes toxic shock, which can be deadly.

In 1998, septicaemia was the cause of more than 1200 deaths in the UK. But fresh hope lies in a new drug from America called drotrecogin alfa activated. It's being sold in the US under the brand name Xigris.

How it works One early damaging effect of septicaemia is the decrease in the levels of a naturally occurring protein called activated protein C, which helps to stop the blood-clotting process and controls inflammation. Since clotting in the blood vessels destroys organ tissues by blocking their blood supply and thus depriving them of oxygen, the protein's absence is disastrous. Xigris – administered as an intravenous infusion over a period of 48 to 96 hours – is essentially genetically engineered activated protein C. It retards the progress of septicaemia by inhibiting blood clotting.

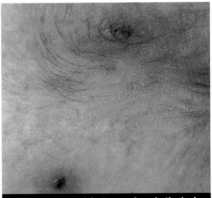
Septicaemia can originate anywhere in the body, such as the kidneys, lungs or skin (as seen here).

Availability The approval of the drug in the USA in early 2002 means that Xigris is now a treatment option there, but its use is limited to septicaemia cases that have reached the life-threatening stage. Where septicaemia is not seen as life-threatening, Xigris is not recommended, since it can cause uncontrolled bleeding. It is likely that a licence for the drug will be applied for soon in the UK, too.

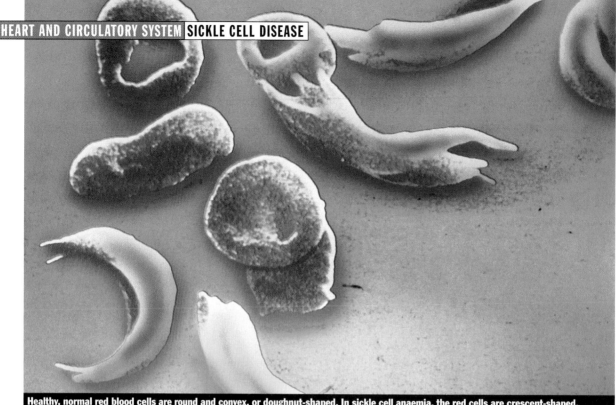

Healthy, normal red blood cells are round and convex, or doughnut-shaped. In sickle cell anaemia, the red cells are crescent-shaped.

Drug development

Experimental drug eases sickle cell crises

A cure for sickle cell disease is still elusive. But researchers have discovered a new drug that promises to cut down on the excruciating 'crises' that periodically strike people with this genetic blood disorder. This will be welcome news for Britain's 10,000 sufferers.

Carriers of sickle cell disease are primarily of African descent. They inherit a gene that results in deformed red blood cells, the iron-based cells responsible for ferrying oxygen through the bloodstream. The deformed cells are rigid and crescent-shaped, like a sickle. Therefore they have difficulty passing through the smaller blood vessels, sometimes clumping together and obstructing blood flow. Those build-ups are thought to be the cause of sickle cell crises and of the accompanying severe pain in the arms, legs, abdomen, or lower back.

The experimental drug, dubbed PP188, appears to do a better job of shortening these crises, which can last for more than a week, than the current therapy options – hydration, oxygen treatment and pain-relieving medications. That finding was the result of clinical trials at 40 US medical centres in which 127 sickle cell patients undergoing a crisis were given PP188 intravenously. About the same number received a placebo of saltwater. Those who got the real drug had shorter pain episodes than the placebo group, lasting 133 hours (about 5½ days) on average, compared with 141 hours. The scientists said the eight-hour improvement was significant proof that the drug works.

How it works Injected into the bloodstream, PP188 reduces the friction between red blood cells, helping them slip around each other more easily and make their way through the blood vessels. That gets oxygen moving to organ tissues, alleviating pain and inflammation.

Availability PP188 is still in the experimental stage, with more clinical trials planned. Next, researchers want to explore its effect on children under 15, who as a group responded much better to the drug. They also want to find out why people who were also taking another sickle cell drug, called hydroxyurea, did better than other PP188 recipients in the initial trials.

ALSO IN THE NEWS

'Repair cells' to the rescue

Many cardiologists are convinced that the heart can be induced to repair itself after damage from a heart attack. But first researchers need to confirm the existence of adult cardiac stem cells that can rush to the site of damage and multiply into healthy new heart tissue. Recently they found an enticing suggestion that such cells do exist. Scientists examined eight female hearts that had been transplanted into men. Reporting their findings in the *New England Journal of Medicine* in January 2002, the investigators said that the transplanted hearts had grown new heart tissue and blood vessels. What's more, many of the new cells had Y chromosomes – meaning they were male and came from the recipient. That's a strong indication that cardiac stem cells – or something very like them – can migrate to where they're needed and proliferate. If they'll also migrate to sites of cardiac damage, the day may come when hearts can be induced to repair themselves.

A heart helper, with no strings attached

A special kind of mechanical pump implanted near the heart adds years to the lives of very sick patients with congestive heart failure. Unlike a mechanical heart, it doesn't completely take over cardiac duties. Instead, it helps only the left ventricle, the part of the heart responsible for pumping. This left ventricular assist system (LVAS) was originally reserved for patients awaiting a donor heart. But today it can be inserted permanently to bring heart performance and blood flow up to speed. Drawbacks?

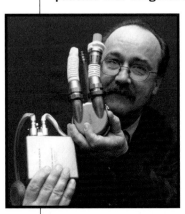

Dr. Walter Pac Jr. holds the Arrow LionHeart left ventricular pump.

Early LVAS models literally bound users to the device's outside power source by wires running through a tube into the body. But the good news is that now there is a new LVAS available that is fully implantable. The pump pictured above, called LionHeart, is soon to hit the market in the USA. It takes in power through the skin from a portable 3.5kg (8lb) power pack worn on a shoulder harness or in a backpack. Rechargeable internal batteries can take over temporarily, which frees the patient from the power pack for 20 minutes. LVADs in use in the UK include the Jarvik 2000 and DeBakely devices.

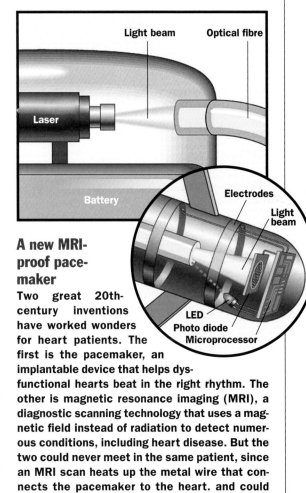

A new MRI-proof pacemaker

Two great 20th-century inventions have worked wonders for heart patients. The first is the pacemaker, an implantable device that helps dysfunctional hearts beat in the right rhythm. The other is magnetic resonance imaging (MRI), a diagnostic scanning technology that uses a magnetic field instead of radiation to detect numerous conditions, including heart disease. But the two could never meet in the same patient, since an MRI scan heats up the metal wire that connects the pacemaker to the heart. and could scar the heart or induce a dangerously rapid heartbeat. But in November 2001, Biophan Technologies in the USA announced the creation of an MRI-proof pacemaker that could make the three million people around the world who have pacemakers eligible for MRI scans.

The prototype – developed by Wilson Greatbatch, the co-inventor of the first pacemaker – uses a semiconductor laser to send electrical signals from the pacemaker to the heart through a fibre-optic cable that won't heat up during an MRI scan. The new model still needs to be tested and approved for use in the USA.

MUSCLES, BONES AND JOINTS

There's never a good time for back or joint pain, but in the past year medical researchers have tapped space-age technology and ancient wisdom to bring you more relief than ever before. Doctors can now repair injured knees by implanting living cells, stop arthritic knee pain with injectable lubrication and may soon be able to strengthen osteoporotic bones with an annual shot that does the work of the daily pills currently prescribed.

At the same time, the practice of a traditional martial art has been found to relieve arthritis symptoms in elderly people, and the age-old belief that weather influences rheumatic pain is getting some respect in scientific circles. Finally, the medical community has opened up new possibilities for pain relief by reconsidering treatments it used to discourage – such as ice treatment for gout attacks, ultrasound therapy for bone fractures, and strength training for fibromyalgia.

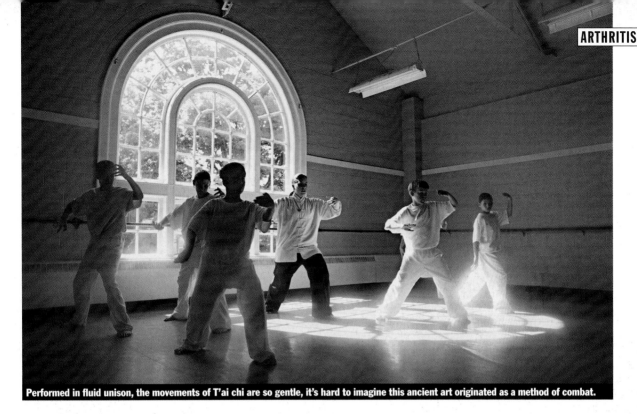

Performed in fluid unison, the movements of T'ai chi are so gentle, it's hard to imagine this ancient art originated as a method of combat.

Key discovery
Ancient remedy for arthritis

The gentle and meditative martial art known as t'ai chi has turned out to be a powerful tool for the elderly. With its emphasis on slow, graceful movements, the traditional Chinese practice is becoming popular in Europe and the USA as more and more older people begin to use it to improve their strength and balance and reduce their risk of falls. Now, there may be even more reason to try t'ai chi, as new research from South Korea indicates that it eases joint pain from osteoarthritis.

This benefit was discovered when investigators put 17 arthritis patients aged 70 and over on a 12-week t'ai chi exercise programme. Twelve weeks later the patient group had much less pain than a control group (which did'nt do t'ai chi), more abdominal muscle strength and better balance.

How it works The Sun-style t'ai chi used in the South Korean study is low-impact exercise that emphasizes fluid but precise movements, such as slowly hugging an imaginary pillar. Its natural, unstressful positions are ideally suited to arthritic elderly people who might find other forms of exercise painful. It can also improve flexibility, posture and balance, reduce hypertension, relieve depression and strengthen muscles, the lungs and the heart.

Availability T'ai chi is an inexpensive pursuit that can be taken up at any age. Studios and classes are increasingly common and training videos are widely available.

PATIENT PROFILE

Pain relief and beyond

When Joyce Keller, 72, moved from Seattle to Santa Cruz, south of San Francisco, she hoped that less rainy weather would ease her osteo-arthritis and osteoporosis pain. Her relief was greater than she could ever have imagined – but it had nothing to do with California sunshine.

The change came when Joyce started taking t'ai chi classes for 'seniors' at the local community centre. 'I started to feel better right away,' she says. When she began to supplement her class sessions with her own daily t'ai chi practice, the pain almost completely disappeared. 'I feel like I have a different body now. I've literally been given a new life.'

Korean researchers have demonstrated that a t'ai chi programme can boost strength and ease arthritis pain. The news comes as no surprise to Joyce. 'I'm very strong now in my arms, my back, and my hands,' she says. 'Before I could barely walk. Now I'm going hiking.'

And she's found one more benefit with t'ai chi. 'My eating habits have changed for the better,' she says. 'For some reason, now that I'm exercising regularly, I don't crave food all the time the way I used to.'

Key discovery
COX-2 painkillers come under fire

A class of breakthrough drugs for arthritis pain came under fire in 2002. Reports stated that the drugs, which include Celebrex (celecoxib) and Vioxx (rofecoxib), were overprescribed in the USA and had potentially dangerous side effects. In addition, a major study used to promote Celebrex was found to have 'serious irregularities'.

The drugs, called COX-2 inhibitors, are pain relievers marketed as having fewer gastrointestinal side effects than most of the non-steroidal anti-inflammatory drugs (NSAIDs), typically prescribed for conditions such as arthritis. NSAIDs include aspirin, ibuprofen, and naproxen.

Celebrex and Vioxx have become blockbusters in Britain and the USA since their approval in the late 1990s. Both are among the top 10 best-selling drugs in the world and are heavily advertised. In 2001, for example, Merck spent about £86 million promoting Vioxxin in the USA, while Pharmacia spent £83 million promoting Celebrex. Yet neither has been found to be better at reducing pain than cheaper drugs such as ibuprofen and naproxen.

A rash of bad news In April 2002, the US Food and Drug Administration announced that Vioxx would require new information on its label noting

> ## Neither has been found to be better at reducing pain than cheaper drugs such as ibuprofen...

that it might be linked to an increased risk of high blood pressure or heart attack. Then, in May, a landmark animal study and an editorial published in the June issue of the US *Journal of Bone and Mineral Research* (JBMR) was released, showing that the COX-2s may impair healing of bone fractures. The drugs are often prescribed for fracture-related pain.

The negative press continued in June as an editorial in the *British Medical Journal* questioned the design of a major clinical trial that convinced the FDA that Celebrex is safer than the NSAIDs ibuprofen and diclofenac because it caused fewer ulcers and ulcer complications.

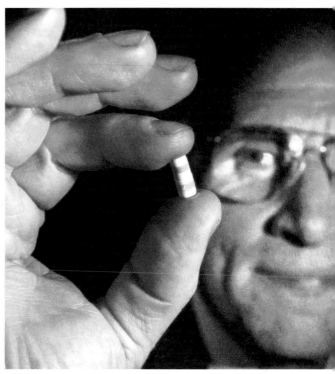

▲ **Dr. Phillip Needleman holds up a Celebrex capsule during a drug company convention.**

Several days later, Express Scripts, one of the largest US pharmacy benefit management companies, released a study finding that the drugs, which are 433 per cent more expensive than the cheaper, generic NSAIDs, are often prescribed when a cheaper alternative would suffice.

In both Britain and the USA, the primary reason for prescribing COX-2s over alternatives, including ibuprofen and naproxen, is when patients are at high risk of developing gastro-intestinal problems such as ulcers. Yet, the study found that 76 per cent of prescriptions were for patients who had no risk of gastro-intestinal problems. The study also found that although the drugs were approved only for the relief of signs and symptoms of rheumatoid arthritis and osteoarthritis (Celebrex) or osteo-arthritis, acute pain (after surgery, for instance) and menstrual pain (Vioxx), 29 per cent of users were taking them for low back pain.

The other side of the story Company officials for both drugs defended their medicines, saying it's best to prescribe them because more than 100,000 people are hospitalized each year in the United States as a result of adverse reactions to NSAIDs. Pharmacia officials also disagreed with the BMJ article, and said that the company stands by its conclusions that Celebrex is safer than NSAIDs as it causes fewer ulcers and ulcer complications.

Key discovery
Risk of osteoarthritis is higher for bow-legged or knock-kneed

Osteoarthritis in the knee can remain a relatively mild hindrance over the years – its pain more aggravating than agonizing. Or, it can progress rapidly into an extremely debilitating condition. Now new research has uncovered a key to predicting which way it will go. That key is the alignment of your hips, knees, and ankles.

The research, from the Northwestern University Medical School in Evanston, Illinois, is the first to identify poor alignment as a risk factor for the progression of knee osteoarthritis. If your legs bow outward at the knees ('bow-legged') or curve inward ('knock-kneed'), you're much more likely to lose some degree of function. And the worse the alignment, the steeper the decline will be.

The researchers made their discovery by observing the condition of 237 people with primary osteoarthritis of the knee over a period of 18 months. They recorded data marking the disease's severity and also measured hip-knee-ankle alignment. People whose alignment was off by 5 degrees or more showed considerably more functional deterioration than those with no or minimal misalignment.

It all has to do with load distribution. Poor alignment increases the weight on either the inner side or outer side of the knee, which boosts the chances of the arthritis progressing on the side bearing the most stress. The study is the first to demonstrate that knee alignment is a factor in the progression of arthritis, and one day its findings may lead to improved treatment based on reducing the stress caused by the poor alignment, says Dr. Leena Sharma the study's lead author.

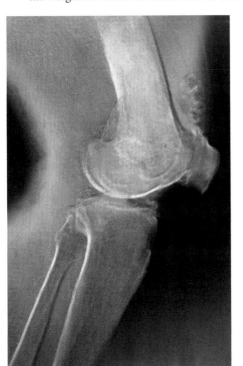

◄ Knee osteoarthritis is, by itself, the cause of more disability in people age 65 and over than any other medical condition.

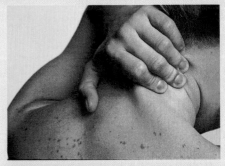

RESEARCH ROUND-UP

Painful joints may be 'under the weather' after all

People often say that they know when the weather is changing because they can 'feel' it in their aching bones and joints. Medical experts have long dismissed the connection as just a superstition. But at least one new study confirms what plenty of arthritis and fibromyalgia sufferers have maintained all along – weather does indeed affect the severity of joint pain.

In fact, the researchers were able to correlate specific weather features with specific joint ailments. In osteoarthritis sufferers, high humidity appears to be associated with pain. In those with fibromyalgia, high atmospheric pressure is a problem. For rheumatoid arthritis patients, it's both. And low temperature is a pain provoker for all three conditions.

How they found out The intriguing study came from the Centro Reumatologico Strusberg in Cordoba, Argentina. Here investigators questioned 151 arthritis or fibromyalgia outpatients about their pain over a year and then correlated their reports with climate conditions over the same period. The connection between the two was clear. And significantly, there was no correlation between weather and pain for 32 healthy people who were also tracked for comparison.

The study, although small, could spark renewed interest in investigating the effect of weather on joint pain. But the issue is still controversial. A small Norwegian study released at the same time concluded that weather does not affect fibromyalgia-related joint pain.

Drug development
'Oiling' the joints: injectable lubrication relieves knee pain

A Canadian study has given a boost to a new osteoarthritis treatment that reduces pain in the knee by replacing its lost joint-cushioning fluid. The procedure, called viscosupplementation or joint fluid therapy, is wonderfully simple. Doctors inject a substance called hyaluronate sodium directly into the knee, where it relieves pain for six months or more by acting as a lubricant.

Published in February 2002, the research confirms that hyaluronate sodium is better at relieving arthritic knee pain than the anti-inflammatory drugs traditionally prescribed.

Canadian researchers gave one group of arthritis patients one weekly injection of hyaluronate sodium for 4 weeks, and another group twice-daily oral doses of diclofenac and misoprostol (a non-steroid anti-inflammatory drug combined with a drug to prevent stomach irritation) for 12 weeks. A third group received both the pills and the shots, while a fourth group received placebo (dummy) pills and placebo injections.

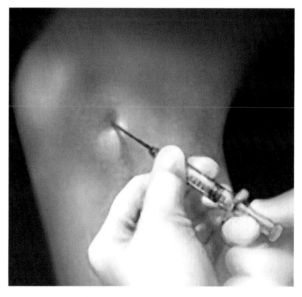

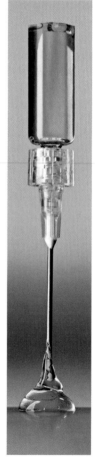

◀ Synvisc involves a series of three injections delivered over 15 days; Hyalgan requires five injections spaced over 10 to 14 days; Supartz, five injections, each a week apart.

... confirms that hyaluronate sodium is better at relieving arthritic knee pain than the anti-inflammatory drugs traditionally prescribed.

After four weeks, all test groups reported feeling better when not moving. But as more time passed, only those receiving the hyaluronate sodium injections reported improvement both at rest and during physical activity.

How it works With arthritis, the joint fluid in the knees loses its gel-like quality, or viscosity, over time, compromising its cushioning effect and causing pain and stiffness. One of the reasons for the thinning of the liquid (called synovial fluid) is the loss of hyaluronic acid. Hyaluronate sodium is an injectable form of hyaluronic acid. It lubricates the knee and restores the cushioning quality of the joint fluid.

Availability Joint fluid therapy, approved in Britain and the USA, has become more popular in the past year or so. Three brands of hyaluronate sodium (or hyaluronan)

products have been licensed for use in viscosupplementation: Hyalgan, Synvisc and Supartz.

The American College of Rheumatology recommends the treatment for sufferers who fail to get knee pain relief from anti-inflammatories. But joint fluid therapy is not a cure for arthritis in the knee and in Britain patients are advised that it may be associated with a short-term increase in knee inflammation. The therapy can, however, alleviate pain and can help to postpone more aggressive therapies such as joint replacement.

Surgical solutions

Back pain: is the answer spare parts for the spine?

Anyone who has experienced excruciating pain from a slipped (herniated) disc craves relief. But is major surgery the answer? There is considerable excitement at present in the USA, about a relatively new surgical technique which can replace a degenerated disc with a fully functioning manufactured version. The procedure, pioneered in Germany and practised at several centres in Britain, is being hailed in the States as 'a tremendous step forward' that may solve many of the problems associated with spinal fusion. But some British specialists have doubts.

How it works The discs that separate one vertebra from the next on your spinal column are made of hard cartilage on the outside with a pulpy middle. The discs strengthen the connection between the vertebrae and absorb shock, while permitting the backbone to move in amazingly flexible ways. When a disc that separates two vertebrae in the lower spinal column degenerates from injury, age, or disease, the pain can be constant and crippling. Spinal fusion ends the pain by removing the damaged disc and fusing the vertebrae together. The relief comes at a price, though. The human backbone is all about motion, and fusing two bones together can disrupt the complex mechanics of the entire back. Nearby vertebrae come under extra stress, and that can mean more pain.

A disc prosthesis may change that. The surgeons go in from the front of the body using small puncture holes in the abdomen so they won't have to move spinal nerves or touch the spinal cord as they take out the bad disc. They then replace it with a polyethylene, steel-plated artificial disc. Instead of fused bones, this is a functioning disc that is designed to restore normal distance between vertebrae, full stability, and natural motion. But does it work?

Availability In Britain and Europe disc prostheses have been implanted in patients for more than a decade although the procedure is still in the final experimental stages in the United States. In Britain, around 100 patients a year with degenerative disc disease have the operation, with varying results. Surprisingly, according to Raymond Ross, consultant spinal surgeon at Hope Hospital in Salford, who has carried out many of these operations, there is currently little proof that either replacing discs or

fusion is particularly beneficial though there is a US study underway comparing the two techniques. Mr Ross firmly believes that the principle of disc replacement is valid but remains concerned about the quality of artificial discs. 'We have to ask ourselves, is this the ultimate technology?'

Those currently approved for use 'still don't mimic the mechanical properties of the human disc,' he says. But soon they may. At least half a dozen companies are currently working to produce a more effective model.

Disc-swapping: How it's done

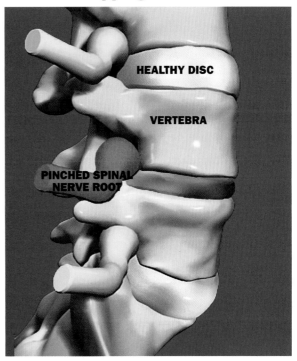

Artificial disc implantation relieves the back and leg pain associated with degenerative disc disease by easing the pressure on pinched spinal nerves. First, the diseased disc is removed. The space between the vertebrae is then widened to relieve pressure on the nerve roots. Metal plates are secured to the exposed faces of the vertebrae, and a polyethylene core is placed in between, replacing the diseased disc.

Key discovery

New steps to secure back pain recovery

It's a painful cycle: back injury, recovery, and injury again. An unusual US study has come up with a good reason that people with previous back problems so often suffer new back injuries. It seems that just about everything the typical back patient does for back protection is wrong.

Researchers at Ohio State University in Columbus asked people with healthy backs and injured backs to do a number of lifts, and then analysed the biomechanics of the movements involved. From this, the researchers determined that people tend to compensate for their injuries by using too many muscles – and the wrong ones, to boot. For example, they might try to protect the injured part of their back by using muscles in the abdomen and sides, as well as uninjured parts of the back, when they would normally use a muscle from the injured area.

That sounds like a reasonable thing to do, but it's actually self-defeating, says William Marras, Ph.D., the biomechanics researcher from Ohio State University who led the study. That's because the more muscles you use, the greater the load you're putting on the spine. The injured group used twice as much twisting force on their spines and one and a half times the compressive force as the healthy group doing the same lifts. Over time, that extra spinal load can cause more back problems.

Trying to protect injured back muscles by lifting extra slowly – another seemingly logical compensation – makes things worse by prolonging the inappropriate muscle use.

To cap it all, the bad habits you develop when your back is injured may persist after the original injury heals, since you may have effectively reprogrammed yourself to lift things in an different (and inefficient) way.

The impact The study, published in the December 2001 issue of the US journal *Spine*, raises the need for reforms in employee safety regulations, according to Dr. Marras. He says that the emphasis should be on minimizing the opportunity for back patients to develop the poor lifting habits revealed in his study. 'The workplace needs to be ergonomically designed to accommodate workers recovering from back injuries,' Dr. Marras says. 'And we've got to make sure we don't send people back to these jobs until they're ready.'

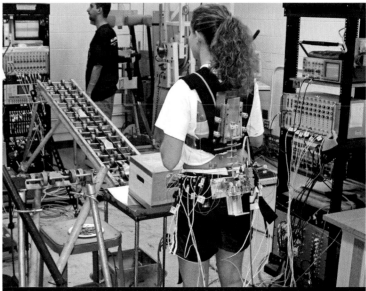

A research volunteer is hooked up to laboratory equipment that records nerve impulses in the muscles and data about back motion in three-dimensional space.

Take action

Correct lifting techniques

Use your legs when you lift ... Don't bend at the waist or lean down and forward to lift ... Strengthen your midsection muscles ... Lose weight if you need to. Those standard back-protection tips still hold. But the latest research suggests some new do's and don'ts:

■ Avoid repetitive lifting Whatever the weight involved, remember cumulative wear and tear causes more back injuries than single heavy lifts.

■ Bend sideways carefully Rapid bending to the left and right leads to back problems.

■ Twist slowly Quick rotation at the torso stresses your spine.

■ Keep this surprising new finding in mind Your load is only slightly reduced – not halved – when someone helps you to carry something.

■ Don't lift at all if it's too painful. Otherwise you may well adjust by using the wrong muscles, inviting more back problems later on.

Alternative answers

Listen to this: sound can heal bones quickly

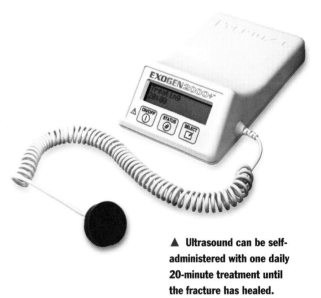

▲ **Ultrasound can be self-administered with one daily 20-minute treatment until the fracture has healed.**

There is good news for people with fractured bones. An extensive medical research review has shown that ultrasound therapy greatly accelerates the healing of bone fractures. The finding is encouraging as the treatment is relatively simple and involves equipment that people can use at home.

Although widely used in other areas of medicine, ultrasound therapy as a fracture treatment is much newer and in the past has been shunned by orthopaedists in the USA on the grounds that it slowed healing rather than advanced it. But Canadian researchers examined medical literature from 1994 to 2000 and concluded that fracture patients who received ultrasound treatment healed on average 64 days sooner than those those who didn't. Their findings were announced in February 2002.

How it works While high-intensity ultrasound generates deep-tissue heat and is a common treatment for tendons, ligaments and other soft tissues, it is low-intensity pulsed ultrasound therapy which appears to accelerate the healing of fractures. The precise action of ultrasound waves on fractures is not fully understood, but the evidence suggests that it is sensed at the cell surface, causing cascades of intra-cellular signalling, which results in

▶ **The X-ray on the left shows a fresh fracture. The one on the right is the same bone after three months of ultrasound therapy.**

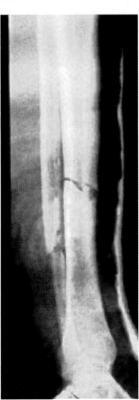

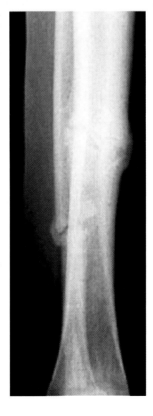

accelerated protein synthesis and therefore enhanced fracture healing. In order for it to work, the pulse has to be aimed through the skin directly at the fracture site.

Availability In Britain, the Exogen ultrasound device – one of several licenced here – has been used since 1998 to treat patients with slow healing fractures. Footballers and other athletes are among those who have used it to accelerate the healing of fractures and their return to sport.

Patients are referred for the treatment either privately or through the NHS and once it has been approved by an orthopaedic surgeon, patients can use the device and treat themselves at home. The Exogen 2000+ model is battery-operated and delivers the ultrasound signal to the fracture either directly through the skin or through a hole in a cast.

Following the Canadian study, the therapy looks set to become increasingly popular both here and in the USA. 'As individual clinicians become more aware of the usefulness of ultrasound for fracture healing, many of them will pursue it as an option,' predicts the study's lead author Dr. Jason Busse.

Key finding

Pumping iron may give fibromyalgia patients a lift

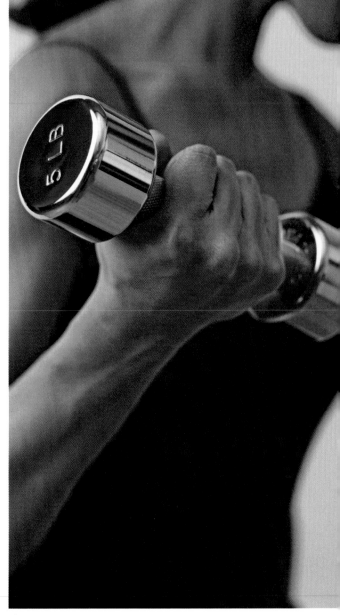

Across the Western world, there are millions of patients who suffer from fibromyalgia, a condition which mostly affects women aged 25 to 55. Seeking relief from their head-to-toe muscular aches and pains, they are usually told to get regular cardiovascular (aerobic) exercise, such as walking or cycling, together with stretching to prevent muscle spasms. Strength training has generally been discouraged by doctors on the grounds that it may cause injury and would exacerbate the symptoms.

New evidence from the USA may change the standard recommendation. Researchers from Harvard found that 15 women who completed a 20-week exercise programme that included a generous amount of strength-training work – the use of hand weights, weight machines and body-weight movements such as pushups, for example – showed significant improvement. Their overall body strength increased and they could walk faster over distance. Most importantly, perhaps, they felt better.

The study is a fair indication that strength training could have a role to play in the treatment of fibromyalgia, the researchers believe. 'These findings demonstrate that an exercise programme that includes strength-training activities can be safe, feasible and beneficial for persons with fibromyalgia syndrome,' notes Daniel S. Rooks, Sc.D., of the Harvard Institute of Medicine.

▲ **A strength-training programme may ease your fibromyalgia symptoms – but be sure to consult your doctor before you proceed with one, then start slowly and gently.**

The results of the pilot study may now lead to larger studies that point to more specific advice regarding strength-training for the relief of the debilitating malady that has a variety of symptoms. It is mainly associated with chronic muscle and joint pain severe enough to disrupt patients' lives and careers, although diagnostic tests reveal that most sufferers show no signs of joint abnormalities or muscle damage. Other symptoms include depression, chronic fatigue, headaches and memory impairment.

'These findings demonstrate that an exercise programme that includes strength-training activities can be safe, feasible, and beneficial for persons with fibromyalgia ...'

Alternative answers

Giving gout attacks the cold treatment

New advice to gout sufferers: keep your ice trays full. Conventional medical wisdom holds that cold treatment for gout pain doesn't work and can even make things worse. But conventional wisdom may be wrong, according to the latest US research. Holding ice packs on the afflicted joint does indeed seem to ease the pain of a gout attack.

Gout, a form of arthritis that affects mostly men, is a metabolic disease. When the body has trouble eliminating a waste product called uric acid, some of the excess can form crystals in the joints, often in the big toe, causing painful attacks. The plant extract colchicine, steroid drugs such as prednisone and nonsteroidal anti-inflammatory drugs (NSAIDs) such as ibuprofen, are the preferred symptom relievers, but rheumatologists have seldom recommended ice therapy.

The misconception is that cooling the joints may increase crystal formation and worsen attacks, says Dr. Naomi Schlesinger who led the study of 19 gout patients at New Jersey Medical School-University of Medicine and Dentistry of New Jersey.

'We even occasionally see clinicians recommending the application of warm packs to gouty joints,' she says.

Rejecting that assumption, Dr. Schlesinger treated two groups of 19 gout patients, one with ice and drugs and the other with drugs only. The 'iced' patients reported less pain than the control group. They also described their attacks as less severe than before.

According to Dr. Schlesinger, it's not too early for gout sufferers to grab an ice pack from the freezer when the next attack hits.

Will the ice therapy work with drugs other than the prednisone and colchicine used in this study? Can it work alone? Larger studies are needed to answer those questions before most rheumatologists will consider recommending ice therapy. But according to Dr. Schlesinger, it's not too early for gout sufferers to grab an ice pack from the freezer when the next attack hits. If by chance ice seems to make your symptoms worse, you should obviously discontinue it.

Take action

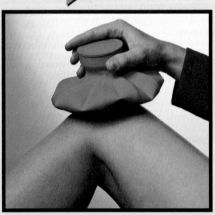

Four ways to put gout pain on ice

Thinking about trying an ice pack on that painful joint – but you don't have an ice pack? Try these alternatives:

1 Use ice cubes in a Ziploc plastic bag, but add some water before you seal it. That way the bag will sit better on the aching joint.

2 Use a bag of frozen vegetables from your freezer. Peas and sweetcorn are best – they're small and round, so they will cover the painful area more evenly than lumpier vegetables.

3 For comfort, wrap a towel around your makeshift ice pack before applying it to the joint. The cold will soon get through.

4 Make a water ice-lolly, or freeze water in a paper cup and peel off the first inch or so of the paper. Massage it directly (with no towel) on the painful area until the ice is melted.

However you fashion your ice pack, apply it for 30 minutes four times a day. That's the schedule that got good results in a study on ice treatment for gout pain.

Surgical solution

Cell therapy paves way to 'pothole' repair in knees

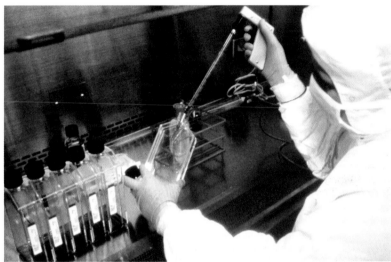

▲ At the Genzyme laboratory, a sample of about 250,000 chondrocytes extracted from the patient can be multiplied to a count of about 12 to 15 million at a cost of about £6,400.

A new surgical technique is bringing faster relief to footballers and other people who suffer the kind of knee injury that creates 'potholes' on the protective knee cartilage of the joint. Until recently, orthopaedic surgeons' best way to repair these potholes was to shave down the joint in order to produce scar tissue, which fills the cavity. The results were usually temporary and often did little to prevent the onset of arthritis. But now specialists in Europe and the USA have an alternative way to 'resurface' damaged knee cartilage.

The procedure is called autologous chondrocyte implantation, or ACI. Healthy cartilage cells, known as chondrocytes, are harvested from the patient, grown in a culture, then implanted in the damaged area, where they grow into healthy new cartilage tissue.

How it works First surgeons examine the damage through an arthroscope, which requires only a tiny incision. If they find a lesion that's a good candidate for ACI, they extract a sample of chondrocytes and send it off to the laboratory to grow. In a few weeks they get back a phial with a few million healthy, living knee cartilage cells.

Then comes the hard part, which involves open-knee surgery. The surgeon first steals from the shinbone a bit of periosteum, a fibrous membrane that covers bones, to use as a patch to hold the new cells in the hole. (The cells are liquid, and they'll spill out if you just squirt them in.) Sewing the patch is a meticulous, time-consuming task requiring many tiny stitches with 'thread' no thicker than an eyelash. The patch is sealed with an adhesive, usually a sticky substance called fibrin that's taken from the patient's own blood or a commercially available product. Next the cells are injected into the lesion through a hole in the patch, which is then sealed tight.

In the past year, much new data has become available from long-term follow-up studies of the original Swedish and other early experimental uses of ACI. The reports show ACI to be highly successful. Around 80 per cent of patients are still experiencing good results, some almost a decade after their surgery.

Availability Among the handful of centres in Britain which perform the surgery is the Robert Jones and Agnes Hunt Orthopaedic Hospital in Oswestry, where the first such operation was carried out in 1996. The centre's surgical team, led by Prof. James Richardson, now performs some 50 ACI operations a year.

To date these reflect the success reported elsewhere. 'We find in general that the knees do improve and that improvement can be maintained for a number of years afterwards,' says Graham Smith, a clinical research fellow at the hospital. Currently, ACI is considered suitable for a select group of patients who have specific knee injuries or cartilage defects such as osteoarthritis dessicans but they plan to extend the treatment to younger patients with localized arthritic conditions. 'We're hoping the surgery could delay or even prevent knee replacement,' he said.

The Oswestry hospital is the only one in Britain where the patients' cartilage cells are grown regularly on site in their own NHS laboratory. In America, Genzyme in Boston operates the only commercial laboratory that is permitted to grow the cultures – at much greater cost.

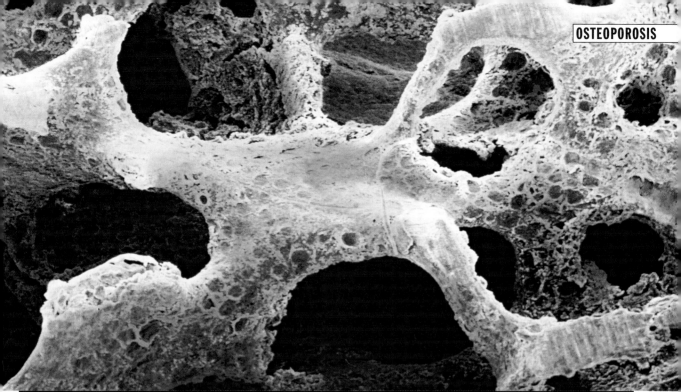

Osteoporosis robs bone tissue of its mineral stores, resulting in porous, fragile, brittle bones. Bisphosphonate drugs help to replenish bone minerals.

Drug development

A once-a-year injection to save your bones

Every day, many people with osteoporosis follow the same routine: They take a Fosamax or Actonel pill first thing in the morning on an empty stomach. They follow it with a full glass of water. Then, for at least a half hour afterwards, they have to stay in an upright position without eating or drinking anything. Not surprisingly, some fail to stick to the regime.

But what if people could get a single injection that would do as much to treat osteoporosis as daily bone-strengthening pills – but only needed the jab once a year? Well, one day it may be possible. A substance called zoledronic acid may prevent as well as treat osteoporosis, which is good news for millions of people – three quarters of them women – who are likely candidates for the disease because of their low bone density.

How it works If zoledronic acid performs in practice the way it did in a New Zealand study, reported in February 2002, that evaluated its effectiveness, a single 4mg dose delivered intravenously will increase bone density and help to prevent bone loss. Most significantly, it will continue to promote bone density for a year or more before another injection is required.

Zoledronic acid belongs to the same class of drugs (bisphosphonates) as the most common once-a-day osteoporosis oral medications – alendronate sodium (Fosamax), now also available as a weekly tablet, and risedronate sodium (Didronel) – but it's much more powerful. Bisphosphonates work by interfering with the body's natural, ongoing cycle of building up bone, then breaking it down, a process known as bone remodelling, which keeps bone tissue healthy and strong. The drugs limit the breakdown phase of remodelling but let the formation phase proceed unimpeded, thus tilting the balance in favour of bone growth and density.

Availability Zoledronic acid is available under the brand name Zometa but is only licenced to treat bone cancer. But several large studies are planned in the USA and elsewhere to confirm that intravenous zoledronic acid really can prevent fractures as well as increase bone density – a move welcomed in the UK by the National Osteoporosis Society. 'The prospect of a once-a-year injection is a very interesting development and one that we will want to watch', said a spokesman.

High-tech help

Mechanical leech: blood flow, minus the 'yuck' factor

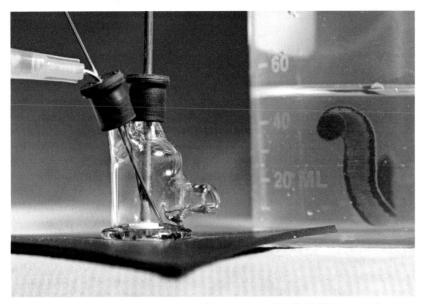

▲ The mechanical leech (left) has a number of distinct advantages over its living counterpart (on the right), especially for the squeamish.

Leeches are ugly little suckers. But because of their phenomenal comeback as a medical tool in the past few decades, patients and their doctors have learned to appreciate the little beasts.

In their heyday in the early nineteenth century, leeches were used for drawing blood. Now, they are used to remove stagnant blood that accumulates where reconstructive surgery has been performed and have become popular again across Europe and America, because of the boom in plastic and reconstructive surgery. When a severed finger is re-attached, for example, the blood may not flow smoothly through the site. If there is no surgical solution, something else may be needed to steadily remove the pooled blood so that fresh blood can move in to keep the tissue alive. That's exactly what leeches are good at.

Leeches can take in up to five times their body weight in blood. They can get blood out of vessels too small for a syringe. And the creatures can get it out slowly and steadily because they prevent blood from clotting by secreting a natural anticoagulant called hirudin.

Usefulness aside, most people would prefer a more appealing alternative. Now, some fine minds at the University of Wisconsin at Madison in the USA have come up with a mechanical device that does everything a real leech can do and is less repellent.

The new mechanical leech also reduces the risk of infection and offers more efficient blood collection. And it is much better behaved. When a leech attaches itself to the skin, its goal is to get a satisfying meal of fresh blood, which may be more or (usually) less than what is required therapeutically. And while the creature works at a pace that suits its own needs, rather than those of the patient, the new mechanical device can be manipulated to handle the requirements of any therapeutic situation. When all is said and done, it is easier to train a machine than a worm.

RESEARCH ROUND-UP

Leeching away arthritis pain

When leeches suck blood, they give as well as take. Their saliva is a virtual pharmacopoeia of potentially useful secretions, including natural painkillers. Those painkillers may explain why leech therapy reduced osteoarthritis pain and inflammation in a recent German study. The researchers treated 10 of 16 osteoarthritis patients with leeches by letting four of the creatures go to work for 80 minutes on the patients' inflamed knees. Only those 10 patients reported significant pain relief soon after – and they still felt relief 28 days later. In modern times, homeopathic practitioners have used similar treatments, but conventional doctors may soon be taking a closer look at leech therapy for arthritis symptoms. Further studies are planned.

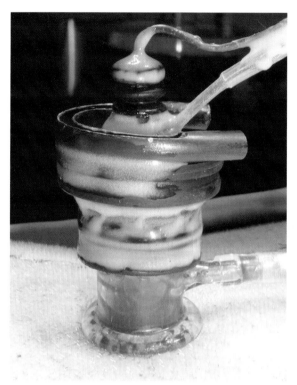

▲ The mechanical leech's glass vacuum chamber maintains suction and irrigation of the wound.

How it works The mechanical leech is bigger, but still small enough to fit in the palm of a hand. It uses suction to get the blood out, just as a real leech does, but then it sends the blood through tubes to storage. The device's suction action creates a kind of mechanical turbulence that helps prevent clotting. It does not release hirudin, but the technician irrigates the wound with the anticoagulant heparin to further inhibit clotting.

Availability Just the fact that the mechanical leech works in the lab with animals is a major breakthrough. 'We've created a device that can draw much more blood than a medicinal leech and can dramatically improve tissue health,' says Dr. Gregory Hartig, the University of Wisconsin otolaryngologist who invented the device. There's more work to be done, however, before live leeches are made redundant.

Dr. Hartig wants to perfect the machine's ability to regulate its suction. A feedback system that's under development will enable the device to automatically draw more or less blood as needed. His team is also working on a new industrial prototype better suited for real-world use. The current experimental model uses glass parts and other features that would cause problems in a hospital setting. Finally, the device needs to be tested sufficiently on humans before the US and other governments will grant the approval required for clinical use. Dr. Hartig guesses all that won't take more than two or three years.

ALSO IN THE NEWS

A quicker way to find hidden tumours.

Patients with a painful bone-softening disease have often had to wait years for surgeons to find and remove the tumours that cause the condition, known as oncogenic osteomalacia. But a team of US researchers at the Johns Hopkins Medical Institutions in Baltimore has reported in the British medical journal *The Lancet* that they've found a way to smoke out the hidden tumours with radiation-detecting gamma X-rays. The breakthrough came when the investigators found a radioactive agent called pentetreotide, which binds to a hormone receptor in the tumours, revealing their hiding place under X-rays. Once the tumours are removed, the condition is reversed and the pain is gone. Onco-genic osteomalacia is very rare, but the researchers think that it's often misdiagnosed as arthritis.

Tidying up during hip surgery saves lives.

Running a vacuum cleaner during hip-replacement surgery could save lives, according to a New Zealand study reported in the *Journal of Bone and Joint Surgery*. During the procedure, tiny particles of fat, bone marrow, and the cement used to attach the new hip are unavoidably loosened. Some find their way into the bloodstream, where they can cause blood clot formation known as deep vein thrombosis. If the clots travel and block the blood supply to the brain, heart or lungs, they can be deadly. According to the study, using a special vacuum to suck out the particles not only removes most of them but also reduces the incidence of deep vein thrombosis. The vacuum device has been available for some time but isn't always used.

The best remedy for tennis elbow? Do nothing.

Tennis elbow (officially, lateral epicondylitis) is a repetitive stress injury marked by pain on the outer elbow resulting from tiny forearm muscle tears caused by wielding tools or swinging rackets. The ailment is usually treated with a corticosteroid shot or physical therapy. But in Holland the treatment of choice is to simply wait for the injury to heal on its own. And a Dutch study published in *The Lancet* indicates that the wait-and-see approach works at least as often as the others do. The researchers found that those who received injections got the most immediate relief, but their recurrence rate was high. The physical therapy and wait-and-see groups came out more or less the same in the long run, with both of them reporting less pain and more general improvement than the injection group.

REPRODUCTION AND SEXUALITY

Last year the brave new world of reproductive technology hit the headlines as a Yorkshire couple were given the go-ahead to create a healthy child whose bone marrow might be able to save a desperately sick sibling while another couple were refused. Read about the cases and the ethical controversies surrounding 'designer babies' on page 218.

A new improvement to in vitro fertilization may make the technique less controversial by cutting down on the incidence of multiple births. And for women wishing not to become pregnant, there will soon be two new methods of birth control to choose from.

If you're facing the menopause, you'll be interested in news of an antidepressant drug that may significantly ease hot flushes – a boon to those who don't want to take oestrogen. Speaking of hormones, turn to page 216 to find out why one pharmaceutical company is pushing the idea of testosterone replacement for middle-aged men.

Drug development

Slow and steady contraceptive ring wins broad approval

The NuvaRing, one of the first new contraceptive methods to receive official approval in years, should be available in Britain by 2005. Developed by the Dutch-based pharmaceutical company Organon Inc. and licensed in the USA and four European countries in 2002, it is a thin, plastic ring about the size of a bracelet that releases a steady, low dose of oestrogen and progesterone, altering the reproductive cycle and preventing pregnancy.

It also provides the lowest dose of hormones of any other available hormonal contraceptive, says Nancy Alexander, Ph.D., director of medical services for contraception at Organon. The device contains just 15mcg of oestrogen, while the lowest amount in birth control pills is 20mcg. Despite the lower hormone dose, the ring is just as effective in preventing pregnancies as the birth control pill, she says, with just one or two women out of every hundred becoming pregnant while using the ring.

'Its low, but steady oestrogen dose should mean fewer oestrogen-related side effects,' Dr. Alexander says. The hormones are mixed into the polymer that is used to make the ring, and an outer 'skin' over the ring's core helps to regulate their release, she explains.

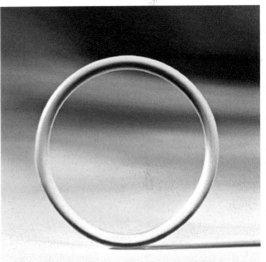

▲ THE FLEXIBLE transparent NuvaRing is about the size of a small bangle. Exact positioning is not essential, so it cannot be inserted incorrectly.

How it's used Women insert NuvaRing just as they would a tampon, and the ring remains in place for three weeks. Then the woman removes it, has her period and, after a week, inserts a new ring. The ring will stay in place even during intercourse, says Dr. Alexander. In studies, around two-thirds of men reported that they rarely or never felt it during intercourse and if it slips out, says Dr. Alexander, women can just wash it off and reinsert it. However, if the ring is out of your body for more than three hours, you should use a back-up birth control method for the next seven days. In clinical tests, side effects, although not common, included vaginal discharge and irritation. Like oral contraceptives, NuvaRing may increase the risk of blood clot formation, heart attack and stroke.

No more periods? NuvaRing may one day be used to help women skip their periods altogether. Clinical trials testing the ring as a form of 'continuous contraception' began in the United States in the summer of 2002. The trials will test the safety and efficacy of allowing women to use the ring continuously, inserting a new ring immediately after finishing with the old one. A growing number of women are turning to continuous contraception – often using birth control pills – to avoid painful or unusually heavy periods.

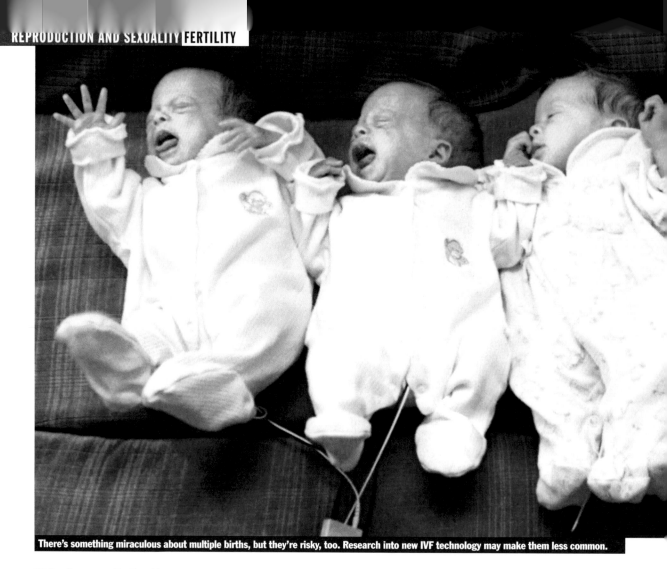

There's something miraculous about multiple births, but they're risky, too. Research into new IVF technology may make them less common.

High-tech help

Better 'bath' means fewer multiple births

One of the biggest problems with assisted reproductive techniques such as in vitro fertilization (IVF) is the high number of multiple births that result. Doctors implant several fertilized eggs in the mother, hoping that at least one will result in a pregnancy, but often more than one succeeds. Since assisted conception became popular, the incidence of multiple pregnancy has increased, from 10-15 per 100,000 maternities in 1981 to more than twice that in 1991. In addition to the strain these pregnancies place on families and the health service, they also carry increased risks, such as a greater chance of premature labour and delivery complications.

But IVF may be getting safer. Changes to the culture in which fertilized eggs are grown (think of it as their food source) are being tested and promise to revolutionize the procedure, enabling eggs to stay in the culture longer and grow larger, say reproductive endocrinologists. This increases the chance of each egg resulting in a pregnancy, and enables doctors to place fewer fertilized eggs in the mother – which should reduce the multiple birth rate.

How it works The new 'high-test' culture medium, which is used to grow the eggs, has specific amino acids and carbohydrates added. This makes it more closely mimic the

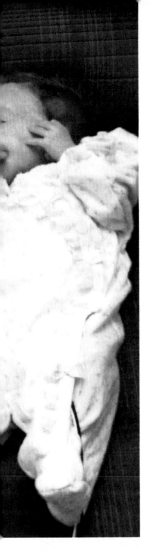

environment in which a naturally developing embryo finds itself from days 3 to 5. This allows the fertilized egg to spend up to five days in its Petri dish 'bath', compared with 3 days in the medium currently used. So instead of returning a 2 or 8-cell embryo to the mother, doctors can implant a 100 to 120-cell embryo, called a blastocyst, significantly increasing the odds of a pregnancy.

Generally, 25 per cent of all embryos transferred at the 8-cell stage on day 3 will survive uterine implantation, while 50 per cent of those transferred on day 5 will continue to thrive, says David K. Gardner, Ph.D., scientific director of the Colorado Center for Reproductive Medicine in Englewood, Colorado. Research in the UK, conducted at the Assisted Conception Unit of Guy's and St Thomas' Hospital, London, agrees that the benefits of transfer at the blastocyst stage include better embryo selection, enabling doctors to identify those embryos which have poor developmental potential. And it also makes other procedures possible, such as genetic testing before the embryo is implanted (see the article on page 218).

There's another exciting benefit to this technology, says Dr. Gardner. Studies are finding that the blastocysts are heartier and freeze well for future implantation, something that wasn't possible when researchers first tried growing embryos beyond the eight-cell stage.

Availability Use of the new culture is now widespread among fertility clinics in the United States, where the rate of triplet and other higher-order multiple births is now in decline. The new procedure is, however, used much less in the UK. An overview of blastocyst culture and transfer, published in 2001 by researchers working at the Assisted Conception Unit, Guy's and St Thomas' Hospital in London, conceded that the procedure's potential benefits included 'better embryo selection, higher implantation rate and lowering of the multiple pregnancy rates by transferring fewer embryos'.

But the researchers added, 'doubts over the safety of extended culture as well as efficacy of the procedure in various patient groups are yet to be resolved before blastocyst transfer can be routinely practised.'

TEST-TUBE TECHNIQUES ALSO DELIVER SOME RISKS

In vitro fertilization (IVF) suffered some negative publicity in early 2002. Three papers were published finding significant rates of birth defects or low birth-weights in babies conceived with the help of IVF and other assisted reproduction techniques. A Swedish study published in the February 2002 issue of *The Lancet* suggests that children born after IVF could be at increased risk of neurological problems, particularly cerebral palsy. In March, two studies published in the *New England Journal of Medicine* in the USA, also indicated similar problems.

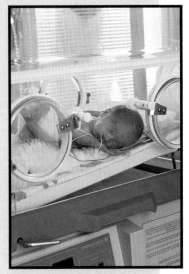

Babies conceived using IVF often have special medical needs right from the start.

'Researchers in Australia found the rate of birth defects in infants conceived with either IVF or intracytoplasmic sperm injection (in which a single sperm is injected into an egg) to be slightly more than double that of children conceived naturally (about 9 per cent compared to 4.2 per cent). And researchers at the Centers for Disease Control and Prevention in the United States, found that test-tube babies have twice the risk of being underweight when born, mainly because of the high number of multiple births associated with the procedure.

'Infertility is a disease,' says Dr. Jamie Grifo, Ph.D., president of the Society for Assisted Reproductive Technology. 'We have known for years that patients who have trouble getting pregnant can often have difficult pregnancies, which can affect their children.' Other risk factors include the advanced age of the mother (women often try to get pregnant naturally for years before turning to assisted techniques), medications used to induce ovulation or maintain the pregnancy early on and factors associated with the procedures themselves.

Provisional figures from the Human Fertilization and Embryology Authority show that in the UK, too, more women aged 38 or older are starting IVF treatment. But the general success rate is still increasing – up from 19.5 per cent for each treatment cycle in 1998-1999 to 21.8 per cent in 2000-2001.

High-tech help

Worried about your biological clock? Wear this watch

P icture the scene – a romantic dinner for two with your husband and suddenly your watch beeps. Did you miss an appointment? Forget to take a pill? No. It's time to have sex. You're wearing the PSC Fertility Monitor, a black wristwatch-like monitor that measures the acidity of your sweat to determine when you're ovulating.

It may *sound* like an episode from 'Sex and the City' (and, in fact, the popular television programme used the monitor in an episode), but it's no fantasy. Made in Canada, the monitor is real, and received approval in the United States last autumn.

How it works The device predicts ovulation by measuring acidity levels in sweat, which are determined by hormone levels. The 'watch' should be worn for only six continuous hours each day from early in the menstrual cycle (starting on days 1 to 3) until the device announces that ovulation will occur. In one study of 105 women, it correctly predicted the time of ovulation to within two days before or after the actual time (which was determined by blood tests) in 73 per cent of participants.

Availability The PSC Fertility Monitor is due to be launched in Britain this year and should soon be available from chemists and pharmaceutical outlets. It is likely to cost between £100 to £150. At present the nearest available alternative is 'Persona', a contraceptive device that measures hormone levels in urine samples to identify fertile and non-fertile days and pinpoint when ovulation is likely to occur. This can help users to avoid unwanted pregnancies and also benefits couples who want to conceive.

◄ More than a fashion statement for hopeful mothers-to-be. The PSC Fertility Monitor will tell you when you're ovulating.

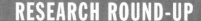

RESEARCH ROUND-UP

Fertility drugs don't increase cancer risk

For years, fertility specialists warned women that the drugs used to increase the number of eggs their ovaries produce could also increase their risk of ovarian cancer. But a study in the February 2002 issue of the *American Journal of Epidemiology* puts that concern to rest. Researchers at the University of Pittsburgh reviewed eight studies involving 5,207 women with ovarian cancer and 7,705 without. They found 'no statistically significant link' between the use of fertility drugs and over-all risk of ovarian cancer.

Study finds no link between the pill and breast cancer

Until recently, researchers believed that taking oral contraceptives raised a woman's risk of developing breast cancer. But now the balance of evidence may be shifting. A new study of more than 9,000 women between ages 35 and 64 found that those who had used oral contraceptives in the past were no more likely to develop breast cancer than women who never used the pill. The study was reported in the *New England Journal of Medicine* in June 2002.

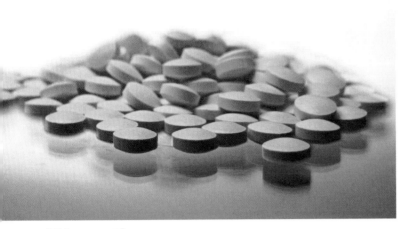

◄ BOOSTING YOUR INTAKE of folic acid and zinc just might boost your chances of becoming a father.

Alternative answers
Supplements for your sperm

Women hear plenty of advice on what they should – and shouldn't – eat and drink even when they're just *considering* getting pregnant. For instance, they're supposed to start taking supplements of folic acid, a vitamin found to prevent spinal deformities in fetuses. Now comes news that the same supplement, paired with the mineral zinc, can also help men plagued by fertility problems.

Dutch researchers compared 107 fertile men with 103 'subfertile' men, giving them either zinc, folic acid, a combination of the two or a dummy pill (placebo) for 26 weeks. In the men who received the zinc (66mg a day) and folic acid (5mg a day), the total sperm count increased by 74 per cent, with only a minor increase (just 4 per cent) in abnormal sperm. Unfortunately, even with that huge increase in sperm count, the sub-fertile men were still subfertile. But, as the lead researcher Régine Steegers-Theunissen, associate professor in obstetrics and gynaecology, told *New Scientist* magazine, 'The more you have, the greater your chances ... You only need one'.

There's no need to take supplements, because you can get plenty of zinc and folic acid through your diet. Good sources of folic acid (also called folate and folacin) include asparagus, broccoli, Brussels sprouts, cabbage, pinto beans, okra, spinach and whole grains. Because the nutrient is destroyed by heat, more than half the folic acid in foods can be lost in cooking, so enjoy your spinach in a salad instead of cooked. Good sources of zinc include oysters (just one serving of six oysters provides more than five times the recommended daily amount of zinc), lean minced beef, sirloin steak, liver, turkey thighs and drumsticks, eggs, and lentil soup.

ALSO IN THE NEWS

Contraceptive skin patch coming soon

To the pills, creams, rings, and other methods used to prevent conception, now add Ortho Evra, a contraceptive skin patch. The sticky patch, about the size of a 50p piece, has already been licensed in the USA and throughout Europe and should be available in the UK later this year. Each patch delivers a 7-day supply of the hormones progestogen and oestrogen through the skin. After wearing the patches for three weeks, a woman takes a one-week break, when she has her period, and then starts a new patch.

Studies find that the patch stays put even in the bath and humid weather. It is thought to be as effective as birth control pills and has been welcomed by the Department of Health as 'an extra contraceptive choice'.

Gel protects against STDs

A new gel that may protect against some sexually transmitted diseases (STDs) began clinical trials in the USA in early 2002, to determine whether it can also protect against pregnancy when coupled with a diaphragm. The gel, called BufferGel, is applied vaginally before intercourse. By increasing the mild acidity in the vagina, it creates a hostile environment for sperm and helps to kill most germs. Tests for its capacity to block transmission of HIV, genital herpes, and other STDs are due to begin in 2003. Aci-Jel, a similar product available in the UK, works in a similar way to restore vaginal acidity, and is currently marketed to protect against thrush.

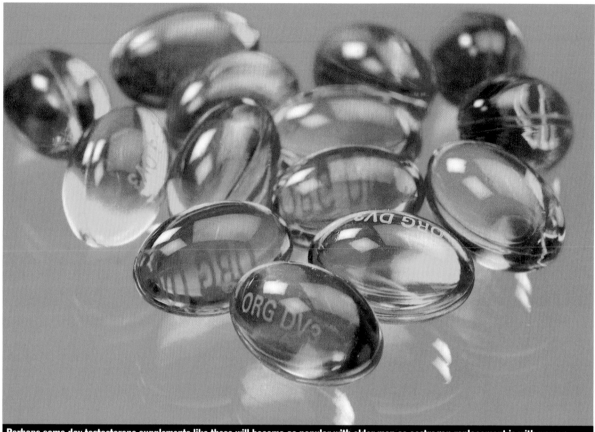

Perhaps some day testosterone supplements like these will become as popular with older men as oestrogen replacement is with women.

Drug development

Men get a turn at hormone replacement

Has your man been acting a little tired lately? Has he lost interest in sex? Seemed to forget things? Complained of general weakness? Give him a break – he might be in the throes of male menopause or, to use the more appropriate term, andropause.

In a study of 302 men, most of whom were 60 or older, 46 per cent said they had problems with impotence, 41 per cent with general weakness, and 36 per cent with memory loss. Most identified the age of onset of andropause as between 51 and 60. Typical symptoms include diminished sexual desire and impotence, memory loss, fatigue, depression, muscle loss, skin changes, decrease in body hair, more fragile bones and increase in abdominal fat. The study was published in the Nov/Dec 2001 issue of the *Archives of Andrology*.

The medical establishments in the UK and United States do not acknowledge andropause as a condition and so there are no drugs officially approved to treat it.

'Other countries, especially Canada, have embraced the idea of male menopause,' says Nancy Alexander, Ph.D., medical services director for contraception at the Dutch-based pharmaceutical company Organon, Inc. Organon markets the only testosterone replacement pill, Andriol, in more than 80 countries worldwide.

But the testosterone replacement products available, such as the gel AndroGel, made by Unimed Pharmaceuticals, are currently approved only for medical conditions associated with low levels of testosterone. These conditions, collectively called hypogonadism, include Klinefelter's syndrome (a chromosomal disorder) and the failure of the testicles to produce sperm or male hormones. Testosterone replacement may also be prescribed for breast cancer, delayed puberty and, in conjunction with HRT, to treat the female menopause.

How it works Men's levels of testosterone tend to decline with age, just as women's levels of oestrogen do. In general, Dr. Alexander says, studies find that treating older men with supplemental testosterone results in a reduction of fat, particularly abdominal fat, the kind known to increase the risk of cardiovascular disease. In one study, men's abdominal fat declined from 27cm to 24.6cm in eight months.

Testosterone replacement therapy increases bone density, reducing the risk of hip fractures due to osteoporosis. New studies suggest that testosterone may also help to protect against atherosclerosis (a narrowing of the arteries). However, like oestrogen replacement for women, it's not without risks. For instance, testosterone supplements may fuel the growth of any existing prostate tumours, so men undergoing the therapy need to have regular prostate examinations.

Availability Research into andropause is near the level research into menopause was 20 years ago, says Dr. Alexander. UK medical professionals are divided in their opinion of the condition, although the possibility that testosterone therapy may help to treat the natural symptoms of ageing in men is increasingly supported. In the US, a large clinical trial of testosterone replacement therapy is currently in progress, exploring androgen (male sex hormone) therapy overall, as well as the effects of testosterone on the risk of fractures.

RESEARCH ROUND-UP

Viagra OK for heart patients

The first study to test the use of sildenafil (Viagra) in men with heart disease that was not funded by the drug's manufacturer has found that many such men can safely take the drug for impotence. Using ultrasound images of the heart during exercise, researchers at the Mayo Clinic in the USA showed that Viagra did not adversely affect blood flow to the heart in men with stable coronary artery disease who are not taking nitrates.

The men rode a bicycle while lying on their backs to mimic the stress sex puts on the heart. For those men, said lead investigator and cardiologist Dr. Patricia Pellikka, 'the study should provide reassurance that sildenafil is not likely to increase their heart attack risks'. Funded by the American Heart Association and the Mayo Foundation, the study was reported in the *Journal of the American Medical Association* (Feb. 2002).

Drug development
New ways to cool hot flushes

Nearly every woman over 50 can describe it – that feeling which begins as a small pulse of warmth, then explodes into a burning throughout her entire body that leaves her red-faced and dripping in sweat. They're hot flushes and they're the most common complaint that women have about the menopause.

The most commonly prescribed medication to treat hot flushes is hormone replacement therapy (HRT). Yet many women avoid HRT because they are concerned about a slightly increased risk of breast cancer, are loathe to introduce supplemental hormones into their bodies or have a history of breast cancer, stroke, or blood clots.

Now there may be a choice of new options. A growing number of studies find that the newer antidepressants – ones that work on specific neurotransmitters in the brain, such as venlafaxine (Efexor) – may significantly ease hot flushes. In one American study, published in February 2002, 102 postmenopausal women suffering from hot flushes received 75mg of Efexor over eight weeks. The women experienced a 60 per cent reduction in their symptoms. An earlier, four-week study showed similar results.

Side effects included mild appetite loss, dry mouth and, in some women, nausea. But one of the study's authors, Mayo Clinic oncologist Dr. Charles Loprinzi noted an unusual, and positive, side effect. Contrary to the typical reaction to Efexor (and most other antidepressants), these women seemed to have improved sexual desire.

In the UK an 'alpha blocker' drug – clonidine – used to treat migraine and high blood pressure is also now licensed for the successful treatment of menopausal flushes.

Further studies are testing other antidepressants, including fluoxetine (Prozac) and paroxetine (Seroxat). As to why the antidepressant seems to affect hot flushes, Dr. Loprinzi can only speculate. 'It has something to do with the pituitary/hypothalamus area of the brain and brain stem, and something to do with serotonin and norepinephrine,' both important brain chemicals, he says. Efexor works for depression by lengthening the amount of time serotonin and norepinephrine are available to the brain.

BEHIND THE BREAKTHROUGH

Flushed with success

Why would a cancer specialist decide to take an interest in hot flushes? Because they are a major problem for women who have survived breast cancer, says Charles Loprinzi, the Mayo Clinic doctor who first investigated antidepressants as a potential treatment for hot flushes.

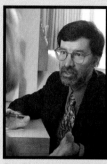

Dr. Charles Loprinzi

Many of the treatments for breast cancer, including high-dose chemotherapy and anti-oestrogen drugs such as tamoxifen, can send pre-menopausal women into menopause prematurely and often abruptly. Yet these women, because of their breast cancer experience, don't want to take replacement oestrogen.

So more than a decade ago, Dr. Loprinzi began the search for something to help his patients with hot flushes. Since then, he's put more than 1,000 women through placebo-controlled trials (in which some women receive a placebo) to test drugs such as clonidine (Catapres) and megestrol (Megace), and natural alternatives such as vitamin E and soy. In the early 1990s, a doctor told him that a patient who was taking Prozac (fluoxetine) had reported that her hot flushes had improved.

'I asked a psychiatrist or two about this; they didn't know anything about it,' remembers Dr. Loprinzi. 'Then we tried it on a patient and it didn't work, so we shelved the idea.'

But a couple of years ago, during a round-table discussion with some fellow physicians, he heard about a few women on Efexor who seemed to have less trouble with hot flushes. Around the same time, a colleague called about a patient suffering from hot flushes and asked if Dr. Loprinzi had any studies under way. He didn't, but he did suggest putting the woman on a very low dose of Efexor – 25mg, less than a quarter the standard dose used to treat depression.

'She had a fabulous reduction in hot flashes (flushes),' Dr. Loprinzi recalls. So he tried it with another patient, who experienced the same result. 'I said, "OK, let's study it."' And the rest, as they say, is history.

High-tech help
Screening techniques in 'designer baby' controversy

Genetic screening may soon be used to help British women with a history of miscarriages achieve successful pregnancies, it was announced in September 2002. The technique – preimplantation genetic screening (PGS) – would screen embryos created in the lab during IVF treatment for the genetic abnormalities that can lead to miscarriage.

Doctors believe that PGS could reduce miscarriages dramatically – particularly in women over 40 who are at greatest risk. But the move was immediately condemned by opponents as unethical and a step towards 'designer babies'. A spokesman for the Society for the Protection of Unborn Children told one newspaper, 'It really does seem to be the next step on the road to eugenic selection.'

The 'designer baby' controversy became particularly poignant in the course of the year. First a Yorkshire couple Raj and Shahana Hashmi were granted permission by the Human Fertilisation and Embryology Authority (HFEA) to use a related technique – preimplantation genetic diagnosis (PGD) – to help them create a sibling whose umbilical cord blood might save their three-year-old Zain who suffers from a rare genetic blood disorder beta thalassaemia major. Developed over the past 10 years and now available at five licensed UK centres, PGD is already used in the UK to test for nearly 50 gene mutations responsible for diseases such as cystic fibrosis, muscular dystrophy and sickle cell anaemia.

But in August, a second couple were refused permission to use the screening technique to find an embryo which would be a perfect tissue match for their three-year-old son who also suffers from a rare blood disorder. In this case the Human Fertilisation and Embryology Authority determined that because this blood disorder was not genetic and any potential child was not at risk of contracting the disorder but was only being selected for suitability as a donor, permission could not be granted. One academic called this 'quibbling over a minor distinction'.

The Government's Select Committee on Science and Technology has called for new legislation, which the HFEA says 'is desperately needed' to take into account the complex ethical issues and the massive scientific advances that have taken place in the past 10 years. A consultative green paper on genetics has been published recently to air the ethical, clinical, scientific and economic issues involved.

RESEARCH ROUND-UP

Push when ready

It's the emotional high point in any TV show about birth – the woman, her face red as she strains to get the baby out, her partner supporting her from behind, and everyone saying 'Push! Push!' But if she's not ready to push, perhaps she shouldn't, suggests a study published in the January/February 2002 issue of the US *Journal of Midwifery & Women's Health*.

The study finds that women who push without the 'urge' to do so may experience more complications, including physiological stress in the mother and acidosis (in which the blood becomes too acidic) in the baby. These women may also need more help from instruments such as forceps during the baby's delivery.

Instead, author Joyce Roberts, C.N.M., Ph.D., of Ohio State University School of Nursing, recommends that the second stage of labour (when women typically push) should be redefined and the time during which pregnant women are instructed to push should be decreased.

Genetic clue to repeat miscarriages

New research reveals that some otherwise healthy women have a trait on their X chromosome that can prove lethal to male foetuses, leading to multiple miscarriages. Eric Hoffman, Ph.D., of Children's National Medical Center in Washington DC, discovered the fatal flaw.

He is still estimating the frequency of this cause of spontaneous abortion, but thinks it exists in about 1 per cent of all women and up to 15 per cent of women with recurrent miscarriages.

Dr. Hoffman offers a free test for the defect through his lab in Washington DC as part of his research. To find out more, see the X-chromosome Inactivation Study on the internet at: www.cnmcxcis.org

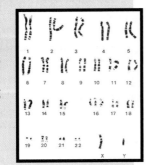

The 23 pairs of chromosomes that make up a human.

Key discovery

Older mothers risk low-birthweight babies

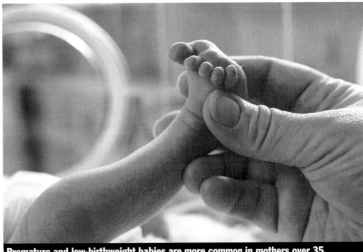

Premature and low-birthweight babies are more common in mothers over 35.

One of the beauties of the sexual revolution and dependable birth control is women's ability to postpone childbearing. Since the late 1970s, birth rates for women in their late thirties and forties have increased dramatically, despite the fact that older women have a higher risk of infertility, miscarriage, and giving birth to a baby with a birth defect. Now, the largest-ever population study of older mothers and their babies, also suggests that women aged 35 or older have a significantly higher risk of having a low-birthweight infant.

The study, published in the March 2002 issue of the US journal *Pediatrics*, analysed the weights of 283,956 infants born to women aged 35 and older in Alberta, Canada, from 1990 to 1996. During those years, more than 75 per cent of the increase in the low-birthweight rate was due to births among these older women, says the study's lead author, Suzanne Tough, Ph.D., assistant professor in the department of paediatrics and community health science at the University of Calgary.

Low-birthweight and pre-term babies are more likely to require neo-natal intensive care and to have more long-term medical complications, Dr. Tough says. The babies are also more likely to experience delays in motor and social development and increased risks of cerebral palsy, learning disability, deafness and blindness.

'This study is in no way designed to tell women at what age they should have children or to discourage women over the age of 35 from having children,' Dr. Tough emphasizes. Instead, it should encourage healthcare providers to explore in greater detail how they can identify women who may be at risk for low-birthweight babies or pre-term deliveries.

Key discovery
Episiotomy falling from favour

For years, doctors have 'helped' women during delivery by enlarging the vaginal opening with a quick 'snip'. The 2.5cm–5cm incision in the perineum, the area of skin and muscle between the vagina and the rectum, is intended to make more room for the baby's head and thereby hasten slow labours and prevent tearing. Called an episiotomy, that small cut is falling out of favour.

A growing body of studies in Europe and the USA finds that episiotomy offers little benefit to mother or baby but its risks include infection, painful recovery and incontinence. 'Episiotomy should not be a routine part of labor,' advised the American College of Obstetricians and Gynecologists (ACOG) in March 2002.

Episiotomy rates in Britain dropped from 51 per cent of all vaginal deliveries in 1975 to 19 per cent in 1995, according to NHS statistics. Maternity units in Britain have moved away from the routine use of the procedure but still perform it for specific reasons, such as to speed up the birth when there is evidence of foetal distress or, less commonly, if the mother is exhausted or to reduce the maternal effort required to deliver the baby if the mother has a history of heart disease or high blood pressure.

In the USA, episiotomy rates have not dropped quite as sharply – down from 56 per cent in 1979 to 31 per cent in 1997 – and prominent obstetricians are saying that the procedure is still overused.

In Britain, where it was once standard medical procedure, episiotomy is being openly questioned by more and more obstetricians. And midwives are equally vocal. In an article published in the *Journal of Midwifery*, March 2001, Joan Cameron and Karen Rawlings-Anderson, two lecturers from St Bartholomew School of Nursing and Midwifery, likened the procedure to female circumcision. 'If mutilation implies injury without conferring any benefit, then routine use of episiotomy can be considered a form of genital mutilation,' they wrote.

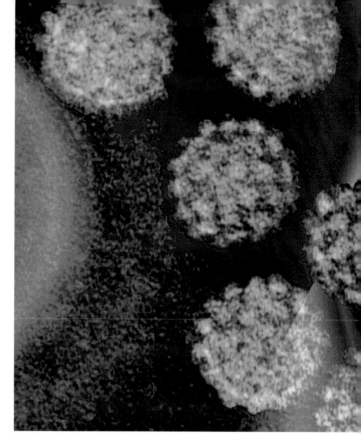

Key discovery
First sexual experience may result in HPV

Infection with the most common sexually transmitted disease – the human papillomavirus (HPV) – which can result in cancer in 20 to 30 years' time, may occur during a woman's first experience with sexual intercourse, British researchers report in the January 2002 issue of *BJOG: An International Journal of Obstetrics and Gynaecology*.

Reported cases of sexually transmitted diseases (STDs) have soared in Britain in recent years, particularly among young people. In 2000, 66,000 new cases of genital warts – a direct result of HPV infection – were diagnosed. Studies find that

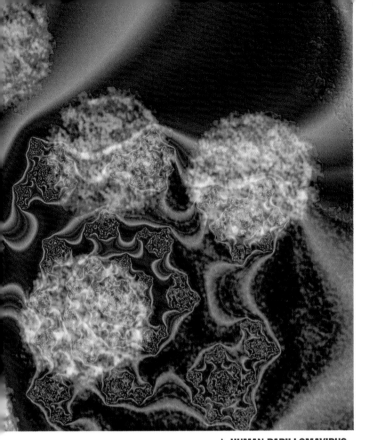

RESEARCH ROUND-UP

Reason to circumcise?

New research suggests that male circumcision may protect women from cervical cancer by reducing the risk of human papillomavirus (HPV). The study, published in April 2002 in the *New England Journal of Medicine*, evaluated nearly 3,800 women in five countries. Half of them had cervical cancer and half did not. Overall, women whose partners were sexually active early (before age 17) and often (having had at least six partners) were more likely to have cervical cancer than those whose partners had been less sexually active. But among women with high-risk partners, the ones whose partners were uncircumcised were five times more likely to develop cervical cancer than those with circumcised partners. The researchers suggest that the inner lining of the foreskin may be particularly susceptible to HPV, which can lead to cervical cancer.

A downside to using the Pill

For all the good that birth control pills do – reducing risk of ovarian cancer, regulating menstruation, clearing up acne – a new study has found one negative aspect. Using birth control pills for five years or longer increases the risk of cervical cancer in women infected with the human papillomavirus. Compared with HPV-infected women who never used oral contraceptives, those who used birth control pills for less than five years had no increased risk of cervical cancer. Those who used them for between 5 and 9 years were about three times more likely to develop cervical cancer. And those who used the pills for 10 years or more were about four times more likely to have the cancer.

certain strains of the virus cause almost all forms of cervical cancer which kills around 1,250 women in the UK each year.

▲ HUMAN PAPILLOMAVIRUS, which causes genital warts as well as cervical cancer, is the most common sexually transmitted disease.

The researchers collected data on 242 women attending a family planning clinic who reported having had sexual intercourse for the first time within the last 6 months. The women were between the ages of 15 and 19 years and had had only one sexual partner. In half the women, the infection was detected within about three months of their first sexual intercourse. The women's overall risk of HPV infection during the first three years after becoming sexually active was 46 per cent.

Preventing transmission of the virus is notoriously difficult, as the *BJOG* study found. Nearly three-quarters of the infected women (74 per cent) were using barrier contraception, such as condoms, during their first relationship. While using a condom may help prevent the spread of HPV, the virus is very sneaky, and infections can occur in genital areas that the condom doesn't cover or protect. Because HPV often has no symptoms, many people don't know they're infected.

Given these facts, and the results of their study, the British researchers suggest that 'perhaps cervical human papillomavirus infection should now be considered an inevitable consequence of sexual activity. Certainly, no stigma should be attached to its acquisition.'

The best way to detect HPV and catch cervical cancer in its earliest stages – when it's most easy to cure – is with regular cervical smears.

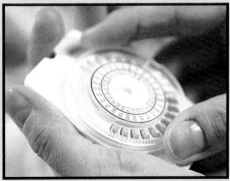

Using the Pill for more than five years can be risky for women with HPV.

RESPIRATORY SYSTEM

This year brings good news for people suffering from various respiratory ailments. For people plagued by hay fever, a vaccine under development appears to eliminate some pollen allergies in just six weeks. A recent study shows that a new form of meditation can help make your lungs less sensitive to asthma triggers. And new understanding of cystic fibrosis may explain why the lung infections that go with it are so difficult to control with antibiotics: a discovery that could pave the way for more effective treatments.

But not all the news is positive. One of the most important findings of 2002 was that lung reduction surgery for emphysema doesn't work as well as surgeons hoped in patients with the most advanced disease – and may make some patients worse. For nasty winter coughs, don't put your faith in cough syrup: British scientists claim that they don't work. And finally, are the new, low-nicotine cigarettes really safer than conventional brands? The answer depends on whom you ask.

Alternative answers
Yoga is in a position to relieve asthma

Doctors have known for a long time that anxiety and emotional stress can trigger an asthma attack and make it harder to breathe once an attack is under way. Now a recent study, published in the February 2002 issue of the medical journal *Thorax,* shows that a relatively new form of meditation known as sahaja yoga, developed in 1970, appears to make asthma attacks less frequent as well as less severe.

How it works Scientists at the Institute of Respiratory Medicine in Sydney, Australia, divided 47 asthma patients into two groups. All the participants were taking moderate to high doses of inhaled steroids to control their asthma, but still had symptoms from time to time. Those patients in the first group practiced the yoga-based form of meditation, which involves focusing on positive mental thoughts in order to reach a state of 'mental silence'. The second group performed non-yoga relaxation techniques, such as visualization and progressive muscle relaxation. People in both groups were required to attend weekly two-hour sessions for four months and were also encouraged to practise the techniques at home.

At the end of the study, standard lung tests showed that patients in the yoga group displayed less airway hyper-responsiveness, or 'twitchiness', than those in the comparison group. This is important because hyper-responsiveness is what causes tiny airways in the lungs to narrow in response to common asthma triggers, such as pollen or dust. People in the yoga group also showed improvements in mood

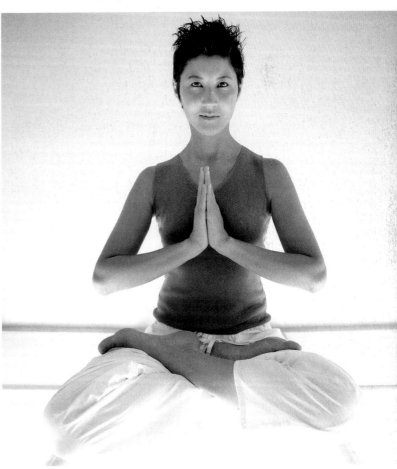

▲ The calming effect that yoga has on the mind and body can help to make asthma more manageable.

and overall quality of life, reporting that they felt less tense and less fatigued. Furthermore, their airways responded more positively to their medications than they had before. According to the researchers, the yoga technique helped every bit as much as inhaled steroids.

Availability Researchers aren't sure why yoga should be more beneficial than other relaxation techniques. Earlier studies have shown that a wide range of relaxation techniques, such as deep breathing, mental imagery and massage, can improve breathing and reduce the severity of asthma attacks. However, the benefits of yoga and other techniques appear to be short-lived. When the Australian researchers looked at the lung function of participants two months after the study, they found no difference between the two groups.

PATIENT PROFILE

More yoga, fewer hospital visits

Barbara Benagh was nearly the perfect asthma patient. She always took her medication when she was supposed to. She watched what she ate, was physically active and did her best to avoid common asthma triggers. Yet, despite her best efforts, her condition kept getting worse.

'I was hospitalized an average of five times a year,' says Barbara, 52, owner of the Yoga Studio in Boston, USA. 'In 1995, I went into full respiratory failure. That's when it really hit me that this disease was going to kill me if I didn't get better control of it.'

Some specialists suspect that asthma is largely caused by disturbed breathing patterns. Asthmatics tend to breathe two or three times faster than normal, even when they're not having attacks. Benagh found herself wondering whether the breathing techniques used in yoga might help her asthma.

She started practising rechaka, a technique in which you breathe in through the nose and slowly exhale through the mouth. 'You want the period of exhalation to be twice as long as the inhalation,' Barbara explains. 'This slows down your breathing and breaks the pattern of hyperventilation.'

She also got into the habit of setting aside 10 to 20 minutes daily to practice savasana, a relaxation technique in which you lie on your back, put a pillow under your head and concentrate on the sounds and rhythms of your breathing.

Hers is not the same style of yoga recently studied by Australian researchers for its ability to reduce asthma symptoms, but she's finding considerable relief nevertheless. 'Since doing the exercises, I'm taking a lot less medication than I used to, and I need it less often,' Barbara says. 'Yoga isn't a cure for asthma, but for me, it's been an excellent way to manage the disease.'

Barbara Benagh in an advanced hatha yoga posture known as Eka Pada Rajakapotasana, Sanskrit for 'One Legged King Pigeon Pose'.

Key discovery
Cough syrup can't hack it

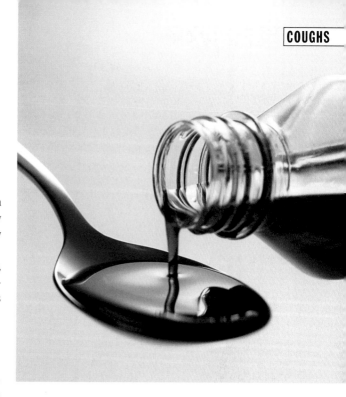

When you're coughing so hard that you feel as though you might break a rib, your first instinct is probably to reach for the cough syrup. But according to new research, it's unlikely to make much of a difference.

That's the conclusion of scientists at Bristol University, who reviewed hundreds of scientific studies on over-the-counter cough medicines. They found that most studies didn't meet the optimal standards of medical science – and the few that did showed that taking cough syrup is usually no more effective than taking nothing at all.

▶ Evidence suggests that cough syrup may be no more effective than honey and lemon.

How it works – or doesn't. There are two main types of cough medicine. Antitussives, for 'dry' coughs, usually contain dextromethorphan, a drug related to codeine, that suppresses coughs. For 'productive', or 'chesty' coughs there are expectorants. These contain guaifenesin, which dilutes mucus, making it easier to expel from the lungs.

The Bristol researchers, led by GP Dr. Knut Schroeder, looked at 328 studies on both types of cough medicines. They found that only 15 had been randomized, controlled trials (the gold standard of scientific research) in which the medicines were compared to placebos (dummy treatments) without the participants knowing which they were taking. Of these 15 studies, 9 showed that cough syrup was no more effective than a placebo. The remaining six studies produced some evidence that cough medicines made a difference, but only just. Patients who took them might have coughed one or two fewer times in the course of a night, an improvement that hardly justifies the cost – or the bad taste – of the medicines, says Dr. Schroeder.

Not surprisingly, representatives of pharmaceutical companies vehemently dispute the study. They argue that an abundance of existing research has compared cough syrups favourably with codeine, a proven cough remedy. Yet these studies, because they weren't placebo-controlled, were excluded from the British researchers' review.

Meanwhile, however effective cough syrup may or may not be, it won't do any harm, so if you feel it helps, there's no reason not to use it.

Of 15 studies, 9 showed that cough syrup was no more effective than a placebo.

Take action

Simple ways to beat a cough
If over-the-counter medicines aren't effective, what can you do to ease a cough?

■ **Drink plenty of water** Try to drink at least eight full glasses a day. Water moisturizes the throat, reduces irritation, and helps flush cough-causing germs from the body.

■ **Get plenty of rest** Vigorous activity can make coughs worse.

■ **Take honey and lemon** These traditional remedies may help to reduce throat irritation. You can mix them in a mug of hot tea or stir them into a glass of warm water.

■ **Sit it out** Most coughs will disappear within two to three weeks and cough syrups won't speed recovery. For a severe cough, see your doctor to check you don't have a more serious problem.

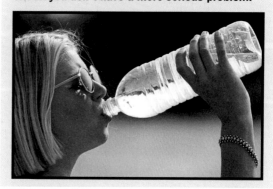

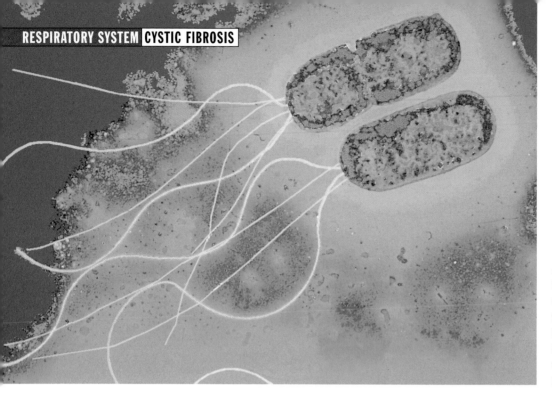

◀ *Pseudomonas aeruginosa* bacteria thrive in warm, damp environments – such as the human intestine and in hospital machinery, like incubators and ventilators – and require little to no oxygen.

Key discovery
Taking aim at deadly bacteria

Every week in the UK, three young people die of cystic fibrosis. The disease affects more than 7,500 children and young adults, causing the body's normally slick, wet secretions to become sticky, creating an oxygen-deficient environment in which bacteria thrive, and making infections much more likely. Lung infections are the most common cause of death in people with cystic fibrosis (CF).

Antibiotics have never worked well at fighting these infections, but researchers now think they may know why, and hope to use this information to create drugs that will be effective. A team at the University of Carolina, led by Ute Schwab, Ph.D., found that a dangerous bacterium, *Pseudomonas aeruginosa*, which can adapt to survive in the low-oxygen mucus, does so by generating protective features that may also help it to resist antibiotics.

How it works Cystic fibrosis affects the glands that produce mucus, sweat and other lubricating fluids, including those in the lungs. In CF sufferers, a defective gene causes cells lining the airways to remove too much salt and fluid from the secretions, making the mucus sticky. The overworked cells in the airways demand huge amounts of oxygen to function, leaving an oxygen-poor environment. 'We found that *Pseudomonas* moved into these low oxygen zones and, to our surprise, grew very well there,' says Dr. Schwab.

Adapting to this new environment, the bacteria generate a protective sugar coating and stick together in clusters known as biofilms, which allow them to evade the body's natural defences and resist conventional antibiotics. The study's results, reported in the February 2002 issue of the *Journal of Clinical Investigation,* suggest that the key to fighting the bacteria is to develop drugs that will stop them adapting to the low-oxygen mucus.

Pseudomonas is thought to contain enzymes that allow it to produce adenosine triphosphate – a fuel that drives cellular functions – even in the absence of oxygen. Designing an antibiotic that targets these enzymes may prevent the organisms from surviving in the absence of oxygen and begin to reduce the high infection rate in cystic fibrosis sufferers.

Key discovery

A blow for lung reduction surgery

The medical treatments for emphysema, a life-threatening lung disease usually caused by smoking, aren't very effective. However, a procedure called lung volume reduction surgery raised the hopes of thousands of sufferers. The technique was pioneered in the 1950s, but it had a poor rate of survival and was abandoned until new surgical procedures brought it back onto the agenda in the 1990s. But early optimism may have been premature, as studies, including a report commissioned by Exeter University, suggest that the operation doesn't work for the patients with the greatest need.

How it works Emphysema destroys air sacs, called alveoli, in the lungs, which makes it increasingly difficult for patients to breathe. Surgeons have reported that lung volume reduction surgery, in which up to 30 per cent of the damaged lung is removed, allows the healthier portions of the lung to expand, letting the patient breathe more readily.

Several UK trials failed to establish a significant difference in survival rates between emphysema patients who had undertaken the lung reduction surgery and those relying on conventional medical treatment. And a 1996 study conducted by the US National Heart, Lung, and Blood Institute identified no improvement in the quality of life among the 69 patients who had the operation. Sixteen died in the month following the surgery, but there were no deaths in the non-surgical group.

Availability The tentative findings don't necessarily mean that lung volume reduction surgery has no place in the treatment of emphysema. In fact, several surgeons in the UK offer the treatment to private patients. It's possible that patients with less severe emphysema than those so far featured in the trials might fare better than people with more developed symptoms.

The Safety and Efficacy Register for New Interventional Procedures in Britain has not yet published any guidance on the procedure. However, a large trial began recruiting in 2000 to measure the costs and effectiveness of the treatment in a UK context.

> **There was no improvement in the quality of life among the 69 patients who had the operation.**

The ravages of emphysema

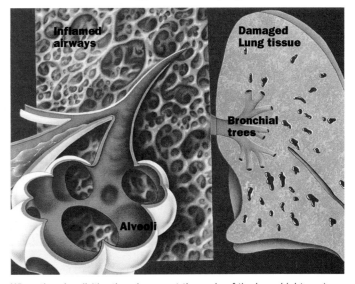

Inflamed airways

Damaged Lung tissue

Bronchial trees

Alveoli

When the alveoli (the tiny air sacs at the ends of the bronchial trees) are damaged by emphysema, the lungs become less able to transfer oxygen to the bloodstream, causing shortness of breath. Inflammation of the airways is also a symptom and may inhibit the entry of air into the alveoli.

Drug development

New vaccine is not to be sneezed at

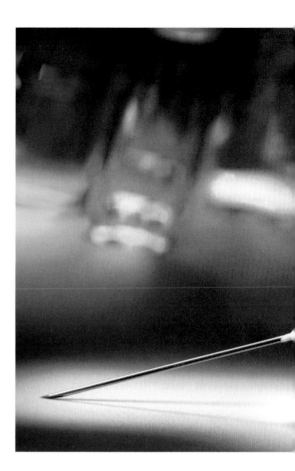

Around 20 per cent of the UK population suffers from hay fever: that's close to 10 million people plagued every spring and summer with runny eyes, blocked noses and sneezing. But getting relief is a hit-and-miss business. Antihistamines and decongestants don't work for everyone, and they may cause uncomfortable side effects, such as drowsiness. The other option, immunotherapy (allergy shots), is often effective, but it requires six months of weekly or monthly injections, followed by regular 'maintenance' jabs for three to five years.

▶ **Instead of years of allergy shots that have limited success, hay fever sufferers may soon get relief with just six shots in six weeks.**

Finally, a better solution may be on the horizon: a vaccine that virtually knocks out ragweed allergies (among the ones that cause hay fever symptoms) in only six weeks.

How it works The vaccine, known as AIC (Amb a 1-ISS Conjugate), was created by attaching immunity-boosting molecules to the ragweed pollen protein. The drug boosts the body's production of IgG (immuno-globulin G) antibodies, a sign of robust immunity, without elevating levels of the 'bad' antibodies that stimulate allergic reactions.

In a study of 25 adults with ragweed allergies, reported at the March 2002 meeting of the American Academy of Allergy Asthma and Immunology, participants were given weekly injections of AIC for six weeks. Scientists measured their response to ragweed pollen before and after the injections. They found that people who took the drug had a significant reduction in symptoms, along with a comparable reduction in the need for medication during peak hay fever season.

'None of the individuals experienced any serious allergic reactions,' says Dr. Peter S. Creticos, associate professor of medicine at Johns Hopkins University in Baltimore and lead scientist of the study – nor any other detrimental side effects.

Availability AIC is still in its experimental stages; it could take several years for the drug to gain approval and reach the market. In the UK, hay fever is more often caused by an allergy to grass pollen than to ragweed, but AIC could pave the way for vaccination against other hay fever allergies.

RESEARCH ROUND-UP

Herbal relief for hay fever

The traditional approach to hay fever is to take antihistamines. The drugs work, but often cause drowsiness, and they're better at preventing symptoms than treating them once they occur. Now a recent Swiss study, published in January 2002 in the *British Medical Journal*, has shown that butterbur (pictured right), a herb, similar to coltsfoot, that's said to have the biggest leaves in Britain, works just as well as a leading antihistamine. Researchers looked at 125 hay fever patients. Half were given four daily doses of butterbur extract, standardized to contain 8mg of petasine, the active ingredient. The other half were given Zirtek, the so-called non-sedating antihistamine also known as cetirizine.

After two weeks, people in both groups reported similar benefits, but those in the group taking butterbur were less drowsy and fatigued. Butterbur also works more quickly than the long-acting antihistamine used in this study, relieving allergy symptoms in 20 to 30 minutes. This means

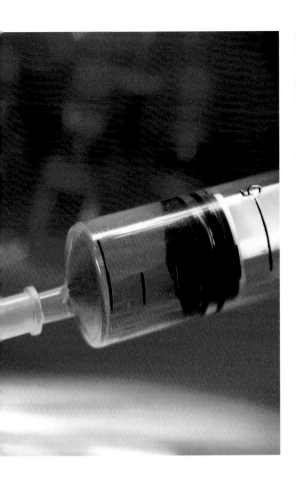

that it could be taken only as needed, rather than daily as a preventative measure. One potential drawback to taking butterbur is that it contains pyrrolizidine alkaloids, compounds that can damage the liver. The safest way to use the herb is to look in healthfood shops for supplements that have had the toxic compounds removed.

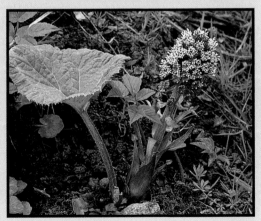

ALSO IN THE NEWS

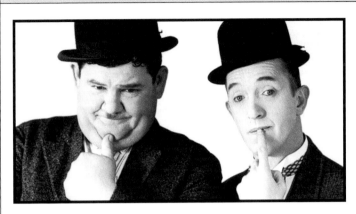

Snoring: it's all in your head

If you find snoring a turn-off, size up potential mates' heads. Researchers in the United States have proved that it's possible to predict snoring – or at least a sleep-related breathing problem that often causes it – by measuring the face. The researchers took 25 measurements and used them to create a 'craniofacial risk index' for snoring. With other factors, such as body mass index and age, this can rate how likely people are to have obstructive sleep apnoea, a potentially life-threatening condition that often causes snoring and has been shown to increase the risk of heart disease and stroke. Even without a pair of calipers, you can guess someone's snore potential just by looking at their head: people with round heads are more likely to snore than those with long, thin heads.

No such thing as a cure for colds and flu?

An experimental cold treatment, pleconaril, or Picovir, has failed to win approval in the USA. Experts agreed that the drug eased symptoms, but it was tested only in a narrow range of patients – mostly female and white with an average age of 36 – and the risk of side effects outweighed the benefits. More than 3 per cent of women who took pleconaril with over-the-counter cold remedies experienced menstrual disorders and two women fell pregnant, suggesting that the drug may interfere with oral contraceptives. Pleconaril worked only when it was given in the first 24 hours of a cold – when few people would visit their doctor – and reduced the cold's duration for no more than one day. Cardiff's Common Cold Centre acknowledges that it is one of the few drugs to work, but cost would probably rule it out as an NHS treatment.

The flu drug Relenza, which can relieve flu if taken within 48 hours of the onset of symptoms, has a similar history in the UK. In recommending it the National Institute for Clinical Excellence noted that 'a small increase in GP workload' could be anticipated. Doctors imagined a stampede: 'If everyone with flu-like symptoms contacted us there is no way the system could cope,' said Cambridge GP, Dr. Ian Dumbleton in the journal *Pulse* in October 2002. What's more, the annual cost of prescribing the drug in England and Wales could be as high as £11.7 million, estimated *Pulse* in January 2002. To limit this, guidelines recommend its use only with high-risk patients, and only during a flu epidemic, when 50 or more patients in every 100,000 visit their doctor in a week.

High-tech help

When the smoke clears, will 'safer' cigarettes prevail?

Smoking is bad for you – everyone agrees, even the tobacco companies. There are 15 million adult smokers in the UK – around a third of the adult population – and they spend an annual £12.5 billion on tobacco products. Cancer Research UK estimates that smoking kills 120,000 people here each year. So can there be such a thing as a safe, or safer cigarette? New brands, such as Omni, Eclipse, and Quest, being launched in the US but not yet available in Britain, claim to reduce the amount of harmful substances that smokers suck into their lungs, potentially making them safer to smoke than conventional brands.

The makers of these cigarettes have a two-pronged strategy: to appeal to consumers who want to reduce the risks associated with their smoking habit, and to deliver a taste that's rich enough to compete with the traditional brands: 'an important step in the right direction,' claims Brown & Williamson Tobacco, sister company to British American Tobacco, and makers of a new reduced-toxin cigarette called Advance Lights.

Advance Lights features a three-part 'Trionic' filter that is supposed to reduce the levels of toxins found in many 'light' cigarettes and uses tobacco cured by a special process designed to reduce carcinogenic compounds. The product was launched in the US in November 2001.

At about the same time, Vector Tobacco released its Omni brand, promising that its new processing technique can also reduce the levels of four known carcinogens. Eclipse, a brand of cigarette being tested by R.J. Reynolds, is also said to be less toxic, because it heats the tobacco rather than burning it. But the latest development is Vector Tobacco's new nicotine-free cigarette, Quest, which was due to hit American shops in late 2002.

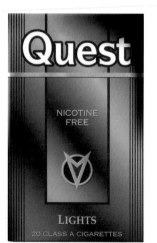

▲ Reduced-nicotine cigarettes may be less deadly than their conventional counterparts, but they're not entirely harmless.

None of these new products is currently available in Europe but if they were, the manufacturers would be limited by strict European marketing guidelines. Adverts and promotions may not make health claims for tobacco products, so promoting a less toxic cigarette would be difficult, if not impossible. However, advocates of 'safer' cigarettes say that for people who are unable to kick their addiction, the products might play a useful role in helping smokers to manage their habit. Detractors counter that smokers may compensate by drawing more deeply on such cigarettes, and they worry that such 'safe' cigarettes may ultimately attract new smokers, especially younger ones, who will later graduate to more harmful brands.

RESEARCH ROUND-UP

Less sticky alternative to the patch

The hardest part about giving up cigarettes is breaking the addictive grip of nicotine. Until they get out of the habit of lighting up, many smokers turn to nicotine gum, patches or inhalers to tide them over, but a new nicotine substitute may be both more convenient and more effective.

Researchers at Duke University in the USA have developed some nicotine drops that can be added to beverages like coffee to disguise their taste. A small study showed that 20 per cent of those who used the drops remained smoke-free after six months. That's about the same success rate found with other nicotine substitutes. What makes the drops attractive is their fast action and the ease of customizing the dose required to control each individual smoker's craving.

Some health experts worry about the toxic effects of nicotine drops. Unlike gums and patches, which release predetermined amounts of nicotine, the drops are entirely controlled by the user, and an overdose can be harmful. Larger studies still have to be done before the drops can be submitted for approval in the US and only then will they be considered for use in Europe, so it is likely to be several years before they reach our shelves.

FOR/AGAINST

A safer cigarette: just a lot of hot air?

In late 2002, an American company called Vector Tobacco planned to introduce a new cigarette in the USA that contains about one-twentieth the normal amount of nicotine.

Supporters say that the cigarette, called Quest, may be less hazardous as well as less addictive. But sceptics insist that there is no such thing as a safer cigarette.

For

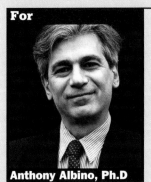

Anthony Albino, Ph.D

a cancer and public health researcher in the USA, is Vector's vice president for public health affairs.

Q. What are the main health advantages of removing nicotine from tobacco?
Dr. Albino We know nicotine is a powerfully addictive drug. Removing the nicotine from tobacco, or lowering it to below addictive levels, will cause cigarette dependence to drop dramatically. Also, nicotine increases heart rate and blood pressure and plays a real role in cardiovascular disease. Losing nicotine will reduce these problems.

Q. Will low-nicotine cigarettes reduce addiction?
Dr. Albino It is nicotine that makes people addicted to cigarettes. But below a certain level – say, 0.2mg per cigarette – nicotine is unlikely to be addictive. A 'Quest' has between 5 and 10 times less nicotine than that.

Q. Won't people smoke differently to compensate for the low nicotine levels?
Dr. Albino We have found that something called 'smoking compensation' occurs when people smoke low-tar, or 'light' cigarettes – that is, they smoke more deeply, or faster, or both. But because the Quest cigarette has a rich taste, people don't compensate by changing they way they smoke.

Q. Who will buy low-nicotine cigarettes?
Dr. Albino These cigarettes are geared toward long-time adult smokers who want to reduce their dependence on nicotine. They are unlikely to attract new smokers, especially young people, for whom nicotine is calming. Without the nicotine, they won't get this physiological effect.

Q. Can low-nicotine cigarettes help smokers quit?
Dr. Albino We're working to get government approval for low-nicotine cigarettes – by themselves or in combination with other nicotine replacements, like the patch – to help smoking cessation. The American Lung Association and other groups have suggested removing nicotine from tobacco products. This could allow millions of smokers to quit more easily.

Against

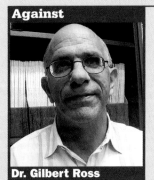

Dr. Gilbert Ross

is medical director of the American Council on Science and Health in New York City.

Q. What are the health advantages of removing nicotine from tobacco?
Dr. Ross It isn't likely to change any of the devastating health effects of smoking, such as cardiovascular disease, or cancers of the lung, pancreas, bladder and cervix. Tobacco contains hundreds, possibly thousands, of chemicals and science has not yet discerned which are potent carcinogens and which are relatively innocuous.

Q. Will low-nicotine cigarettes reduce addiction?
Dr. Ross Nicotine is one of the most important elements in cigarettes that cause addiction, but it's not the only one. Many people smoke for the oral gratification, to do something when they're anxious, or to fit in around other smokers. Removing nicotine won't affect the behavioural aspects of smoking.

Q. Won't people smoke differently to compensate for the low nicotine levels?
Dr. Ross People smoke for the nicotine, not the tar. I see them smoking more and inhaling more deeply to get the kick of nicotine they crave. I suspect that if you eliminate nicotine from a cigarette, you'll have a very short-lived product.

Q. Who will buy low-nicotine cigarettes?
Dr. Ross I worry that young people, who make up 90 per cent of new smokers, might be tempted to take up smoking if they believe the new cigarettes are less addictive. They could then move on to standard high-nicotine brands.

Q. Can low-nicotine cigarettes help smokers quit?
Dr. Ross Shifting to a very low nicotine cigarette might help people withdraw from nicotine if they also cut down on the number of cigarettes they smoke. This needs to be studied. You could compare the success rate of people who smoke regular cigarettes and use a nicotine patch with those using very low nicotine cigarettes and the patch. I would take this kind of data into account to assess which approach is best.

SKIN, HAIR AND NAILS

It's not painless, nor cheap but it's fast becoming fashionable. The wrinkle-reducing procedure known as Botox injection has been licensed for cosmetic use in the USA, and though still off-licence in the UK, it has become increasingly available.

If you have 'sun spots' like the ones George W. Bush had removed in December 2001, you'll want to read all about a new gel that can actually undo the damage – without the need for painful, time-consuming procedures. The gel stops the pre-cancerous lesions, which often start as innocent-looking flat red spots, from turning into skin cancer. Researchers have also discovered that an eczema cream, licensed in Britain in 2002, is also effective for treating vitiligo, the skin disorder that destroys the skin's pigment cells, leaving unsightly white patches.

In other news, scientists report on a new way to make topical nail fungus treatments work better and researchers sound another alarm about hair dye (turn to page 237 to find out what they say).

Drug development

New gel and cream to head off skin cancer

P resident George W. Bush had four skin lesions removed from his cheeks and forehead in December 2001 – just four months after three others had been removed. His press office assured everyone, 'They're harmless'. But the US Skin Cancer Foundation warns that this is not always the case.

Millions of people have these precancerous lesions, called actinic keratoses or 'sun spots'. Unfortunately, about 10 per cent of them will see their lesions turn into squamous-cell carcinoma, the second most common form of skin cancer.

Actinic keratoses often first appear as innocuous-looking flat red spots. But over time, they can evolve into thicker, scaly, wart-like bumps, indicating that the genetic mutations which lead to cancer may already be happening.

The best way to prevent this is to wear a UVA/UVB-protecting sunscreen of SPF 15 or higher when outdoors. But undoing the damage has never been quite as simple. Traditional treatments can be expensive, time-consuming and painful, and involve minor surgical procedures. Now science has produced two new topical drugs that offer the best solutions yet.

■ **Solaraze Gel** Licensed in Britain in the late Nineties and approved in the USA in January 2002 , Solaraze Gel is a revolutionary treatment that removes actinic keratosis lesions using a nonsteroidal anti-inflammatory drug (NSAID) called diclofenac sodium. The clear prescription gel is surprisingly powerful and actually kills precancerous, or mutated, cells when applied twice daily for two to three months. And it's amazingly safe. Because very little of the drug gets into the patient's system, the only adverse effects noted by researchers have been various skin irritations. People who are allergic to NSAIDs (the class of drugs that includes aspirin and ibuprofen) should tell their doctors before using the gel.

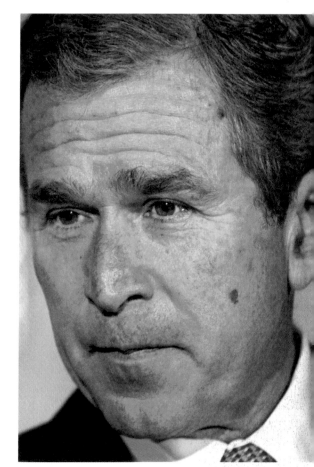

▲ **WHEN PRESIDENT BUSH** had seven benign skin lesions removed in 2001, it was an opportunity for the US press to stress the importance of using sunscreen and consulting a doctor about suspicious moles or spots.

The clear prescription gel is surprisingly powerful and actually kills precancerous ... cells when applied twice daily for two to three months.

■ **Dimericine** A potentially major advance in skin-cancer prevention, this cream actually helps skin to repair the genetic damage caused by over-exposure to the sun. It is not yet available in the USA, but is in the late stages of clinical trials, after which it will undergo trials in Europe. Dimericine contains an enzyme that penetrates the outer layer of skin cells and speeds up the process of DNA repair. (The body is able to repair damaged DNA naturally, but as people age, this ability declines.)

Timing is critical. If Dimericine isn't applied early enough to prevent the chemical changes caused by sun exposure – which can take months or years to develop – then the damage converts into permanent genetic mutations that could lead to cancer.

The cream was recently tested on patients with a rare disorder that makes them excessively sensitive to sunlight and prone to skin cancer. After a year of applying it twice daily, the patients had a 68 per cent decrease in the number of actinic keratoses and a 30 per cent decrease in the number of basal cell carcinomas, a type of skin cancer that often appears as fleshy nodules on the hands, neck, or head. New research began in 2002 to test the lotion on 600 more subjects – people who don't have the light sensitivity disorder but have had one skin cancer lesion removed already and are at high risk for more – in three sun-drenched US cities: Los Angeles, San Diego and Jacksonville, Florida.

Dimericine may also be of interest to those who worry about the ageing effects of tanning, as previous research on animals suggests that it may help prevent sun-induced wrinkling, too.

Repairing the sun's damage

The sun's ultraviolet light rays penetrate the epidermal layer of the skin and damage cells. This is how the experimental cream, Dimericine, may prevent certain skin cancers by repairing the genetic damage that causes them.

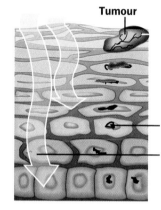
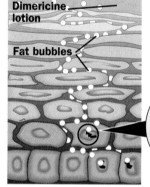
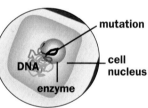

Tumour

Damaged cells
Ultraviolet rays damage DNA inside the nuclei of skin cells. Most of the damage is repaired. naturally. However, over time, a build-up of gene mutations can lead to cancer.

Build-up of DNA damage

Ultraviolet rays

Repaired cells
The cream is absorbed into the skin. It has a special enzyme placed within microscopic fat bubbles that slip inside skin cells. The enzyme then binds to the DNA mutation and initiates repair.

Dimericine lotion

Fat bubbles

mutation

cell nucleus

DNA

enzyme

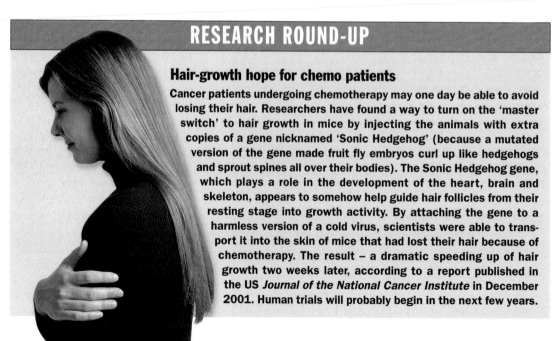

RESEARCH ROUND-UP

Hair-growth hope for chemo patients

Cancer patients undergoing chemotherapy may one day be able to avoid losing their hair. Researchers have found a way to turn on the 'master switch' to hair growth in mice by injecting the animals with extra copies of a gene nicknamed 'Sonic Hedgehog' (because a mutated version of the gene made fruit fly embryos curl up like hedgehogs and sprout spines all over their bodies). The Sonic Hedgehog gene, which plays a role in the development of the heart, brain and skeleton, appears to somehow help guide hair follicles from their resting stage into growth activity. By attaching the gene to a harmless version of a cold virus, scientists were able to transport it into the skin of mice that had lost their hair because of chemotherapy. The result – a dramatic speeding up of hair growth two weeks later, according to a report published in the US *Journal of the National Cancer Institute* in December 2001. Human trials will probably begin in the next few years.

Drug development

Eczema cream treats vitiligo, too

A leopard can't change its spots, but people with vitiligo may soon be able to. About 2 out of every 100 people have this skin disorder, which causes a loss of pigment-producing cells. The resulting white spots – most noticeable on dark skin – may spread over the face and body or be limited to certain areas.

Until now, the most common treatments have been steroid creams and a light therapy called PUVA, a combination of a substance called psoralen (P) and long-wave ultraviolet radiation (UVA). PUVA involves taking a light-sensitizing pill and regular use of a UVA-tanning machine as a hospital out-patient. The therapy comes with potentially serious side effects, including skin thinning, high blood sugar, weak bones and cancer.

Now, there's a new option: an ointment called tacrolimus (brand name Protopic). It made headlines in December 2000 as the first new drug in some 40 years for the itchy-skin disorder eczema, but researchers are finding that it works for vitiligo as well.

How it works Like eczema, vitiligo stems from an immune system glitch that makes the body attack its own tissues – in this case, pigment cells in the skin. Tacrolimus, derived from a rare soil bacterium found in Japan, is already commonly used in oral and intravenous forms to prevent the body from rejecting tissue in organ transplant recipients. As a topical cream, it targets immune cells in the skin, disrupting the abnormal chemical messages that cause the misguided attacks and allowing pigment cells to grow and reproduce.

In her own study, Dr. Pearl Grimes, director of the Vitiligo and Pigmentation Institute of Southern California in Los Angeles, found that nearly half the vitiligo patients treated with tacrolimus regained pigment in their skin, to

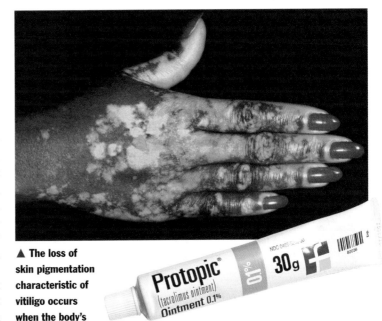

▲ **The loss of skin pigmentation characteristic of vitiligo occurs when the body's own immune system mistakenly attacks pigment-producing cells. Protopic cream inhibits these assaults, allowing pigment to reappear.**

varying degrees. And, with nearly five years of research on tacrolimus showing no link to skin cancer or other serious side effects, the drug appears to be the safest treatment yet because it is not readily absorbed into the bloodstream or body, says Dr. Grimes. She presented her findings in May 2002 at the Society for Investigative Dermatology meeting in Los Angeles.

Availability In Britain tacrolimus was first licensed as an immunosuppressant to prevent organ rejection after transplantation, and in February 2002 was approved as an ointment (brand name Protopic) for the treatment of severe eczema. But, if other studies repeat Dr. Grimes's results, the medication could one day win approval in the USA and Europe as a standard treatment for vitiligo.

Nearly half the vitiligo patients treated with tacrolimus regained pigment in their skin, to varying degrees.

Surgical solution

The 'beauty poison' gets a green light in the USA

I magine paying hundreds of pounds to have poison injected into your skin, all to get rid of a couple of wrinkles. It sounds crazy but it's a growing trend. In the States, Botox has become the most popular cosmetic treatment ever, and it's catching on so fast here that in 2002 four Boots' stores began offering the treatment.

Botox, officially called botulinum toxin injection, is used cosmetically to smooth furrowed brows, creased foreheads, and crow's feet. In 2001, more than 1.6 million people in the USA got the injections, a 46 per cent increase since 2000. And that may be just the beginning, because in April 2002, Botox was finally approved for cosmetic purposes. The British office of its manufacturers, Allergan, said it was their intention to seek a licence for cosmetic purposes in the UK at some time, but could not say when.

In fact, for years Botox has been approved to treat medical conditions such as involuntary muscle spasms, but currently any British doctor who gives Botox injections 'off-licence' for cosmetic reasons must take personal responsibility for the treatment.

How it works A Botox procedure involves injecting minute amounts of the botulism toxin into facial muscles, typically into the ones that cause deep vertical grooves between the eyebrows or horizontal 'worry lines' on the forehead. The toxin blocks the transmission of impulses between nerve cells and muscles, temporarily weakening the muscle so that it can't contract. With the muscle no longer able to contract, the existing furrow, or wrinkle, goes away. Some dermatologists even believe this may prevent more lines from forming. On average, the effect lasts for four to six months, so patients must become repeat customers in order to retain the results.

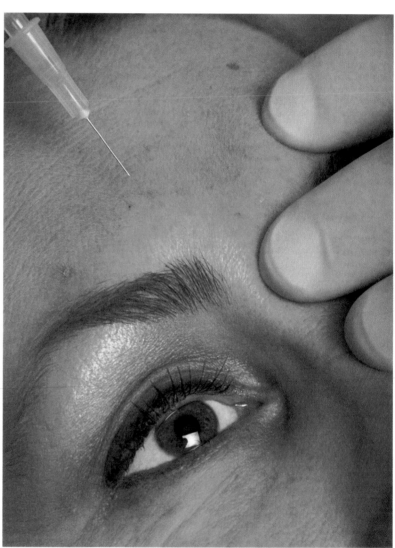

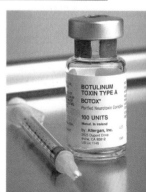

▲ **BOTOX INJECTIONS contain a purified form of the toxin that causes botulism, a deadly type of food poisoning. Botulism occurs when large amounts of the toxin are ingested – usually more than 3,000 units. The injections involve only about 20 to 40 units.**

Side effects vary. It's not unusual to encounter numbness, swelling, bruising or burning in the injection site afterwards. There's also the risk of mild to moderate drooping of one or both eyelids, lasting for about two weeks. And some people experience temporary nausea or headaches. But others find that frequent migraines get better after the Botox procedure, possibly because it blocks nerve signals that contract the muscles causing the headaches.

Availability As Botox injections become increasingly available at clinics and high street beauty salons, prospective customers are advised to check that the drug is always given by personnel with the right medical training or supervision. At the four Boots clinics launched in May 2002 – two in London, one in Manchester and a fourth in Milton Keynes – the doctors administering the injections are all qualified GPs with at least one year's experience of using Botox, said a spokesman. Prices vary; at Boots in late 2002, injections cost £200 for one area, £265 for two and £320 for three.

PATIENT PROFILE

Killing two birds with one stone

Christin Kilmetz, a San Francisco receptionist, was fed up with hearing the same question, 'Why do you look so worried?' It seemed as if everyone zeroed in on the deep furrows between her eyes.

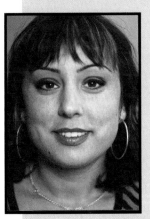

Says Christin, 'I began to notice that my eyebrows were always squashed together'. So two years ago, at the age of 29, Christin began doing what many women twice her age are just beginning to consider – getting Botox injections. After she had undergone her first round of injections, the results became noticeable in a little over three days, which is typical.

Christin had two particular incentives to try Botox. She worked for a plastic surgeon who would do the procedure free of charge, and she suffered from recurrent migraines that, she knew from working in the office, might go away as an added bonus. And they did. Her almost-daily pounding headaches became a rare occurrence after the first treatment. She also attained the worry-free look she wanted. Christin was hooked.

Like all other Botox patients, Christin has to go back under the needle every six months for an injection that feels like a bee sting. 'It's worth it because I'm also preventing new wrinkles from forming,' she says, subscribing to the theory that if you can't move the muscles that make the skin crease and furrow, there's no way that wrinkles can form.

ALSO IN THE NEWS

Getting rid of nail fungus

If you've ever had a thick, yellow, crumbly nail – the telltale sign of a fungal infection – you know how hard it is to get rid of. Part of the problem lies in the nail bed, which works as a protective shield between the fungus and any topical medica-

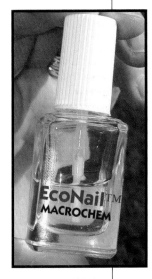

tion. Scientists in the USA have now developed a way to help brush-on treatments penetrate better and, as a result, work better. The technology is called SEPA – soft enhancement of percutaneous absorption. In a study published in the US *Journal of Pharmaceutical Sciences* in late 2002, researchers found that a SEPA-containing topical treatment called Eco-Nail penetrated nails six times better than an identical antifungal nail lacquer that didn't contain SEPA.

If topical treatments work, doctors won't have to prescribe as many oral drugs, which have been linked to serious side-effects, including liver disease. EcoNail should be available in the next few years in the USA. Its maker MacroChem is in discussions with several companies interested in introducing it in Europe.

Hair dye danger?

Women who use a permanent hair dye for 20 years or more may almost double their risk of developing rheumatoid arthritis, says a study published in the US *Annals of the Rheumatic Diseases* in October 2001. The Swedish researchers speculate that the ingredient paraphenylenediamine may be to blame, as it can prompt allergic reactions on some skins and, like allergies, rheumatoid arthritis is a result of overactive cells in the immune system. An earlier American study showed an increased risk for bladder cancer in women who used a permanent hair dye every month for 15 years – but no links with cancer have been found for semi-permanent or temporary hair dyes.

URINARY TRACT

The 180,000 Britons with some form of kidney disease will welcome two important new discoveries. Kidney patients often lose muscular power as a result of their condition and the low-protein diet that may go with it. Now it turns out that a simple strength-training programme using weight machines can reduce muscle wasting. And two relatively new drugs for high blood pressure have been found to have an extra bonus: they can also slow the progress of kidney disease. If you have kidney failure, you probably undergo the blood-cleansing process called dialysis three times a week. But researchers now believe that having the procedure done every day would result in fewer complications, a lower risk of death and a higher quality of life. Finally, a new vaccine that comes in the form of a vaginal suppository may put an end to the recurring urinary tract infections that plague millions of women.

Drug development

Blood pressure drugs rescue diabetics' kidneys

An American baseball legend, Jackie Robinson, died aged 53 from an all-too-common triple threat – diabetes, high blood pressure and kidney disease. He's not alone. Of the 150 million people in the world with Type 2 diabetes (the non-insulin-dependent type that tends to develop after the age of 40), 20 to 30 per cent develop kidney disease as a complication of their diabetes. And high blood pressure has a way of making both conditions worse. Blood pressure drugs can solve one of the problems, but it is uncertain how much they help the kidneys. Until recently, no drug had been approved for treating diabetes-related kidney disease. But now a drug called irbesartan has been approved in the EU for diabetics with that lethal combination – high blood pressure and kidney disease.

Irbesartan was developed as a blood pressure-lowering drug. A study published in the *New England Journal of Medicine* in September 2001 showed that a special class of drugs, designed to reduce blood pressure, also slow down the progression of kidney disease in diabetics. The two drugs tested, losartan and irbesartan, worked so well in clinical tests that they promise to make dialysis and transplants less likely in the future for perhaps millions of kidney disease patients.

How it works Losartan and irbesartan are in a fairly new class of drugs that lower blood pressure by preventing a vessel-constricting hormone called angiotensin II from doing its work. While an older class of drugs, called ACE inhibitors, limit the angiotensin production, the newer drugs – called angiotensin-II receptor blockers (ARBs) – use a different tactic. They occupy the hormone's sites on cells so that angiotensin-II can't get there.

That strategy works better inside the kidneys than the ACE inhibitor approach, the study showed, improving blood flow. Good blood flow is vital for kidney function, since blood nourishes the organs and also delivers waste products to the kidneys' filtering sites. Here, wastes and toxins are filtered out of the blood as it passes through the tiny capillaries of the glomerulus. The ability of losartan and irbesartan to work inside these capillaries may be what sets them apart from other blood pressure drugs. Losartan and irbesartan are marketed under the brand names Cozaar and Aprovel.

Chronic kidney failure

In kidney failure, the kidneys cannot filter waste products from the blood properly, maintain the body's balance of water and salt, or regulate blood pressure. Chronic kidney failure develops gradually, causing progressive and irreversible damage.

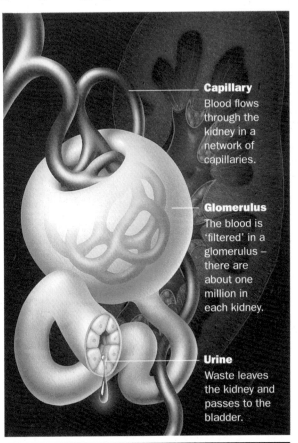

Capillary
Blood flows through the kidney in a network of capillaries.

Glomerulus
The blood is 'filtered' in a glomerulus – there are about one million in each kidney.

Urine
Waste leaves the kidney and passes to the bladder.

Key discovery

Weight training benefits kidney patients

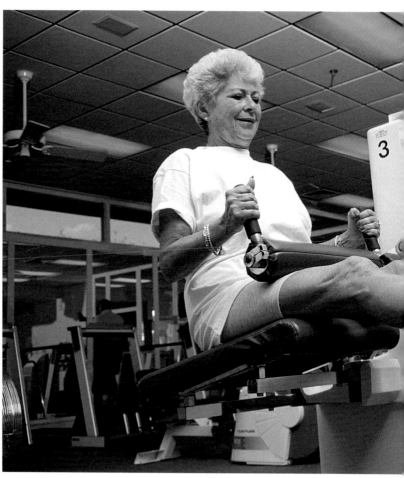

▲ Weight training just three days a week appears to help prevent and even to reverse the muscle wasting that so often occurs with impaired kidney function.

Patients with kidney disease suffer from muscle wasting that can turn everyday activities into demanding tasks. This muscle wasting is caused by the combined effects of impaired kidney function and a low-protein diet. Kidney patients are advised to reduce their protein intake because poorly functioning kidneys are unable to process high-protein foods. The trouble is, that while the body can store fats and sugars, it cannot store excess protein. So when dietary protein is restricted, the body takes the amino acids it needs from the only place protein is available – the muscles. Now new studies suggest that exercise may combat muscle-wasting.

In March 2002, researchers at Manchester Metropolitan University published the results of an investigation into the effects of aerobic exercise on kidney patients. They randomly divided 18 patients into two groups. One group cycled regularly under supervision; the other group maintained their normal daily routine. After three months the stamina of the patients in the cycling group was significantly improved when compared to members of the control group.

Researchers at Tufts University in Boston, USA tell a similar, though slightly different, story. They divided 26 kidney patients (all over 50) into two groups. Both groups were put on a low-protein diet. One group did supervised weight training three days a week. The other followed a much gentler exercise routine of bends and stretches. After 12 weeks, those who pumped iron had increased their muscle strength by one-third, while the other group actually got weaker.

Both studies suggest that some form of controlled, vigorous exercise may combat muscle-wasting and help kidney patients live more normal lives.

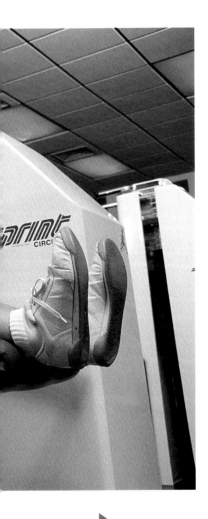

RESEARCH ROUND-UP

Discovered: polycystic kidney disease gene

Polycystic kidney disease (PKD) is the most common life-threatening genetic disease on the planet. Some 12.5 million people worldwide have PKD, an inherited condition in which multiple sac-like growths, or cysts, develope within the kidneys. These cysts inhibit the kidneys' function and cause the kidneys to grow to three or four times their normal size. There is a 50 per cent chance that a person with PKD will pass it on to his or her children. And at the moment there is no cure. But in February 2002 hopes were raised when Japanese and American researchers announced that they had identified the gene responsible for a rare form of the disease, called autosomal recessive PKD, which often kills infants shortly after birth. The investigators hope that identifying the gene will pave the way for further study that may eventually lead to treatment for all forms of PKD, as well as earlier and more conclusive diagnosis.

A computed tomography (CT) scan of PKD in a 32-year-old woman.

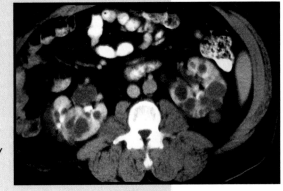

Take action

Waste not, want not

Do you feel ready to pump a little iron to combat muscle wasting? This routine got good results in the Tufts University study. But talk to your doctor before starting any exercise programme and make sure a trained expert teaches you how to use the weight machines safely.

Exercise on three days each week, leaving at least one day between sessions. For each of the exercises below, perform three sets of eight repetitions. (In other words, do the movement eight times, rest, do it eight more times, rest, and then do it a final eight times.) Start with light weights, and increase the resistance as you get stronger. So once you are able to complete three sets of equal repetitions, you can increase the weight slightly.

■ **KNEE EXTENSION** Sit with the front of your ankles against the footpad. Raise the footpad by straightening your knees (but don't lock them) and then lower it slowly. Muscles worked: the quadriceps at the front of your thighs.

■ **LEG CURL** Sit with your legs stretched out and the back of your heels on the footpad. Push the pad down and towards you by bending your knees. Let it rise back up slowly. Muscles worked: the hamstrings on the back of your thighs.

■ **LEG PRESS** Sit with your knees bent and your feet flat on the plate. Push the plate out by straightening your legs, and then let it return slowly. Muscles worked: quadriceps, hamstrings and buttocks.

■ **CHEST PRESS** Sit and grip the handles in front of you at chest level. Push them straight out in front of you by straightening your arms, then let them return slowly. Muscles worked: chest (pectorals) and the triceps at the backs of your upper arms.

■ **LAT PULL DOWN** Sit facing the machine holding the long handle at either end with a wide overhand grip, your arms fully extended above you. Pull the handle down to your chest and then let it rise back up slowly. Muscles worked: upper back and biceps.

Key discovery

Dialysis works better when it's done every day

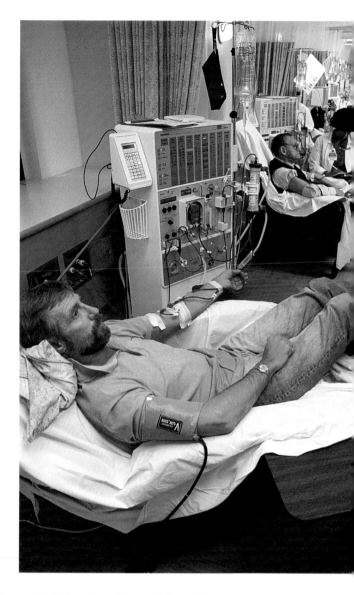

▶ A patient undergoing kidney dialysis in a New York hospital. New research shows that daily dialysis treatments are more beneficial than normal treatment schedules – but NHS funding means that we are unlikely to see daily dialysis in the UK for years.

If three-times-a-week dialysis improves – and indeed saves – the lives of patients with kidney failure, then wouldn't a daily version of the blood-cleansing procedure help even more? Absolutely, say German researchers at Munich University, who compared daily dialysis with the conventional every-other-day schedule and published their results in January 2002.

They found that more frequent dialysis means fewer complications from kidney failure, a lower risk of death and a higher quality of life. The study looked only at patients with acute kidney failure – those whose kidney function declined suddenly, often after injury, such as in a car accident. But it is thought that people with the slower-progressing chronic disease would also benefit from daily dialysis.

Both chronic and acute kidney disease mean that the kidneys can no longer do their job, so the patient's blood has to be filtered by dialysis.

Daily dialysis offered other benefits, too. For example, patients on a daily regimen had lower levels of toxins in their urine than the non-daily group. They were also less likely to suffer from low blood pressure during dialysis, systemic (whole body) inflammation, gastric bleeding and blood infection.

Nonetheless, in the UK, where most kidney patients have dialysis two or three times a week, daily dialysis would be prohibitively costly. The NHS simply couldn't cope. So implementing these findings in Britain is only likely if further research discovers that, in the long term, the cost savings are huge – and that could take years.

Key discovery
Training your bladder to behave

Bladder control isn't a topic high on most women's list of things to talk about. Even GPs rarely bring up the subject with their patients, despite the fact that 3 million people in the UK suffer from some degree of urinary incontinence – including as many as half of all post-menopausal women – and only one in ten asks for advice. But recent research shows that talking about the problem and learning how to tackle it may be an effective way to solve it without drugs or surgery.

A study published in *Obstetrics & Gynaecology* in July 2002 showed that simple behaviour therapy reduced episodes of urinary incontinence by half for most of the female subjects and even eliminated the problem completely in some.

How it works The behaviour therapy took place during six weekly sessions in which the women learned the basics of how the urinary process works. They were asked to perform regular exercises to strengthen the pelvic muscles. They also maintained a journal that included keeping track of their urinary habits in order to learn to go to the toilet regularly. After six weeks, the women discussed their condition at support group meetings and worked on gradually increasing the time they could wait until urinating. The bonus was not so much in terms of fewer trips to the toilet, but better control and fewer embarrassing accidents.

> ## The bonus was not so much in terms of fewer trips to the toilet, but better control and fewer embarrassing accidents.

The motivation to take control of your condition is a key factor in the success of a drugless treatment programme. The first step is simply telling your doctor about the problem and, if necessary, asking for a referral to a specialist. The study leaders hope their results will encourage more doctors to offer behaviour therapy as a first line of treatment when appropriate, but the patient may still have to be the one to take the initiative and ask about it.

Take action

Five questions to ask your doctor about urinary incontinence

Embarrassed to talk about your bladder control problems? Many people with urinary incontinence hesitate to seek help for this reason. Don't be one of them. Your doctor can make sure there isn't a medical problem, such as infection or pelvic abnormalities, causing loss of bladder control. And he or she can offer treatment advice. Here's a good icebreaker and suggested follow-up questions:

1. Since my last visit there have been several occasions when I couldn't control my bladder. Should I be worried?
2. What might be causing the problem?
3. What treatments can help me to regain bladder control? Which one is best for me?
4. What can I do about the smell and rash?
5. Would it be worth my seeing a specialist, like a urologist or gynaecologist?

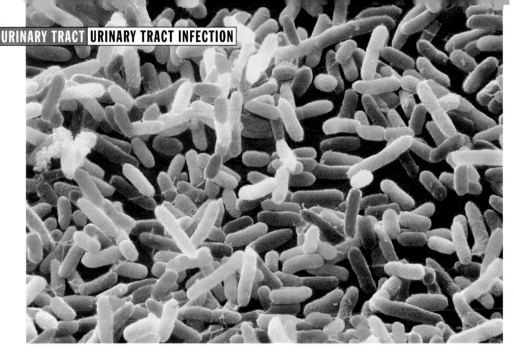

◄ An electron micrograph of *Escherichia coli* bacteria, commonly known as *E. coli*. Strains of *E. coli* are responsible for about 80 per cent of all urinary tract infections.

Progress in prevention

Simple suppository protects against cystitis

More than half the women in the UK will have cystitis at some time in their lives, with many suffering from repeated attacks. Men can get cystitis too, but the infection is 50 times more common in women.

Cystitis is an infection of the bladder but the term tends to be more broadly used to cover a range of infections and irritations in the lower urinary system. Symptoms are a painful burning sensation during urination and a frequent need to urinate. There may be pain directly above the pubic bone and the urine may be cloudy and foul-smelling.

Most urinary tract infections are simple cystitis, and most are treated with antibiotics. But that treatment isn't without its problems. For one thing, bacteria are becoming increasingly resistant to antibiotics, in part because of their widespread use over many years. Amoxycillin,

for example, now has resistance levels of 50 per cent in the general community, and many doctors are reluctant to prescribe this and other powerful antibiotics as a first resort.

In addition, because bladder infections often recur, this means repeated courses of antibiotics, which can further contribute to increased drug resistance. A patient is also more likely to have an allergic reaction as different antibiotics are used over time to avoid a build-up of resistance.

But an alternative may be on the horizon – a prevention rather than a cure. Vaccines to combat cystitis have been undergoing clinical trials in the Netherlands and the USA over the past few years. Now a vaccine candidate has emerged that may be the most promising yet. Researchers at the University of Wisconsin announced in December 2001 that they had successfully tested a vaccine that will shield women from 10 different infection-causing microbes, six of them strains of the usual suspect in urinary tract infections – the notorious *E.coli* (*Escherichia coli*) bacterium, which is present in high numbers in everyone's intestinal tract. While other research is looking into oral or injectable vaccines that target only *E. coli*, this vaccine's broader protection will come in the easy-to-use form of a vaginal suppository.

How it works Some vaccines use harmless parts of the targeted bacterium to prompt the immune system to mount a defence against the mock invaders – as well as against the genuine article, should it attack. But the vaccine suppository accomplishes the same thing by using whole bacteria that have been killed by heat. When released from the suppository, the billions of dead microbes come into direct contact with the lining of the vagina, activating antibodies that target the same mucous membrane occupied by the infectious bacteria.

The Wisconsin researchers tested the vaccine on 54 women who suffered from recurring urinary tract infections – some coming down with as many as 20 infections a year. All were taken off the long-term antibiotic regime they

More than half of those [women in the study] who received the vaccine plus boosters were infection-free [after 14 weeks].

had been using to suppress their infections and were given either three weekly doses of the vaccine, three weekly doses plus three subsequent boosters, or a monthly placebo suppository with no vaccine in it. All but two of the women who received the placebo developed another infection after 14 weeks, while more than half of those who received the vaccine plus boosters were infection-free. Those who had the vaccine without the boosters were protected only while they were using the suppositories.

Availability The next step is a bigger clinical trial to test the vaccine on more women. That study is due to begin in America in 2003 and will take about two years to complete. If the vaccine reaches the market, it will be aimed primarily at women who suffer from three or more urinary tract infections each year.

RESEARCH ROUND-UP

Dealing with bladder infections

Anyone with a bladder infection needs a high fluid intake. Alkaline substances, such as diluted lemon barley water, can improve symptoms by making the urine more alkaline, which discourages bacterial growth and improves the results of antibiotic therapy.

Antibiotics are the main treatment for urinary tract infections. Under a variety of brand names, the antibiotic trimethoprim is the most widely prescribed drug for cystitis in the UK. There are three reasons for this: it is cost-effective, it has few reported side effects and it works in 80 per cent of all cases. Few women are likely to complain about a drug that successfully clears up their cystitis, and it is fortunate both for women with cystitis and for the NHS purse that one of the least expensive antibiotics happens to be the most effective.

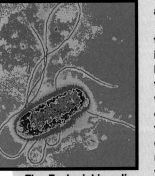

The Escherichia coli *bacterium that often causes cystitis.*

Reach out and cure someone

Getting yet another urinary tract infection is miserable enough. But you also have to rearrange your day, trek down to the surgery and give a urine sample just to confirm what you already know – that you've got cystitis again and you need an antibiotic. Wouldn't it be great to be treated over the phone?

Researchers in the USA have now investigated the viability of telephone prescribing. They compared the outcomes for 36 women with symptoms of cystitis who visited their doctor with 36 others who simply phoned in, answered a series of questions from a checklist and were issued a prescription immediately. They found that the two approaches were equally effective. This may lead to a wider availability of 'phone cure' for bladder infections – in the US anyway.

But in the UK, while many GPs do this in practice, telephone prescribing, unless for repeat prescriptions, is strongly opposed by the insurance companies responsible for paying out if a doctor were sued by a patient. The General Medical Council would blame a doctor for a missed diagnosis if he or she had not gathered all the information needed to make an accurate diagnosis, by seeing the patient and testing their urine.

Credits

Index

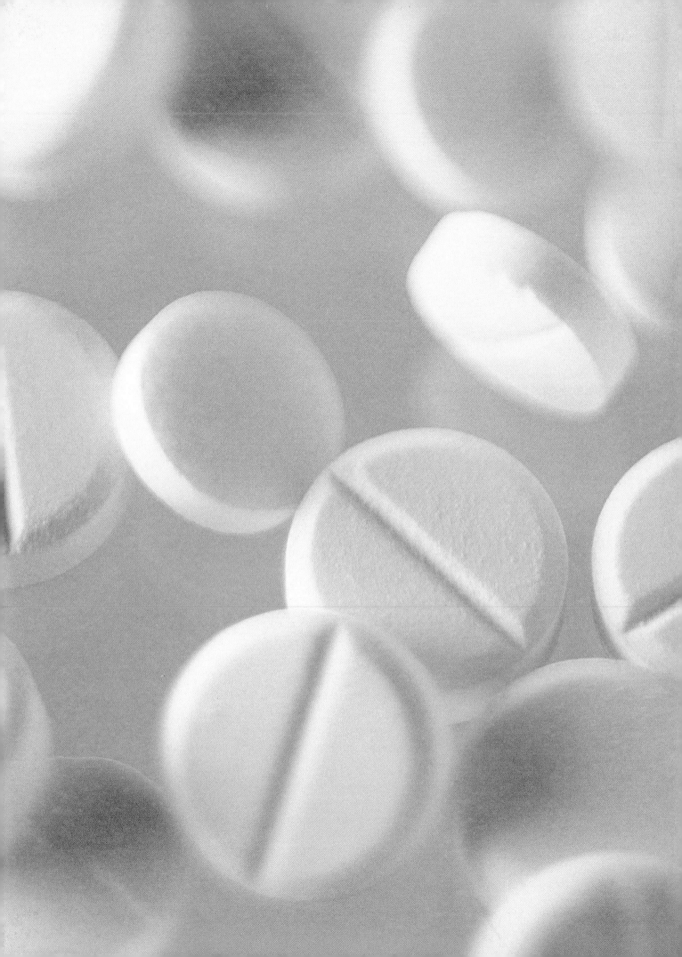